HEMODYNAMICS IN DAILY PRACTICE

HEMODYNAMICS IN DAILY PRACTICE

edited by

ERIK ANDRIES

Department of Cardiology
O.L.V. Hospital, Aalst, Belgium

and

ROLAND STROOBANDT

Department of Cardiology
St. Jozef Hospital, Oostende, Belgium

Foreword by

BEVERLY H. LORELL

Hardvard Medical School

SPRINGER SCIENCE+BUSINESS MEDIA, B.V.

Library of Congress Cataloging-in-Publication Data

Hemodynamics in daily practice / edited by E. Andries and R. Stroobandt.
p. cm. (Developments in cardiovascular medicine: 111)
ISBN 978-94-010-5698-4 ISBN 978-94-011-3820-8 (eBook)
DOI 10.1007/978-94-011-3820-8
1. Hemodynamic monitoring. 2. Heart–Pathophysiology.
I. Andries, E. (Erik) II. Stroobandt, R. (Roland) III. Series
RC670.5.H45H46 1990 90–4260
616.1'20754–dc 20

ISBN 978-94-010-5698-4

Printed on acid-free paper

Table of contents

Foreword

This book is an edited compilation of the scientific presentations given at a symposium on cardiovascular hemodynamics and the contemporary practice of cardiology which was organized in Malta, April 1989. The field of cardiovascular medicine has undergone an extraordinary explosion of knowledge regarding the basic biology of the heart and circulation in health and disease, as well as technologic innovations for probing and assessing cardiac geometry and physiology. This edition addresses such issues which are key problems in current management of patients with heart disease. For example, the classic notion that severe myocardial ischemia is invariably followd by either recovery of normal function or the progression to cell death has been challenged by experimental studies and clinical observations of patients undergoing thrombolysis and revascularization. This growing body of observations clearly indicates that the consequences of ischemia and reperfusion are much more complex and variable, and include several states of abnormal metabolism and contractile function which are distinct from either 'health' or 'death'. This book presents current issues of both consensus and controversy regarding the effects of myocardial ischemia and reperfusion, including irreversible cell loss (infarction), myocardial stunning, and myocardial hibernation. Particular attention is paid to the assessment and differentiation of such patients in the coronary care unit, catheterization suite, or following surgical revascularization.

Secondly, this book addresses the hemodynamic evaluation of the patient with valvular heart disease in today's cardiology practice. What are the important differences in the pathophysiology of aortic stenosis versus regurgitant valvular lesions? How does the assessment of loading conditions modify the evaluation of left ventricular function in the patient with a depressed ejection fraction? What are the consequences of valve replacement versus percutaneous valvuloplasty? The importance of factors such as the type of hypertrophic adaptation (pressure vs. volume overload resulting in concentric vs. eccentric hypertrophy) are clearly presented. Building on this fresh synthesis of current knowledge in the field, the authors develop contemporary invasive

E. Andries & R. Stroobandt (eds.), Hemodynamics in Daily Practice, vii–viii.

and noninvasive approaches for the assessment of the severity of valvular heart disease. The focus of these discussions is to maximally prepare today's clinician for the difficult decision regarding the optimal timing of valve replacement.

Third, this book addresses the problem of the clinical syndrome of heart failure, which is a problem of increasing importance as the population becomes more aged. The relevance and clinical implications of current basic science knowledge regarding those intracellular processes that control myocardial excitation-contraction coupling and metabolism, neurohumoral adaptations, and receptor-second messenger coupling (including beta adrenergic receptor down-regulation) are clearly discussed. At the nest level, current information regarding the biologic basis and clinical discrimination of systolic versus diastolic dysfunction as the physiologic basis for the clinical syndrome of heart failure is presented. Included as a superb discussion of evolving concepts regarding the pathophysiology and management of dilated and hypertrophic cardiomyopathies. These considerations are developed into clear conceptual and methodological approaches for the sophisticated and practical assessment and treatment of patients with congestive heart failure. The authors also address the evaluation and management of heart failure patients who are candidates for or recipients of cardiac transplantation.

In summary, this book will prove to be stimulating and highly informative during the first reading, and then be savored again and again as a reference. This book invites the cardiology clinician who is already committed to excellence in both scholarship and patient care to participate in an intimate discussion with experts. For the reader, this volume will serve as a guide for more expert and insightful hemodynamic assessment of the patient with heart disease, and as a stimulus for future clinical investigations.

Beverly H. Lorell, M.D.
Harvard Medical School

Preface

This book aims at being a manual on hemodynamic problems for the practicing clinician, who faces an ever increasing amount of information on cardiac hemodynamics.

In the past few years extensive research resulted in the development of important pathophysiological concepts, which have proven to be relevant for correct patient care in different clinical settings.

With the advent of reliable non-invasive techniques such as echocardiography, Dopplerechocardiography and radionuclide angiography, and also with the widespread use of flow directed balloon catheters in the coronary care unit, hemodynamic data can be obtained outside the catheterization laboratory.

Hemodynamic evaluation of left ventricular function revealed systolic and diastolic etiologies of left ventricular failure in patients with coronary artery disease, valvular heart disease and cardiomyopathies.

In the setting of valvular heart disease, concepts of pressure and volume overload resulted in a clear understanding of adequate or inadequate adaptation of the myocardium to the overload state and guided optimal timing for surgery.

The early effects of thrombolytic therapy on vessel patency have been extensively studied but effects on left ventricular function need further investigation.

Hypertrophic cardiomyopathy continues to be a subject of fascination and frustration. Multiple pathophysiological mechanisms are operative mainly consisting of impaired diastolic relaxation and in some patients of outflow tract obstruction. Therapeutic interventions should be guided by assessment of those mechanisms.

Major advances have been achieved in the pharmacological treatment of congestive cardiomyopathy (unloading agents and new positive inotropic drugs). Cardiac transplantation can be offered to the patient with endstage disease.

E. Andries & R. Stroobandt (eds.), Hemodynamics in Daily Practice, ix–x.

This book focuses on the clinical application of new hemodynamic pathophysiological concepts in daily practice. It is the result of a workshop organized in Malta, April 1989.

The support of G. De Vriese, MD and his staff at ICI Pharma in organizing this symposium, is highly appreciated.

Erik Andries & Roland Stroobandt

List of authors and editors

Erik ANDRIES, MD
Department of Cardiology, O.L.V. Ziekenhuis, Moorselbaan, B-9300 Aalst, Belgium
Editor

Robert O. BONOW, MD
National Institute of Health, Building 10, Room 7B15, Bethesda, MD 20892, USA
Chapter 10 co-authors: Barry J. Maron, MD, Martin B. Leon, MD, Richard O. Cannon III, MD and Stephen E. Epstein, MD

Kenneth M. BOROW, MD
Cardiac Noninvasive Physiology Laboratory, The University of Chicago Medical Center, 5841 S. Maryland Avenue, Box 44, Chicago, IL 60637, USA
Chapter 2 co-authors: Alex Neumann, BS, Daniel David, MD, Roberto M. Lang, MD
Chapter 4

Johannes BRACHMANN, MD
Medizinische Klinik, Abteilung Innere Medizin III (Kardiologie), Medizinische Universiteitsklinik, D-6900 Heidelberg, Germany
Chapter 10 co-authors: Claus Schmitt, Thorsten Beyer, Bernd Waldecker, Thomas Hilbel, Mark Schweizer and Wolfgang Kübler

Blase A. CARABELLO, MD
Cardiology Division, Medical University of South Carolina, 171 Ashley Avenue, Charleston, SC 29425, USA
Chapter 3

W. FLAMENG
Department of Cardiac Surgery, University Hospital Gasthuisberg, Herenstraat 49, B-3000 Louvain, Belgium
Chapter 7

E. Andries & R. Stroobandt (eds.), Hemodynamics in Daily Practice, xi–xii.

Guy R. HEYNDRICKX, MD
Cardiovascular Center, O.L.V. Ziekenhuis, Moorselbaan, B-9300 Aalst, Belgium
Chapter 5

Wolfgang KÜBLER, MD
Department of Internal Medicine III, University of Heidelberg, Bergheimer Strasse 58, D-6900 Heidelberg, Germany
Chapter 9

H.F.J. MANNAERTS, MD
Thorax Center, Erasmus University, P.O. Box 1738, 3000 DR Rotterdam, The Netherlands
Chapter 13 co-authors: Jos R.T.C. Roelandt, MD, George R. Sutherland, MD, FRCP, A.H.M.M. Balk and J.H. Smyllie

Walter J. PAULUS, MD, PhD
Cardiac Catherization Laboratory, Cardiovascular Center, O.L.V. Ziekenhuis, Moorselbaan, B-9300 Aalst, Belgium
Chapter 1 co-author: Erik Andries, MD

Philip A. POOLE-WILSON, Professor
National Hart and Lung Institute & National Heart and Chest Hospitals, Dovehouse Street, London SW3 6LY, UK
Chapter 8

Jos R.T.C. ROELANDT, MD
Thorax Center, Erasmus University, P.O. Box 1738, 3000 DR Rotterdam, The Netherlands
Chapter 12 co-authors: Foltert J. ten Cate, MD and George R. Sutherland, MD, FRCP

Roland STROOBANDT, MD, PhD
Department of Cardiology, St. Jozef Hospital, Nieuwpoortsesteenweg 57, B-8400, Oostende, Belgium
Editor

Frans VAN DE WERF, MD, FACC
Division of Cardiology, University Hospital Gasthuisberg, Herestraat 49, B-3000 Louvain, Belgium
Chapter 6

F. WELLENS, MD
Department of Cardiovascular Surgery, O.L.V. Ziekenhuis, Moorselbaan, B-9300 Aalst, Belgium
Chapter 14

1. From hemodynamic principles to clinical management

WALTER J. PAULUS & ERIK ANDRIES

The surgical 'Geheimrat' on Forssmann after the first right heart catheterization in man: 'Let him show his tricks in a circus, but not in a respectable German hospital'.

Since the first right heart catheterization in man [1], hemodynamics evolved from scientific observations to a tool for clinical diagnosis and therapeutics in patients with different forms of cardiac failure. Since the advent of reliable noninvasive techniques, such as echocardiography, Dopplerechocardiography and radionuclide angiography, hemodynamic data acquisition occurred not only in the cardiac catheterization laboratory but also in a noninvasive setting. Moreover, the use of flow-directed balloon catheters allowed right heart catheterization to be performed in intensive or coronary care units without cardiac fluoroscopy. A meticulous hemodynamic assessment of cardiac failure unveals the underlying pathophysiology and is a prerequisite for correct clinical management of patients with coronary artery, valvular heart disease and cardiomyopathies.

CORONARY ARTERY DISEASE

Case report 1

A 57 year old white male was admitted to a general hospital for an anteroseptal myocardial infarction one year before his present admission. The hospital stay for the myocardial infarction had been uneventful. He subsequently started to develop progressive cardiac failure and postinfarct angina and was therefore referred for cardiac catheterization and coronary angiography. His admission electrocardiogram showed a regular sinus rhythm at a rate of 80 beats per minute, PQ-interval of 0.20 msec, QS-pattern and ST-segment elevation in anterior leads suggesting anteroapical aneurysm. His chest X-ray showed an enlarged cardiac silhouette with prominent left ventricular and left atrial contour. There was redistribution of bloodflow to the upper lobes and the pulmonary arteries appeared prominent. At cardiac catheterization, left ventricular filling pressures were elevated (left ventricular end-diastolic pressure = 25 mmHg). A left ventricular angiogram showed a dilated left ventricle (left ventricular end-diastolic volume

E. Andries & R. Stroobandt (eds.), Hemodynamics in Daily Practice, 1–20.

index = 160 ml/m²), reduced left ventricular ejection fraction (=35%), and a large anteroapical left ventricular aneurysm. There was no mitral regurgitation. The coronary angiogram revealed two vessel obstructive coronary disease with an occlusion of the left anterior descending artery distal to the first diagonal branch and a severe stenosis on the right coronary artery. Left ventricular aneurysmectomy and coronary bypass grafting of the right coronary artery were performed two weeks later. The postoperative course was uneventful, without signs of cardiac failure or complaints of angina on follow-up.

Case report 2

A 60 year old white female was transferred because of episodes of angina at rest. There was massive left ventricular failure of recent onset. Chest X-ray showed a small cardiac silhouette, redistribution of blood flow to the upper lobes, interscissural and pleural effusions. The electrocardiogram showed left axis deviation of the QRS-complex with widespread and deep ST-segment depression in anterior and inferior leads, ST-segment elevation in lead aVR. The patient underwent immediate cardiac catheterization and coronary angiography, which revealed elevated left ventricular filling pressures (left ventricular end-diastolic pressure = 40 mmHg), a normal left ventricular size (left ventricular end-diastolic volume index = 75 ml/m²), slightly reduced left ventricular ejection fraction (=52%) and hypokinesia of anterior and inferior wall segments. The coronary angiogram revealed a tight distal left main coronary artery stenosis with slow anterograde filling of the left anterior descending and circumflex coronary arteries. The right coronary artery was without significant obstructive lesions. The patient underwent urgent coronary bypass grafting with an internal mammary artery graft to the left anterior descending artery and two venous grafts to the left circumflex artery and first marginal branch.

As obvious from the first two case reports, the cause of left ventricular failure in patients with coronary artery disease can be variable. A previous extensive and transmural myocardial infarct with left ventricular aneurysm leads to symptoms and signs of left ventricular failure because of reduced left ventricular stroke volume, higher end-systolic volume, higher end-diastolic volume and therefore elevated left ventricular filling pressure. This mechanism of cardiac failure can easily be appreciated from the left ventricular end-systolic pressure-volume relation (outlined in Figure 1). The use of the left ventricular end-systolic pressure-volume relation as index of left ventricular systolic performance has received widespread attention over the last decade [1–9]. The left ventricular end-systolic pressure-volume relation is constructed from minimal two unequally loaded pressure-volume loops. A pressure-volume loop is obtained by matching corresponding points of left ventricular pressure and left ventricular volume during a cardiac cycle. In Figure 1 the dashed lines show pressure-volume loops for two unequally loaded beats. By connecting the outer left hand corners of the two unequally loaded beats, the left ventricular end-systolic pressure-volume line can be constructed. The slope of this line

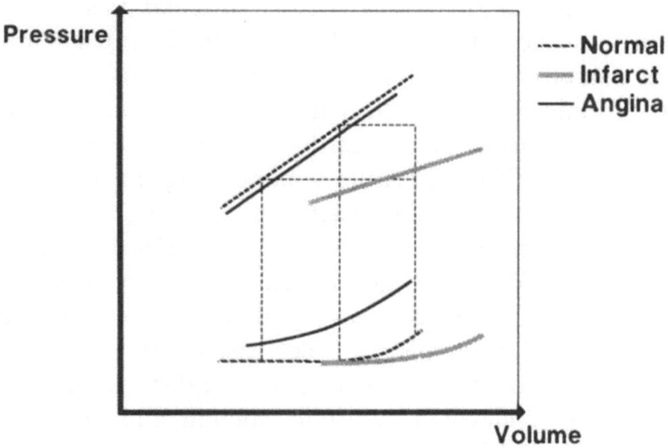

Figure 1. Divergent effects of transmural myocardial infarct and of pacing induced angina on LV end-systolic and diastolic pressure-volume relations. Transmural myocardial infarct causes a downward and rightward shift of the LV end-systolic pressure-volume relation. During pacing induced angina, the LV diastolic pressure-volume relation shifts upward.

provides an index of left ventricular contractility which is independent of left ventricular load. An increase in left ventricular contractility steepens the slope of the left ventricular end-systolic pressure-volume relation. A decrease in left ventricular contractility causes a shallower slope of the left ventricular end-systolic pressure-volume relation. In the patient of case report 1, who suffered a large transmural myocardial infarct, the end-systolic pressure-volume relation was shifted to the right (see Figure 1) [8, 9]. This rightward shift implies in an isovolumically beating left ventricle (i.e., non ejecting left ventricle) a lower peak left ventricular systolic pressure for the same left ventricular volume. Similarly, in an ejecting left ventricle, the left ventricular stroke volume will be smaller for the same end-diastolic volume when the end-systolic pressure-volume relation is shifted to the right.

When cardiac failure occurs during angina pectoris, its mechanism is different from cardiac failure as a result of transmural myocardial infarct. During angina pectoris, systolic performance deteriorates slightly but diastolic performance is greatly impaired because of an upward shift of the diastolic pressure-volume relation (see Figure 1) [10–12]. The diastolic pressure-volume relation is constructed by matching corresponding left ventricular volumes and left ventricular filling pressures during the diastolic portion of the cardiac cycle. An upward shift of the diastolic left ventricular pressure-volume relation implies higher filling pressures for the same left ventricular volume, whereas a downward shift of the diastolic pressure-volume relation implies lower filling pressures for the same left ventricular volume. An upward shift of the diastolic left ventricular pressure-volume relation is described as a decrease of left ventricular diastolic distensibility and a downward shift of the diastolic pressure-volume relation as an increase of left ventricular diastolic distensibility [13]. The notion 'diastolic distensibility' differs from left ventricular compliance, which measures a slope of the diastolic left ventricular pressure-volume relation ($\Delta V/\Delta P$). Other indices of diastolic left ventricular function, such as left ventricular chamber stiffness or myocardial stiffness also relate to the slope of the diastolic left ventricular pressure-volume or stress-strain relation [14]. Decreased left ventricular diastolic distensibility during angina pectoris has been the subject of intense research both in man [10–18] and in different experimental animal models, in which increased myocardial oxygen demand was superimposed on reduced coronary perfusion (low flow/high demand ischemia) [19–22]. The mechanism of decreased left ventricular diastolic distensibility during angina pectoris is related to a disturbance of myocardial inactivation because of elevated cytosolic calcium and persistent diastolic crossbridge interaction [20,23].

Recognition of the different causes of cardiac failure in patients with coronary artery disease is important for correct medical or surgical management. If cardiac failure is secondary to angina pectoris, myocardial revascularization is mandatory whereas cardiac failure caused by transmurally infarcted myocardium will remain unresponsive to revascularization. Medical therapy of patients with cardiac failure due to a previous myocardial infarct will focus on left ventricular unloading and left ventricular remodeling [24] by vasodilators [25] or positive inotropic drugs [26]. Medical therapy of patients with cardiac failure due to angina pectoris should be based on reduction of myocardial oxygen demand preferably by slow calcium channel blockade, which has a beneficial effect on diastolic left ventricular distensibility [27]. A drug such as digoxin, which has been used for centuries in the treatment of heart failure, appears to be contraindicated when heart failure is related to diastolic left ventricular dysfunction of angina pectoris [28].

VALVULAR HEART DISEASE

In valvular heart disease, cardiac failure is caused by malfunctioning of the valve or by inadequate adaptation of the myocardium to the pressure or volume overload. A distinction will therefore be made between hemodynamic problems related to valve malfunctioning or related to pressure or volume overload of the myocardium.

Valvular stenosis: Hemodynamic pitfalls

Definitions of transvalvular gradients. A crosstalk between invasive and non-invasive Dopplerechocardiographic measurements requires a correct use of the different definitions of transvalvular gradient. Three types of transvalvular gradients can be distinguished:

-. Peak gradient is the maximal pressure difference between two pressure tracings (e.g., left ventricular and aortic pressure tracing in aortic stenosis). Peak gradient can easily be derived from the Dopplerechocardiogram as the maximal flow velocity across the valve. In the cardiac catheterization laboratory, measurement of peak gradient is sensitive to proper positioning of catheters on both sides of the narrowed valve. In many procedures on patients with aortic stenosis, the aortic pressure recording is replaced by a femoral artery pressure recording. Femoral artery pressure is delayed with respect to aortic pressure and this offsets an accurate measurement of peak gradient.
- Peak to peak gradient measures the pressure difference between the maximal excursions of two pressure tracings. For aortic stenosis, peak to peak gradient corresponds to peak left ventricular pressure minus peak aortic pressure. Peak to peak gradient is readily obtainable in the cardiac catheterization laboratory but difficult to measure in a noninvasive setting.
- Mean gradient provides a tool for correct comparison of Dopplerechocardiographic and hemodynamic gradients. Mean gradient equals the transvalvular gradient averaged over the ejection period in aortic or pulmonary stenosis and the transvalvular gradient averaged over the filling period in mitral or tricuspid stenosis. Mean gradient can be obtained in the cardiac catheterization laboratory from planimetry of the recorded pressure differences and is calculated on line by most of the newer Dopplerechocardiographic machines. Therefore, in order to achieve a crosstalk between invasive and noninvasive data [29], a transvalvular gradient is preferably reported as a mean gradient.

The small aortic transvalvular gradient. The hemodynamic significance of a small transvalvular aortic gradient in a patient with signs of congestive failure and low cardiac output, is a challenging clinical problem. A representative case report follows.

Case report 3

This is a 74 year old female who had undergone mastectomy and radiotherapy a couple of months prior to hospital admission. She was admitted in cardiac failure (NYHA class IV) *and hypotension (arterial pressure = 90/70 mmHg). There was a late peaking and faint ejection murmur, maximal at R2 and a holosystolic blowing murmur, maximal at the apex. There was no audible S2 sound and there were gallop sounds. The carotids had a faint upstroke and there was prominent neck vein distension. The electrocardiogram showed a regular sinus rhythm at 130 beats/min, a PQ-interval of 0.20 sec, left atrial enlargement, normal QRS voltage and repolarisation disturbances. Because of clinical suspicion of critical aortic stenosis and because of imminent collapse, the patient was transferred for urgent percutaneous balloon aortic valvuloplasty. The hemodynamic recordings before, immediately after and 48 hours after the procedure*

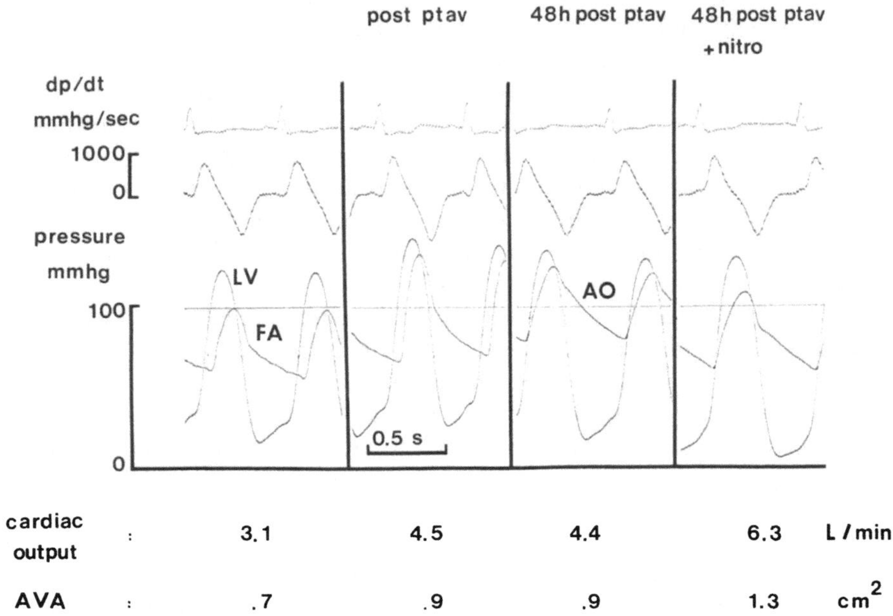

Figure 2. Recordings of LV dp/dt, tip-micromanometer LV Pressure, femoral artery (FA) pressure and aortic (AO) pressure obtained in a patient with a small aortic transvalvular gradient and signs of congestive failure and low cardiac output. Recordings were obtained in control conditions, after balloon aortic valvuloplasty (post ptav), 48 hours after balloon aortic valvuloplasty (48 h post ptav) and during nitroprusside infusion 48 hours after balloon aortic valvuloplasty (48 h post ptav + nitro).

are shown in Figure 2. Figure 2 displays from top to bottom the electrocardiogram, the left ventricular dP/dt, the left ventricular pressure recorded by a tip-micromanometer catheter, femoral artery pressure in the two left hand panels and the central aortic pressure in the two right hand panels. In the two left hand panels, the upstroke of the femoral artery pressure tracing is delayed with respect to the upstroke of the left ventricular pressure tracing. In the two right hand panels, the upstroke of the aortic pressure tracing coincides with the upstroke of the left ventricular pressure tracing and occurs at the crossover of the pressure tracings. In the outer left hand panel, there is a 30 mmHg mean transvalvular gradient, a low cardiac output of 3.1 liters/minute and a calculated valve area of 0.7 cm^2*. Immediately after percutaneous balloon aortic valvuloplasty the mean transvalvular gradient is reduced to 10 mmHg, the upstroke of the femoral artery pressure tracing is faster and the pulse pressure is wider. Cardiac output has risen to 4.5 liters/minute and the aortic valve area calculates to be 0.9 cm*^{2}*. The left ventricular filling pressures remain elevated. 48 hours after percutaneous balloon aortic valvuloplasty, the mean transvalvular gradient is comparable to* *the mean transvalvular gradient recorded immediately after aortic valvuloplasty but the aortic pulse pressure is again narrower. This implicates that the wider pulse pressure observed immediately after aortic valvuloplasty was partly due to aortic regurgitation, related to some reversible fibroelastic compression of the valve leaflets by the inflated valvuloplasty balloon. Cardiac output remains unchanged at 4.4 l/min and the calculated valve area equals the valve area obtained immediately after aortic valvuloplasty. At the time of the repeat catheterization, 48 hours after aortic valvuloplasty, a nitroprusside infusion is started. The infusion rate is gradually increased to 200 μg/minute. Hemodynamic recordings during nitroprusside infusion are shown in the outer right hand panel. There is a small decrease of peak aortic pressure from 130 to 105 mmHg, a small rise of the mean transvalvular gradient to 25 mmHg, a rise of cardiac output to 6.3 l/min and of calculated aortic valve area to 1.3 cm*^{2}*. The patient is discharged on ACE inhibitors (lisinopril) and is doing well* (NYHA class II) *at 1 year follow-up.*

Case report 3 illustrates the problem of a patient with a small aortic transvalvular gradient, signs of cardiac failure and low cardiac output. Is the low output secondary to an afterload mismatch between a severely stenosed aortic valve and the left ventricle [30] or is the low output the cause of insufficient opening of stiff valve leaflets so that a small transvalvular gradient starts to develop? Case report 3 shows both mechanisms to coexist. The immediate beneficial effect of balloon aortic valvuloplasty on cardiac output favors the presence of a fixed obstruction to left ventricular outflow which, although of smaller magnitude, leads to cardiac failure, probably because of afterload mismatch [31]. The beneficial response to vasodilator therapy after balloon

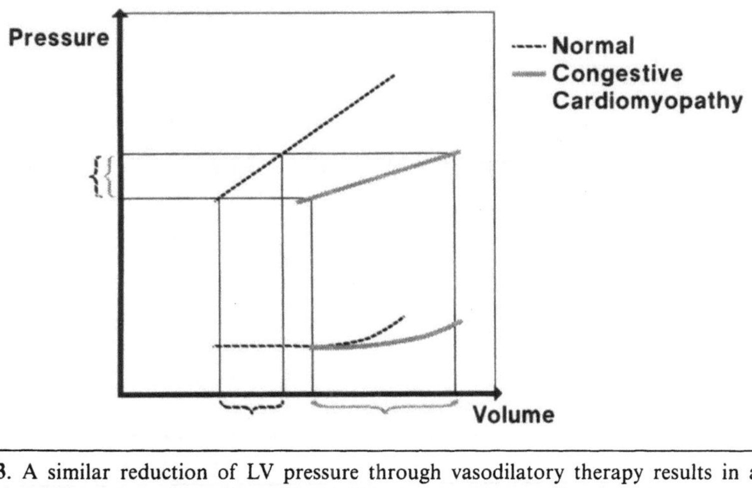

Figure 3. A similar reduction of LV pressure through vasodilatory therapy results in a larger increase of LV stroke volume in a dilated LV of congestive cardiomyopathy compared to a normal LV because of different slopes of the LV end-systolic pressure-volume relation.

aortic valvuloplasty with a striking increase in cardiac output and calculated aortic valve area argues in favor of some orifice variability of the stenotic sclerocalcific aortic valve as function of cardiac output or of transvalvular flow. A higher output or transvalvular flow causes wider opening of the valve leaflets and increases effective valve orifice [32-34].

The doubling of cardiac output in case report 3, after combined balloon aortic valvuloplasty and vasodilator therapy, also illustrates the greater efficacy of left ventricular unloading in a dilated hypocontractile left ventricle compared to a normal left ventricle. The concept is outlined in Figure 3. In contrast to a normal left ventricle a dilated left ventricle has a shallow end-systolic pressure-volume relation. Because of this shallower end-systolic pressure-volume relation, a similar amount of afterload reduction will induce a larger change in end-systolic volume in the dilated left ventricle than in the normal left ventricle. Inversely, reducing left ventricular afterload by vasodilator therapy in a small left ventricle, such as frequently observed in hypertensive cardiomyopathy of the elderly, can induce a precipitous fall in blood pressure and induce fatal hypotension [35].

Dynamic outflow tract obstruction. The distinction between fixed and dynamic gradients across the left ventricular or right ventricular outflow tract is important because of different therapeutic implications. A dynamic gradient across the left ventricular outflow tract is observed in obstructive hypertrophic

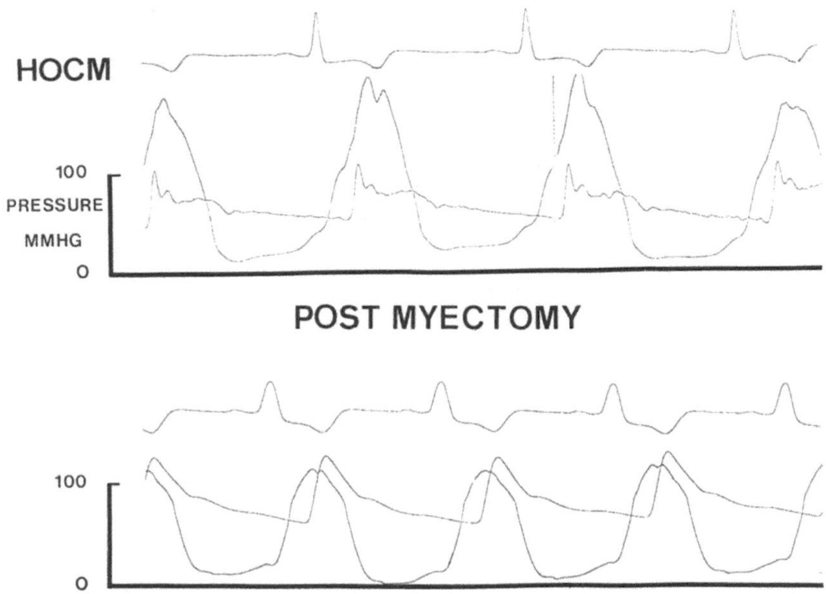

Figure 4. Tip-micromanometer LV and femoral artery pressure tracings recorded in a patient with obstructive hypertrophic cardiomyopathy before (top) and after (bottom) septal myectomy.

cardiomyopathy. Such a dynamic outflow tract gradient of obstructive hypertrophic cardiomyopathy is shown in Figure 4 before and after myectomy. Before myectomy, the peripheral artery pressure tracing differs from the peripheral artery pressure tracing of a patient with valvular aortic stenosis. The peripheral artery pressure tracing in valvular aortic stenosis is characterized by a slow upstroke. The peripheral artery pressure tracing in obstructive hypertrophic cardiomyopathy shows a characteristic spike and dome pattern with a brisk upstroke. When the transmission delay of the peripheral artery pressure tracing is accounted for in Figure 4 by shifting it leftwards so that the upstrokes of the peripheral artery and left ventricular pressures coincide, the absence of a gradient in the initial portion of systole or of ejection is obvious [36]. The gradient across the left ventricular outflow tract appears only after the first third of systole at a time, which corresponds with SAM-septal contact on the echocardiogram [37]. This late onset of the outflow tract gradient in obstructive hypertrophic cardiomyopathy correlates with the Dopplerechocardiographic flow velocity pattern observed in this disease. After myectomy (bottom panel of Figure 4) the outflow tract gradient has disappeared and the spike and dome pattern on the peripheral artery pressure tracing has vanished.

Calculated mitral valve area in mitral stenosis: Effects of percutaneous transluminal mitral valvuloplasty

Case report 4

This 55 year old female had undergone aortic valve replacement for severe aortic stenosis in 1974 and received a Björk-Shiley tilting disc prosthesis. She recently developed recurrent dyspnea with signs of mitral stenosis. She was transferred for percutaneous balloon mitral valvuloplasty. Percutaneous balloon mitral valvuloplasty resulted in a reduction of mean PCW pressures from 25 to 11 mmHg, an increase of cardiac output from 3.8 to 5.2 l/min and an increase of mitral valve area from 1.2 to 2.0 cm^2. Dopplerechocardiograms were obtained before and immediately after balloon mitral valvuloplasty. The Doppler echocardiogram showed the mitral valve area to be 1.3 cm^2 before and only 1.4 cm^2 immediately after balloon mitral valvuloplasty! The patient was discharged from the hospital 2 days after the procedure. On clinical follow-up, six months later, she had greatly improved to NYHA class II.

Case report 4 illustrates the pitfall of calculating a mitral valve area using deceleration of mitral valve flow velocity of the Dopplerechocardiogram [39, 40]. The deceleration of mitral valve flow velocity is sensitive to left atrial driving pressure, left atrial and left ventricular compliance or left ventricular preload [41–44]. The acute reduction of left atrial driving pressure induced by percutaneous balloon mitral valvuloplasty offsets the effect of a larger mitral valve area on the deceleration of mitral flow velocity. The larger mitral valve area as a result of the balloon dilatation fastens the deceleration of mitral flow velocity but the acute reduction of mean PCW pressure counteracts this effect by reducing the deceleration of mitral flow velocity. Because of the balancing effects of a larger valve area and a reduced left atrial driving pressure, the mitral valve area calculated from the deceleration of mitral valve flow velocity on the Dopplerechocardiogram fails to show a significant change after balloon mitral valvuloplasty. This erroneous Dopplerechocardiographic result calls for a cautious use of mitral valve areas derived from Doppler-echocardiograms.

A similar critique applies to the use of the mitral valve Dopplerechocardiogram for assessment of diastolic properties of the left ventricle [45]. At a fixed left atrial driving pressure or a fixed mean PCW, a reduction of left ventricular distensibility will lead to a reduction of the deceleration of early diastolic flow velocity on the mitral valve Dopplerechocardiogram. A reduced diastolic distensibility of the left ventricle also elevates mean PCW or left atrial driving pressure. This augments the deceleration of early diastolic flow velocity, thus partially correcting the changes induced by the reduction of left ventricular distensibility. Assessment of left ventricular diastolic properties from Dopplerechocardiographic mitral valve flow velocity is therefore only valid if left atrial driving pressure or mean PCW is known [46].

Hemodynamic assessment of volume or pressure overload hypertrophy

Pressure overload hypertrophy

Case report 5

This 65 year old female had undergone aortic valve replacement for severe aortic stenosis. She had received a 19 mm Carpentier-Edwards bioprosthesis. Two years after valve replacement she was again highly symptomatic with complaints of dyspnea and angina (NYHA class III). *Her blood pressure was 150/75 mmHg. There was an early peaking ejection murmur, intensity 3/6, maximal at R2. There was a loud S4. The electrocardiogram showed persistent left ventricular hypertrophy. The echocardiogram revealed SAM motion of the mitral valve with late systolic SAM septal contact. Leaflet motion of the bioprosthesis appeared to be normal and there was massive left ventricular hypertrophy. At cardiac catheterization there was only a small protosystolic gradient over the bioprosthesis as evident from left ventricular and peripheral artery pressure recordings (Figure 5). There was no dynamic outflow tract gradient in mid- or late systole. Left ventricular filling pressures were elevated and left ventricular pressure decay was slow. The RAO left ventricular angiogram showed left ventricular hypertrophy of the apical and mid-cavity segments and near total cavity obliteration at end-systole. The LAO left ventricular angiogram confirmed late systolic SAM septal contact. A diagnosis was made of hypertrophic cardiomyopathy of the apical and mid-cavity type post aortic valve replacement. The patient was discharged*

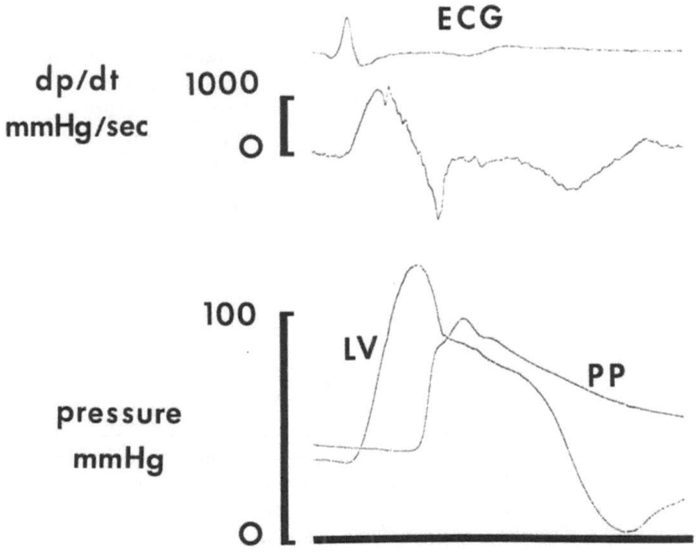

Figure 5. LV dp/dt, tip-micromanometer left ventricular (LV) pressure and peripheral artery (PP) pressure recorded in a patient with a 19 mm bioprosthesis in aortic position.

on a high dose verapamil and a low dose diuretic. There was gradual improvement in symptoms at follow-up.

Case report 5 illustrates persistent hemodynamic problems in pressure overload left ventricular hypertrophy even after removal of the stimulus for hypertrophy. When the left ventricle faces a high left ventricular afterload, myocardial wall stress becomes elevated. To lower the elevated myocardial wall stress, parallel addition of myofibrils will occur leading to increased left ventricular wall thickness [47]. The process of concentric left ventricular hypertrophy therefore tends to normalize myocardial wall stress, whenever the left ventricle faces a high left ventricular afterload. This process of concentric left ventricular hypertrophy can at times be inadequate, causing left ventricular ejection fraction to be lower than predicted by the ejection fraction-myocardial wall stress relationship [30]. This process of left ventricular hypertrophy can at times also exceed a level required for normalization of myocardial wall stress. A lower than normal left ventricular wall stress has indeed been observed in congenital aortic stenosis [47]. A similar finding is present when hypertrophic cardiomyopathy coexists with aortic stenosis [48–49].

After removal of the stimulus for left ventricular hypertrophy, the regression of the myofibrillar hyperplasia and of the altered fibrous skeleton are variable processes [50–51]. In congenital aortic stenosis, there is failure of regression of left ventricular hypertrophy after aortic valve replacement with a persistent

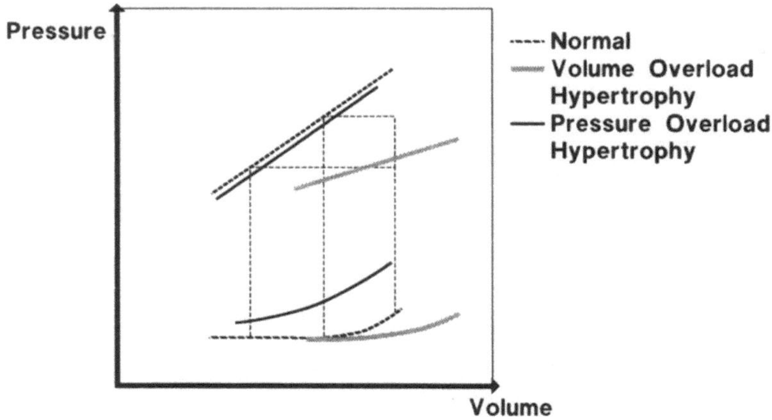

Figure 6. Divergent effects of LV pressure and volume overload on LV end-systolic and diastolic pressure-volume relations. LV volume-overload hypertrophy causes a downward and rightward shift of the LV end-systolic pressure-volume relation. LV pressure-overload hypertrophy induces an upward shift of the LV diastolic pressure-volume relation.

pattern of low left ventricular wall stress [52]. In adult aortic stenosis, regression of myofibrillar hyperplasia after aortic valve replacement is a fast process, whereas the fibrous content of the left ventricular wall remains elevated [50]. This causes persistent reduction of diastolic distensibility of the left ventricle despite removal of the stimulus for left ventricular hypertrophy [53]. Reduced diastolic distensibility is indeed a prominent feature of left ventricular hemodynamics during or after pressure overload hypertrophy [54]. For a pressure overloaded and hypertrophied left ventricle, the diastolic pressure-volume curve is shifted upward as shown in Figure 6, while systolic performance is well preserved because of normalization of myocardial wall stress. In contrast to pressure overload hypertrophy, volume overload hypertrophy secondary to mitral or aortic regurgitation causes depressed systolic performance with increased diastolic distensibility. This pathophysiology is illustrated by case report 6.

Volume overload hyperthophy

Case report 6
This 24 year old female had increasing complaints of dyspnea. There was no history of rheumatic fever. Physical examination showed a blood pressure of 130/80 mmHg, a displaced apical impulse, a loud S1, an opening snap, a short S2 opening snap interval, an apical mitral regurgitation murmur (4/6) and a diastolic rumble (2/4). The electrocardiogram showed a regular sinus rhythm, left atrial enlargement and normal QRS ST-T morphology. Dopplerechocardiographic examination revealed a thickened and amobile posterior mitral valve

leaflet, a localised mitral regurgitation jet and a congenital malformation of the mitral valve with fusion of papillary muscles and chordae to a single structure (parachute type deformity). At cardiac catheterization, mean PCW pressure was slightly elevated to 14 mmHg with a further increase to 21 mmHg after angiography. Mean PA pressure was 19 mmHg with an increase to 26 mmHg after angiography. There was a mean mitral valve gradient of 8 mmHg, 4+ mitral regurgitation on the left ventricular angiogram, and a normal pulmonary vascular resistance. The ejection fraction was 62% and the end-systolic volume index was increased to 55 ml/m^2. Because of the elevated end-systolic volume index, the patient was referred for surgery. Mitral valve reconstruction was performed. After mitral valve reconstruction there was only a trace of mitral regurgitation and, at six months follow-up, there was persistent improvement of symptoms.

Case report 6 illustrates the problem of optimal timing of valve surgery in patients with volume overload hypertrophy due to mitral or aortic regurgitation. On one hand, an eventual valve replacement should be postponed as long as possible because of the inherent risks of valve replacement in terms of anticoagulation, malfunctioning of prostheses and foreign body endocarditis. On the other hand, valve replacement should not be postponed beyond a stage where irreversible left ventricular dilatation has occurred. Over the last couple of years, several criteria of left ventricular performance have been proposed, based on the left ventricular end-systolic pressure-volume relation, to distinguish reversible from irreversible left ventricular dilatation in left ventricular volume overload. The left ventricular end-systolic volume appears to be a useful determinant of long-term prognosis after either mitral or aortic valve replacement for mitral or aortic regurgitation. A left ventricular end-systolic volume index of 60 ml/m^2 [55] or a left ventricular end-systolic dimension of 54 mm [56] have both been proposed as critical values beyond which left ventricular dilatation should not be allowed to progress in order to avoid a poor short-term or long-term surgical outcome. Although other investigators have subsequently challenged these criteria [57], most studies confirm the usefulness of the left ventricular end-systolic volume as a parameter to distinguish reversible from irreversible left ventricular dilatation in volume overload. The precise cut-off value was however gradually displaced towards higher volumes for aortic regurgitation [58], probably because of better surgical technique or improved myocardial protection during heart-lung bypass. In contrast to aortic regurgitation, mitral regurgitation still requires a more cautious approach and probably the continued use of the original 60 ml/m^2 cut-off value beyond which the left ventricular end-systolic volume index should not be allowed to progress. This different appoach for mitral and aortic regurgitation is based on the different wall stress patterns in both forms of left ventricular overload [59]. In mitral regurgitation, the volume overloaded left ventricle ejects part of its stroke volume in a low resistance pathway, i.e., the left atrium. Because of this loading pattern, a normal ejection fraction can still belie left ventricular muscle dysfunction in mitral regurgitation [60]. After mitral valve replacement, the low resistance pathway disappears and left ventricular muscle dysfunction becomes obvious as a larger left ventricular end-systolic volume. Correct timing of mitral or aortic valve replacement in volume overload hypertrophy will lead to early shrinkage of the left ventricular volumes, usually already evident at the time of hospital discharge [61].

CARDIOMYOPATHIES

Case report 7
This 50 year old white male was hospitalized because of symptoms and signs of left ventricular failure. The electrocardiogram revealed regular sinus rhythm at a rate of 80 beats/min, first degree atrioventricular block and left bundle branch block. A bidimensional echocardiogram showed marked left ventricular dilatation with hypokinesia of all left ventricular segments. Despite diuretics and vasodilators, the patient remained symptomatic (NYHA class III) *and was referred for the transplant program. Cardiac catheterization revealed a left ventricular pressure of 100/17 mmHg, a mean PCW pressure of 15 mmHg, an ejection fraction of 11% and a left ventricular enddiastolic volume index of 180 ml/m²^2. The coronary angiogram showed normal coronary arteries and endomyocardial biopsy revealed myocardial fibrosis and hypertrophy without acute cellular infiltrate. Cardiac transplantation was performed and at 6 months follow-up the patient was doing well without signs of rejection on endomyocardial biopsy.*

Case report 8
This 60 year old white female presented with complaints of angina and dyspnea (NYHA class III). *On physical exam there was a loud S4 and an early peaking systolic ejection murmur. There was no neck vein distension and the carotid upstroke was brisk. The electrocardiogram revealed a regular sinus rhythm at 60 beats/min, fist degree atrioventricular block, left ventricular hypertrophy and giant negative T-waves over the precordial leads. The diagnosis of apical hypertrophic cardiomyopathy was suspected and the patient was referred for cardiac catheterization and coronary angiography. At cardiac catheterization, left ventricular pressure was 120/35 mmHg and mean PCW pressure was 30 mmHg. The left ventricular angiogram showed a left ventricular enddiastolic volume index of 70 ml/m^2, a left ventricular ejection fraction of 85% and apical wall thickening with prominent trabeculations and papillary muscles. At endsystole there was cavity obliteration of the apical and mid-ventricular segments and there was no SAM motion of the mitral valve on the LAO left ventricular angiogram. The coronary angiogram revealed normal coronary arteries. The diagnosis of nonobstructive hypertrophic cardiomyopathy of the apical type was confirmed by the left ventricular angiogram* [62-64]. *The patient was treated with high dose calcium channel blockers, which resulted in prompt improvement of symptoms.*

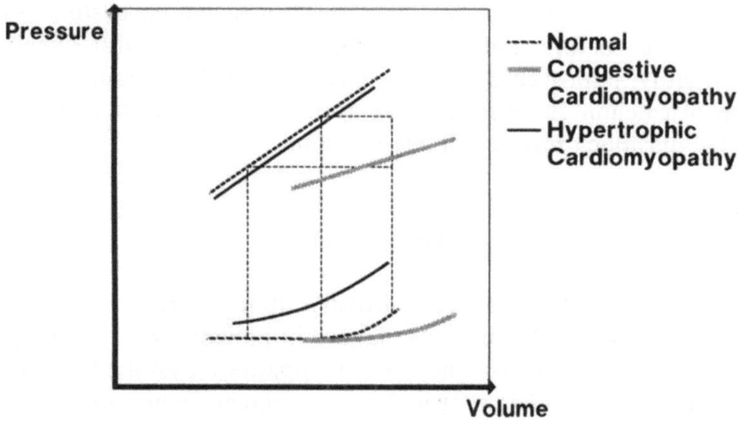

Figure 7. Divergent effects of congestive and hypertrophic cardiomyopathy on LV end-systolic and diastolic pressure-volume relations. Congestive cardiomyopathy causes a downward and rightward shift of the LV end-systolic pressure-volume relation. Hypertrophic cardiomyopathy induces an upward shift of the LV diastolic pressure-volume relation.

Case reports 7 and 8 illustrate the divergent hemodynamic findings of patients with congestive or hypertrophic cardiomyopathy. Congestive or dilated cardiomyopathy [65] is characterized by progressive enlargement of the left ventricular cavity and reduced left ventricular ejection fraction and wall motion. Hypertrophic cardiomyopathy features a normal or small left ventricular cavity with elevated left ventricular ejection fraction and small endsystolic left ventricular cavity size. In both conditions, the left ventricular filling pressures are elevated. As illustrated in Figure 7, these divergent hemodynamic properties can easily be appreciated on left ventricular end-systolic and diastolic pressure-volume diagrams. Congestive cardiomyopathy results in a right and downward shift of the left ventricular endsystolic pressure-volume relation. Hypertrophic cardiomyopathy causes an upward shift of the diastolic pressure-volume relation. Hypertrophic cardiomyopathy features a so-called 'hypercontractile response' with increased left ventricular ejection fraction and endsystolic cavity obliteration. This 'hypercontractile' response is the consequence of inappropriate left ventricular hypertrophy, causing extreme unloading of the left ventricular wall [66]. When this low left ventricular wall stress is taken into account for the assessment of the contractile state, the velocity of myocardial shortening appears to be depressed in hypertrophic cardiomyopathy [67]. The low wall stress for myocardial fibres embedded in a thick hypertrophied left ventricular wall masks an inherent depression of myocardial contractile state. In a later stage of the disease the inherent depression of myocardial contractile state manifests itself through dilatation of the left ventricular cavity and depression of regional wall motion [68]. In patients with congestive cardiomyopathy, the effects of vasodilator and inotropic therapy [69] can be quantitatively assessed by construction of left ventricular endsystolic pressure-volume relations before and after therapy. In patients with hypertrophic cardiomyopathy, improved diastolic left ventricular distensibility after administration of calcium channel blocking agents [70–73] can be deduced from shifts of the diastolic pressure-volume relation.

CONCLUSION

Hemodynamic evaluation of left ventricular function revealed systolic and diastolic etiologies of left ventricular failure in patients with coronary artery disease, valvular heart disease and cardiomyopathies. Systolic left ventricular failure, characterized by left ventricular enlargement, reduced left ventricular wall motion and depressed left ventricular ejection fraction is observed after transmural myocardial infarct, left ventricular volume-overload of mitral or aortic regurgitation and dilated cardiomyopathy. Systolic left ventricular failure can most accurately be assessed by shifts of the left ventricular endsystolic pressure-volume relation. Diastolic left ventricular failure is observed in angina pectoris, pressure-overload hypertrophy and hypertrophic cardiomyopathy. Diastolic left ventricular failure can be appreciated from shifts of the diastolic left ventricular pressure-volume relation. Such a quantitative approach to left ventricular dysfunction has evolved from scientific description into a practical tool for daily clinical management. This evolution was predicted by J. H. Comroe in his Retrospectroscope: 'Although scientific thinking alone is not enough to advance the art of medicine, there will be no advance at all without its rigorous application in everyday medicine'.

REFERENCES

1. Forssmann W (1929) Die Sondierung des rechten Herzens. *Klin Wschr* 8:2085
2. Suga H, Sagawa K, Shoukas AA (1973) Load independence of the instantaneous pressure-volume ratio of the canine left ventricle and effects of epinephrine and heart rate on the ratio. *Circ Res* 32:314
3. Sagawa K, Suga H, Shoukas AA, Bakalar KM (1979) End-systolic pressure-volume ratio: A new index of contractility. *Am J Cardiol* 40:748
4. Grossman W, Braunwald E, Mann T, McLaurin LP, Green L (1977) Contractile state of the left ventricle in man as evaluated from end-systolic pressure-volume relations. *Circulation* 56:845
5. Marsh JD, Green LH, Wynne J, Cohn PF, Grossman W (1979) Left ventricular pressure-dimension and stress-length relations in normal human subjects. *Am J Cardiol* 44:1311
6. Paulus WJ, Claes VA, Brutsaert DL (1980) End-systolic pressure-volume relation estimated from physiologically loaded cat papillary muscle contractions. *Circ Res* 46:20
7. Borow KM, Neumann A, Wynne J (1982) Sensitivity of end-systolic pressure-dimension and pressure-volume relations to inotropic state in humans. *Circulation* 65: 988
8. Sunagawa K, Maughan WL, Sagawa K (1983) Effect of regional ischemia on the left ventricular end-systolic pressure-volume relationship of isolated canine hearts. *Circ Res* 52:170

9. Kass DA, Maughan WL (1988) From Emax to pressure-volume relations: A broader view. *Circulation* 77:1203
10. Dwyer EM Jr (1970) Left ventricular pressure-volume alterations and regional disorders of contraction during myocardial ischemia induced by atrial pacing. *Circulation* 42: 1111
11. Barry WH, Brooker JZ, Alderman EL, Harrison DC (1974) Changes in diastolic stiffness and tone of the left ventricle during angina pectoris. *Circulation* 49:255
12. Mann T, Goldberg S, Mudge GH, Grossman W (1979) Factors contributing to altered left ventricular diastolic properties during angina pectoris. *Circulation* 59:14
13. Grossman W (1988) Relaxation and diastolic distensibility of the regionally ischemic left ventricle, pp 193–203, in: *Diastolic Relaxation of the Heart*, ed. by W Grossman and BH Lorell. Boston/Dordrecht/Lancaster: Martinus Nijhoff Publishers
14. Mirsky I and Rankin JS (1979) The effects of geometry, elasticity and internal pressures on the diastolic pressure-volume and stiffnes-stress relations. How important is the pericardium? *Circ Res* 44:601
15. Bourdillon PD, Lorell BH, Mirsky I, Paulus WJ, Wynne J, Grossman W (1983) Increased regional myocardial stiffness of the left ventricle during pacing induced angina in man. *Circulation* 67:316
16. Sasayama S, Nonogi H, Miyazaki S, Sakurai T, Kawai C, Eiho S, Kuwahara M (1985) Changes in diastolic properties of the regional myocardium during pacing-induced ischemia in human subjects. *J Am Coll Cardiol* 5:599
17. Bronzwaer JGF, Plokker T, Ascoop C, Paulus WJ (1989) Systolic shortening determines diastolic distensibility of ischemic myocardium during pacing induced angina and transluminal coronary occlusion. *J Am Coll Cardiol* 13 (Suppl A): 80
18. Paulus WJ (1990) Upward shift and outward bulge: The divergent myocardial effects of pacing angina and of brief coronary occlusion. *Circulation* 81:1436
19. Serizawa T, Carabello BA, Grossman W (1980) Effect of pacing induced ischemia on left ventricular diastolic pressure-volume relations in dogs with coronary stenoses. *Circ Res* 46:430
20. Paulus WJ, Serizawa T, Grossman W (1982) Altered left ventricular diastolic properties during pacing-induced ischemia in dogs with coronary stenoses: Potentiation by caffeine. *Circ Res* 50:218
21. Paulus WJ, Grossman W, Serizawa T, Bourdillon PD, Pasipoularides A, Mirsky I (1985) Different effects of two types of ischemia on myocardial systolic and diastolic function. *Am J Physiol* 248:H 719
22. Momomura S, Ingwall JS, Parker JA, Sahagian P, Ferguson JJ, Grossman W (1985) The relationships of high energy phophates, tissue PH and regional blood flow to diastolic distensibility in the ischemic dog myocardium. *Circ Res* 57:822
23. Kihara Y, Grossman W, Morgan JP (1989) Direct measurement of changes in intracellular calcium transients during hypoxia, ischemia and reperfusion of the intact mammalian heart. *Circ Res* 65:1029
24. Mc Kay RG, Pfeffer MA, Pasternack RC, Markis JE, Come PC, Nakao S, Alderman JD, Ferguson JJ, Safian RD, Grossman W (1986) Left ventricular remodeling after myocardial infarction: A corollary to infarct expansion. *Circulation* 74:693
25. Pfeffer MA, Lamas GA, Vaughan DE, Parisi AF, Braunwald E (1988) Effect of captopril on progressive ventricular dilatation after anterior myocardial infarction. *NEJM* 319:80
26. Pouleur H, van Eyll C, Hanet C, Cheron P, Charlier AA, Rousseau MF (1988) Long-term effects of xamoterol on left ventricular diastolic function and late remodeling: A study in patients with anterior myocardial infarction and single vessel disease. *Circulation* 77:1081
27. Lorell BH, Turi Z, Grossman W (1981) Modification of left ventricular response to pacing tachycardia by nifedipine in patients with coronary artery disease. *Am J Med* 71:667
28. Cunningham MJ, Apstein CS, Weinberg EO, Lorell BH (1989) Deleterious effect of ouabain on myocardial function during hypoxia. *Am J Physiol* 256:H 681
29. Gordon JB, Folland ED(1989) Analysis of aortic valve gradients by transseptal technique: Implications for noninvasive evaluation. *Cath and Cardiovasc Diagnosis* 17:144
30. Carabello BA, Green LH, Grossman W, Cohn L, Koster JK, Collins JJ Jr (1980) Hemodynamic

determinants of prognosis of aortic valve replacement in critical aortic stenosis and advanced congestive heart failure. *Circulation* 62:42
31. Ross J Jr (1985) Afterload mismatch in aortic and mitral valve disease: implications for surgical therapy. *J Am Coll Cardiol* 5:811
32. Carabello BA (1987) Advances in the hemodynamic assessment of stenotic cardiac valves. *J Am Coll Cardiol* 10:912
33. Paulus WJ, Heyndrickx GR, Andries E (1988) Orifice variability of the stenotic aortic valve: Evaluation before and after balloon valvuloplasty. *Circulation* 78(II): 124 (abstract)
34. Wyman RM, Diver DJ, Lorell BH (1988) The effects of increasing inotropy and transvalvular flow on Gorlin formula aortic valve area calculations in aortic stenosis. *Circulation* 78(II): 124 (abstract)
35. Topol EJ, Traill TA, Fortuin NJ (1985) Hypertensive hypertrophic cardiomyopathy of the elderly. *NEJM* 312:277
36. Criley JM, Siegel RJ (1985) Has 'obstruction' hindered our understanding of hypertrophic cardiomyopathy? *Circulation* 72:1148
37. Wigle ED (1987) Hypertrophic cardiomyopathy: A 1987 viewpoint. *Circulation* 75:311
38. Yock PG, Hatle L, Popp RL (1986) Patterns and timing of Doppler-detected intracavitary and aortic flow in hypertrophic cardiomyopathy. *J Am Coll Cardiol* 8:1047
39. Hatle L, Angelsen B, Tromsdal A (1979) Noninvasive assessment of atrioventricular pressure half-time by Doppler ultrasound. *Circulation* 60:1096
40. Thomas JD, Wilkins GT, Choong CYP, Abascal VM, Palacios I, Block PC, Weyman AE (1988) Inaccuracy of mitral pressure half-time immediately after percutaneous mitral valvotomy. *Circulation* 78:980
41. Murakami T, Hess OM, Gage JE, Grimm J, Krayenbuehl HP (1986) Diastolic filling dynamics in patients with aortic stenosis. *Circulation* 73:1162
42. Choong CYP, Herrmann HC, Weyman AE, Fifer MA (1987) Preload dependence of Doppler-derived indexes of left ventricular diastolic function in humans. *J Am Coll Cardiol* 10:800
43. Thomas JD, Weyman AE: Doppler mitral pressure half-time: A clinical tool in search of theoretical justification. *J Am Coll Cardiol* 10:923
44. Appleton CP, Hatle LK, Popp RL (1988) Relation of transmitral flow velocity patterns to left ventricular diastolic function: New insights from a combined hemodynamic and Doppler echocardiographic study. *J Am Coll Cardiol* 12:426
45. Stoddard MF, Pearson AC, Kern MJ, Ratcliff J, Mrosek DG, Labovitz AJ (1989) Influence of alteration in preload on the pattern of left ventricular diastolic filling as assessed by Doppler echocardiography in humans. *Circulation* 79:1226
46. Lew WYW (1989) Evaluation of left ventricular diastolic function. *Circulation* 79:1393
47. Dorn GW, Donner R, Assey ME, Spann JF Jr, Wiles HB, Carabello BA (1988) Alterations in left ventricular geometry, wall stress, and ejection performance after correction of congenital aortic stenosis. *Circulation* 78:1358
48. Hess OM, Schneider J, Turina M, Carroll JD, Rothlin M, Krayenbuehl HP (1983) Asymmetric septal hypertrophy in patients with aortic stenosis: An adaptive mechanism or a coexistence of hypertrophic cardiomyopathy? *J Am Coll Cardiol* 1:783
49. Panza JA, Maron BJ (1988) Valvular aortic stenosis and asymmetric septal hypertrophy: Diagnostic considerations and clinical and therapeutic implications. *Eur Heart J* 9 (Suppl E): 71
50. Krayenbuehl HP, Hess OM, Monrad ES, Schneider J, Mall G, Turina M (1989) Left ventricular myocardial structure in aortic valve disease before, intermediate, and late after aortic valve replacement. *Circulation* 79:744
51. Bonow RO (1989) Left ventricular structure and function in aortic valve disease. *Circulation* 79:966
52. Assey ME, Wisenbaugh T, Spann JFJr, Gillette PC, Carabello BA (1987) Unexpected persistence into adulthood of low wall stress in patients with congenital aortic stenosis: Is there a fundamental difference in the hypertrophic response to a pressure overload present from birth? *Circulation* 75:973

53. Hess OM, Ritter M, Schneider J, Grimm J, Turina M, Krayenbuehl HP (1984) Diastolic stiffness and myocardial structure in aortic valve disease before and after valve replacement. *Circulation* 69:855
54. Lorell BH, Grossman W (1987) Cardiac hypertrophy: The consequences for diastole. *J Am Coll Cardiol* 9:1189
55. Borow KM, Green LH, Sloss LJ, Braunwald E, Collins JJ, Cohn L, Grossman W (1980) End-systolic volume as a predictor of post-operative left ventricular performance in volume overload from valvular regurgitation. *Am J Med* 68:655
56. Henry WL, Bonow RO, Borer JS, Ware JH, Kent KM, Redwood DR, McIntosh CL, Morrow AG, Epstein SE (1980) Observations on the optimum time for operative intervention for aortic regurgitation, I: Evaluation of the results of aortic valve replacement in symptomatic patients. *Circulation* 61:471
57. Fioretti P, Roelandt J, Bos RJ, Meltzer RS, van Hoogenhuijze D, Serruys PW, Nauta A, Hugenholtz PG (1983) Echocardiography in chronic aortic insufficiency: Is valve replacement too late when left ventricular systolic dimension reaches 55 mm? *Circulation* 67:216
58. Carabello BA, Usher BW, Hendrik GH, Assey ME, Crawford FA, Leman RB (1987) Predictors of outcome for aortic valve replacement in patients with aortic regurgitation and left ventricular dysfunction: A change in the measuring stick. *J Am Coll Cardiol* 10:991
59. Wisenbaugh T, Spann JF, Carabello BA (1984) Differences in myocardial performance and load between patients with similar amounts of chronic aortic versus chronic mitral regurgitation. *J Am Coll Cardiol* 3:916
60. Wisenbaugh T (1988) Does normal pump function belie muscle dysfunction in patients with chronic severe mitral regurgitation? *Circulation* 77:515
61. Bonow RO, Dodd JT, Maron BJ, O'Gara PT, White GG, Mc Intosh CL, Clark RE, Epstein SE (1988) Long-term serial changes in left ventricular function and reversal of ventricular dilatation after valve replacement for chronic aortic regurgitation. *Circulation* 78:1108
62. Yamaguchi H, Ishimura T, Nishiyama S, Nagasaki F, Nakamishi S, Takatsu F, Nishigo T, Umeda T, Machii K (1979) Hypertrophic non-obstructive cardiomyopathy with giant negative T waves (apical hypertrophy): Ventriculographic and echocardiographic features in 30 patients. *Am J Cardiol* 44:401
63. Shapiro LM, McKenna WJ (1983) Distribution of left ventricular hypertrophy in hypertrophic cardiomyopathy: A two-dimensional echocardiographic study. *J Am Coll Cardiol* 2:437
64. Wigle ED, Sasson Z, Henderson MA, Ruddy TD, Fulop J, Rakowski H, Williams GW (1985) Hypertrophic Cardiomyopathy: The importance of the site and the extent of hypertrophy. A review. *Progr. Cardiovasc Dis* 28:1
65. Abelmann WH, Lorell BH (1989) The challenge of cardiomyopathy. *J Am Coll Cardiol* 13:1219
66. Paulus WJ, Heyndrickx GR, Buyl P, Goethals MA, Andries E (1990) Wide-range load shift of combined aortic valvuloplasty-arterial vasodilation slows isovolumic relaxation of the hypertrophied left ventricle. *Circulation* 81:886
67. Pouleur H, Rousseau MF, van Eyll CV, et al (1983) Force-velocity-length relations in hypertrophic cardiomyopathy: Evidence of normal or depressed myocardial contractility. *Am J Cardiol* 52:813
68. ten Cate FJ, Roelandt J (1979) Progression to left ventricular dilatation in patients with hypertrophic obstructive cardiomyopathy. *Am Heart J* 97:762
69. Borow KM, Lang RM, Neumann A, Carroll JD, Rajfer SI (1988) Physiologic mechanisms governing hemodynamic responses to positive inotropic therapy in patients with dilated cardiomyopathy. *Circulation* 77:625
70. Bonow RO, Rosing DR, Bacharach SL, Green MV, Kent KM, Lipson LC, Maron BJ, Leon MB, Epstein SE (1981) Effects of verapamil on left ventricular systolic function and diastolic filling in patients with hypertrophic cardiomyopathy. *Circulation* 64:787
71. Lorell BH, Paulus WJ, Grossman W, Wynne J, Cohn PF (1982) Modification of abnormal left ventricular diastolic properties by nifedipine in patients with hypertrophic cardiomyopathy. *Circulation* 65:499
72. Paulus WJ, Lorell BH, Craig WE, Wynne J, Murgo JP, Grossman W (1983) Comparison

of the effects of nitroprusside and nifedipine on diastolic properties in patients with hypertrophic cardiomyopathy: Altered left ventricular loading or improved muscle inactivation? *J Am Coll Cardiol* 2:879
73. Hess OM, Murakami T, Krayenbuehl HP (1986) Does verapamil improve left ventricular relaxation in patients with myocardial hypertrophy? *Circulation* 74:530

2. The clinical use and accuracy of echo-Doppler techniques for assessing severity of disease in valvular stenotic lesions

KENNETH M. BOROW, ALEX NEUMANN, DANIEL DAVID & ROBERTO M. LANG

1. INTRODUCTION

A. *Historical perspective*

The Doppler effect was described by Johann Christian Doppler in the mid-1800s and first applied to the cardiovascular system in the 1950s. Initial applications were confined to assessment of peripheral vascular blood flow patterns. Subsequent advances resulted in the development of Doppler systems designed to measure blood velocity in humans. In 1972, a direct correlation was shown between left ventricular stroke volume and the integral of blood flow velocity by Doppler study [1]. Three years later, with the advent of two-dimensional ultrasound cardiac imaging, it became possible to accurately determine the site at which blood flow velocity was measured as well as the angle between the flow and the sampling ultrasound beam. By 1980, improvements in transducer technology, image processing and Doppler spectral analysis made accurate quantitation of intracardiac velocities, blood flows and transvalvular gradients feasible for routine clinical use.

B. *Doppler calculation of blood flow*

Attempts at calculating absolute stroke volume (SV) using Doppler echocardiography have been performed using the following formula:

$$SV = (FVI)(CSA)$$

where FVI is the Doppler flow velocity integral in cm and CSA in the cross-sectional area in cm^2 of the orifice through which blood flows [2–5]. Cardiac output in cm^3/min can then be calculated as the stroke volume times heart rate in beats/min. In practical terms, these calculations require an accurate measurement of the cross-sectional area of the orifice or vessel being interrogated, an accurate temporal and spatial representation of the blood flow velocity across the area of interest, and knowledge of the angle of incidence of the Doppler ultrasound beam with respect to the mean vector for blood flow velocity. Use of either pulsed or continuous wave Doppler echocardio-

E. Andries & R. Stroobandt (eds.), Hemodynamics in Daily Practice, 21–41.

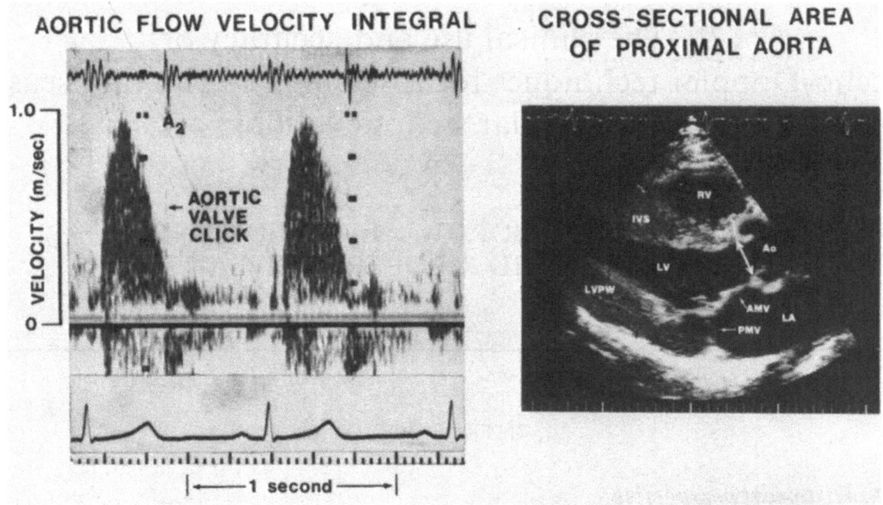

Figure 1. Example of how the continuous wave Doppler flow velocity integral and cross-sectional area (CSA) at the level of the aortic valve annulus can be used to calculate cardiac output and left ventricular stroke volume.

Cardiac output = [(Stroke volume)]) (HR)
= [(Mean flow velocity) (Ejection time) (CSA)] (HR)
[(Flow velocity integral) (CSA)] (HR)

graphy in conjunction with two-dimensional echocardiographic imaging allows these calculations to be performed (Figure 1). Data have been collected from several sites including the LV outflow tract, the ascending aorta, the pulmonary artery, the LV inflow area and the RV inflow tract.

C. *Doppler estimation of pressure gradients*

Years ago, Bernoulli demonstrated that the pressure gradient across a narrowed orifice can be approximated using a complicated mathematical formula. In 1976, Holen and coworkers showed that the Bernoulli equation could be simplified to

$$\Delta P = 4(V_2^2 - V_1^2)$$

where ΔP is the pressure drop across a stenotic valve, V_2 is the high velocity distal to the stenosis, and V_1 is the velocity proximal to the stenosis [6]. In most cases, further simplification is possible if the velocities within the orifice are large when compared to those proximal to the stenosis. Thus, in its simplest form, the modified Bernoulli equation states that the gradient across a stenotic valve can be measured as four times the maximal Doppler-derived blood flow velocity (i.e., $\Delta P = 4V^2$). In high flow states, however, failure to consider elevated velocities proximal to the valve can lead to a gradient overestimation. The realization that a pressure gradient can be reliably quantitated by a simple formulation involving only a determination of the magnitude of velocity increase has had great impact on the role and use of Doppler techniques in clinical cardiology.

II. AORTIC STENOSIS

A. *Invasive techniques for measuring pressure gradients*

The transvalvular pressure gradient in patients with aortic stenosis is ideally measured by simultaneous recordings of phasic pressures on both sides of the diseased valve (Figure 2). The mean gradient measured by planimetry from those tracings is used for the calculation of the stenotic area. The LV peak minus aortic peak pressure value (i.e., peak to peak gradient) is easy to obtain at catheterization but has little physiologic meaning since these pressures rarely occur at the same time in the cardiac cycle.

In many catheterization laboratories, the transvalvular gradient is measured by a catheter in the left ventricle together with a pressure recording from the femoral artery. Because of pressure augmentation secondary to reflected wave effect, this practice may result in as much as a 17-mmHg underestimation of the mean aortic gradient if the femoral and left ventricular tracings are

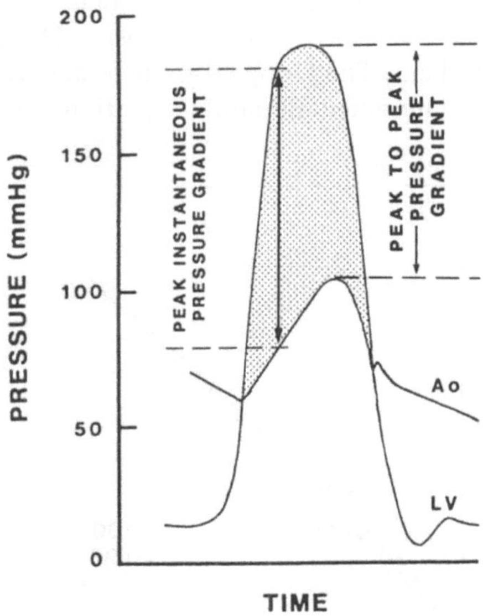

Figure 2. Simultaneously recorded left ventricular and aortic pressure tracings from a patient with valvular aortic stenosis. The shaded area represents the gradient. The temporal difference that exists for the peak instantaneous pressure gradient and the peak-to-peak pressure gradient is depicted. Peak aortic pressure in most patients with aortic stenosis does not occur simultaneously with peak LV pressure.

temporally aligned, and as much as an 18-mmHg overestimation of mean gradient if temporal alignment is not performed [8]. Thus, for accurate estimation of aortic valve area, mean pressure gradients should be measured using simultaneous left ventricular and central aortic pressures [9]. When this is not available, pressure measurements on catheter pullback from the left ventricle (LV) to the aorta are acceptable.

B. *Noninvasive assessment*

1. *Ultrasound imaging.* Traditional two-dimensional echocardiography can provide useful information regarding aortic root size as well as aortic valve thickness, calcification and overall mobility. It can accurately define the level of anatomic obstruction (i.e., supravalvular, valvular or subvalvular). However, it cannot determine reliably the severity of valvular stenosis in the presence of a significantly deformed valve. Recently, Hoffman et al. have suggested that the use of transesophageal two-dimensional echocardiographic imaging can circumvent this problem [9].

2. *Doppler estimation of peak and mean pressure gradients.* Hatle et al. [10] initially demonstrated the clinical applicability of the simplified Bernoulli equation for assessing peak and mean transaortic gradients. Subsequently, several investigators have confirmed a good correlation between Doppler and catheterization measured gradients [11–15]. Currie et al. [15] conducted the largest clinical study of aortic stenosis (100 patients, ages 50–89 years), comparing simultaneously obtained continuous-wave Doppler data and catheterization derived gradient. The Doppler gradient across the stenotic valve was calculated using the modified Bernoulli equation (i.e., $\Delta P = 4V^2$). All

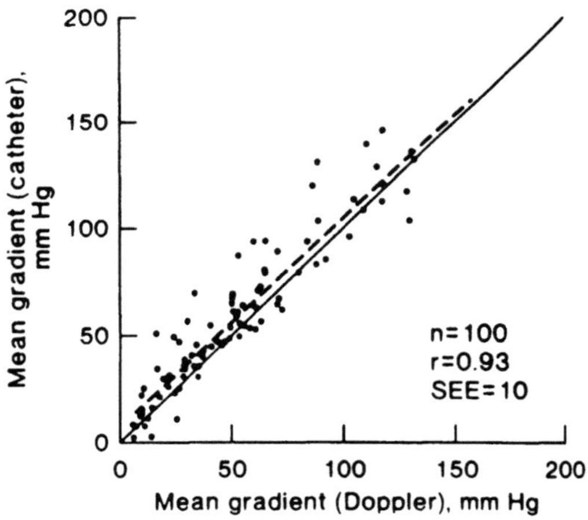

Figure 3. Plot of simultaneous mean Doppler derived and catheter measured pressure gradients in 100 patients (ages 50–89 years) with aortic stenosis (Reprinted from PJ Currie et al. [15].

Doppler data were considered usable with most recorded from an apical transducer position. For their entire study population, there was a high correlation (r = 0.92) between maximum Doppler-determined gradient and the simultaneously obtained maximum instantaneous (not peak-to-peak) catheter gradient. The correlation coefficient for the mean gradient was the same (Figure 3). Accuracy was not affected by cardiac index (0.7–5.3 l/min/m^2), ejection fraction (14–89%) or the presence of coronary disease. Thus, continuous-wave Doppler can be used to reliably predict the pressure gradient in adults with aortic stenosis. The clinical importance of this capability was noted by Tierstein et al. [16] in a study of 30 patients with valvular aortic stenosis. In almost all cases in which the Doppler-determined mean gradient was greater than 50 mmHg, patients had critical aortic stenosis at catheterization. When the Doppler mean gradient was less than 20 mmHg, critical aortic stenosis was rarely present. It is important to note that in the 14 patients with Doppler mean gradients between 30 and 50 mmHg, the distinction between critical and non-critical aortic stenosis could not be made.

3. *Noninvasive determination of LV instantaneous ejection pressures.* In a recent report, Borow et al. [17] demonstrated the ability to accurately determine instantaneous left ventricular pressure throughout ejection in patients with aortic stenosis. Instantaneous LV ejection pressures (P_{LV}) were estimated using the formula

$$P_{LV} = PG_{NI} + PAO_{NI}$$

where P_{NI} is the instantaneous pressure gradient across the valve determined by Doppler and PAO_{NI} is the instantaneous aortic pressure determined from a time-corrected calibrated external carotid or subclavian pulse tracing. Figure 4 illustrates the noninvasive determination of instantaneous LV ejection pressure in a patient with aortic stenosis. In panel A, the Doppler profile obtained from the apex is shown as well as the calibrated carotid pulse tracing and the simultaneous LV pressure measured by catheter. In panel B, the computer generated LV pressure tracing from the noninvasive data (P_{NI}) is shown compared to the simultaneous catheter-obtained LV pressure tracing (P_{LV}). For the study population, the noninvasive determination of left ventricular pressure had less than a 5% error at 20, 40, 60, and 80% of ejection as well as at peak ejection [17]. With the ability to noninvasively determine instantaneous left ventricular ejection pressure in aortic stenosis in conjunction with echo measured LV dimensions and wall thicknesses, it is now possible to calculate peak, mean and end-systolic wall stresses. These measurements are important in patients with valvular aortic stenosis since they are the major determinants of the magnitude of LV hypertrophy, the amount of oxygen consumed by the heart, and overall ventricular performance. The relationship between systolic wall stress and LV performance may also be useful for distinguishing LV dysfunction in aortic stenosis due to abnormal myocardial loading conditions from that due to decreased ventricular contractility.

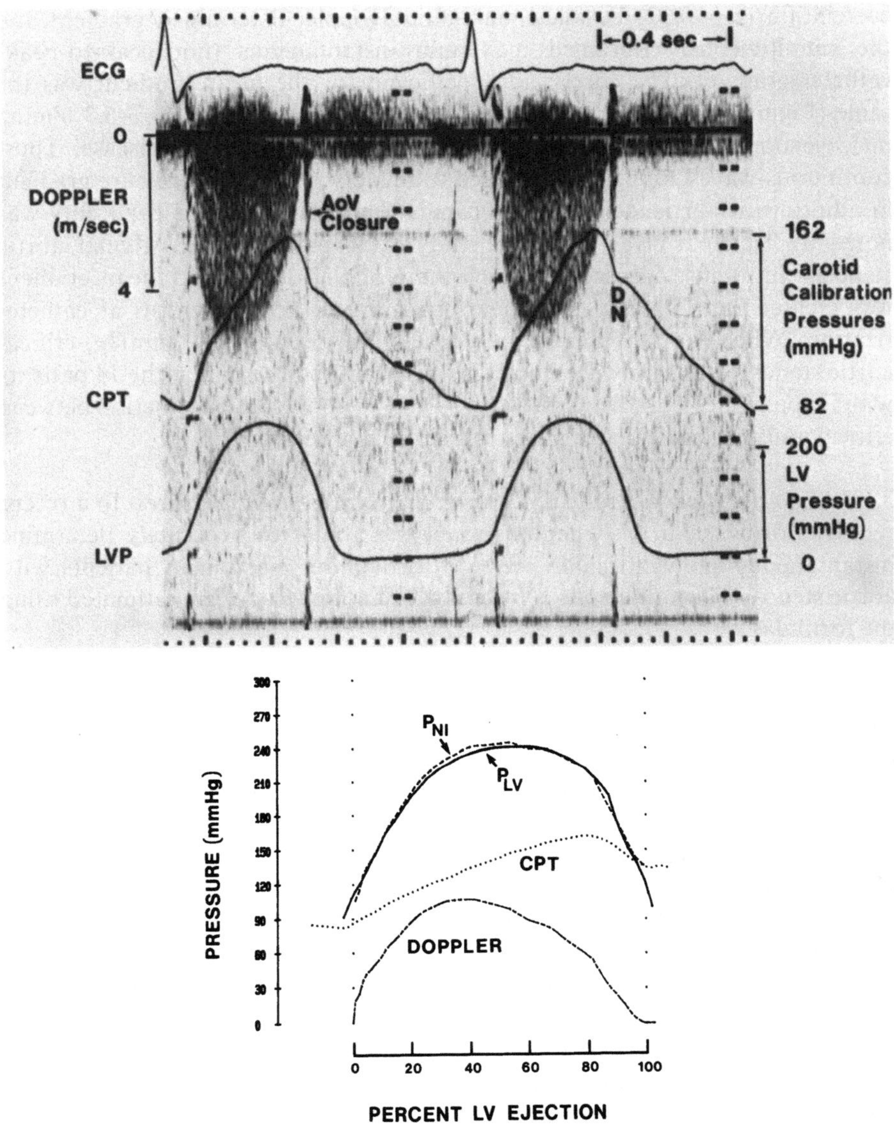

Figure 4. *Upper panel*: Simultaneously acquired invasive and noninvasive data for subsequent digitization.
Lower panel: Example of the digitized data generated from a patient with aortic stenosis. Note the marked similarity between the catheterization measured (P_{LV}) and noninvasively derived (P_{NI}) instantaneous left ventricular ejection pressures.
ECG = electrocardiogram; CPT = carotid pulse tracing; LVP = left ventricular pressure; AoV = aortic valve; DN= dicrotic notch.

4. *Transaortic valve flow and aortic valve area.* Pressure determinations alone do not fully define hemodynamics in aortic stenosis. Since the magnitude of the pressure drop varies with flow, a significant pressure drop may be present with only moderate obstruction when flow is increased (e.g., aortic regurgitation, hyperdynamic state). Similarly, a severe obstruction may be associated with a moderate pressure gradient if flow is reduced. The distinction between hemodynamically critical and non-critical aortic stenosis often requires calculation of the aortic valve area. In 1951, Gorlin et al. [18] reported that aortic valve area (AVA) could be estimated by dividing the quantity of blood crossing the valve per unit time by the velocity of flow across the valve. Until recently, the velocity of flow across the valve could be determined only at specialized research centers. To simplify the calculation of valve area, a constant (K) was derived which, when multipled by the square root of the mean pressure gradient (ΔP_m), estimated transaortic blood flow velocity. Thus, aortic valve area (AVA) can be approximated using the following equation:

$$\mathrm{AVA} = \frac{\text{Flow/Time}}{\text{Velocity of flow}} = \frac{\mathrm{CO/SEP}}{(\mathrm{K})(\Delta \mathrm{P_m})} = \frac{\mathrm{SV/ET}}{(\mathrm{K})(\Delta \mathrm{P_m})}$$

where CO is the cardiac output and SEP is the systolic ejection period. Of note, CO/SEP is the same as stroke volume divided by ejection time (ET).

Examination of the Gorlin equation reveals that all of the variables needed to calculate AVA can be determined noninvasively by combined Doppler measurement of velocity and echo imaging for cross-sectional area. Cardiac output is the product of cross-sectional area of flow, the mean velocity (Vm) of flow through the CSA, and the duration of flow. Systolic ejection period is determined from the Doppler recordings of the stenotic jet as the ejection time per beat multipled by heart rate. The mean systolic gradient is determined by summating a series of individual pressure gradients which are calculated from instantaneous velocities and dividing by the number of observations. Alternatively, the area under the Doppler-determined instantaneous gradient curve can be planimetered and divided by the ejection time. Currently available cardiac ultrasound units provide software that allows this calculation to be performed on line. With the advent of accurate Doppler echocardiographic techniques, it is possible for the first time in routine clinical settings to measure transaortic flow velocities in aortic stenosis. With this capability, AVA area can be calculated without the use of a derived constant of the Gorlin equation:

$$\mathrm{AVA} = \frac{\frac{\mathrm{C.O.}}{\mathrm{SEP}}}{\overline{\mathrm{V_{AV}}}} = \frac{\frac{\mathrm{SV}}{\mathrm{ET}}}{\overline{\mathrm{V_{AV}}}} \qquad \text{Modified Gorlin Formula}$$

where $\overline{V_{AV}}$ is the mean velocity of flow across the stenotic aortic valve. This noninvasive approach allows serial assessment of the severity of aortic valve stenosis independent of aortic regurgitation and other valve disease. In addition, it allows more appropriate selection and follow-up of patients who might be candidates for aortic balloon valvuloplasty or surgical decalcification of the valve.

It is obvious from examining the modified Gorlin formula that a reliable means for determining total LV stroke volume in patients with aortic stenosis is required. As noted earlier, Doppler methods have been used successfully to determine volume flow in the ascending aorta [4,19], and pulmonary artery [20] as well as across the mitral [21] and tricuspid valves [22]. If the flow velocity profile across the interrogated site is flat, integration of the Doppler envelope is equivalent to the mean flow velocity times the duration of flow. However, in valvular aortic stenosis, ascending aortic flow cannot be used to help calculate cardiac output since the recorded velocities reflect the combination of flow and turbulence created as blood passes through the stenotic valve. Technical problems are also present in these patients which preclude reliable use of tricuspid, pulmonary, or mitral methods for flow calculations. In addition, volume flow across any of these cardiac valves cannot be substituted for total transaortic stroke volume in patients with coexisting aortic regurgitation. To circumvent these problems, Lewis et al. [23] estimated total stroke volume utilizing the LV outflow tract just below the aortic valve. They reported data from 39 patients in whom thermodilution-determined cardiac outputs were obtained within minutes of Doppler measurements. A pulsed Doppler velocity profile was obtained from the apical five-chamber view with the sample volume positioned immediately proximal to the aortic annulus. The resultant velocity-time profile was integrated and combined with a cross-sectional area derived from the echo measured diameter of the aortic anulus. The correlation between Doppler and invasively measured stroke volumes was 0.95, with a standard error of the estimate of 6.4 cc.

The fluid dynamics of a stenotic valve suggest that flow proximal to a stenotic valve is laminar with a flat profile [24]. Because of this, the LV outflow tract is particularly well suited for the assessment of transaortic flow in patients with aortic stenosis. Advantages of the LV outflow tract method for flow calculation include: (1) the anulus is a sharply defined area and relatively

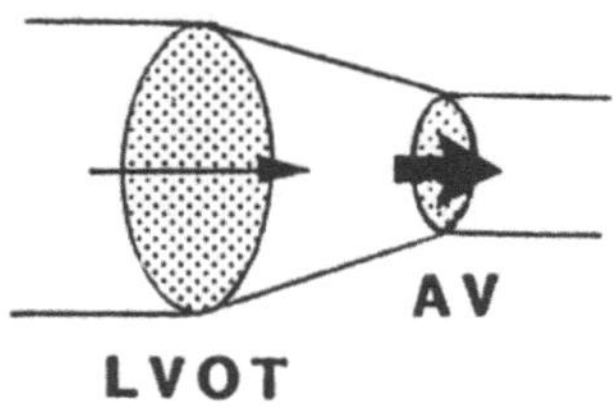

Figure 5. Use of the continuity equation for calculating aortic valve area (AVA). The continuity principle states that flow through the left ventricular outflow tract (LVOT) is equal to flow through the aortic valve (AV). The ratio of the flow velocity integrals (FVI) times the LVOT area (A) yields the AVA.

easy to image by two-demensional echocardiography, (2) the pulsed Doppler signal is easy to obtain from this region, (3) the left ventricular outflow tract diameter remains relatively constant throughout the cardiac cycle and provides highly reproducible measurements [25], and (4) the calculated flow is total LV output per beat and, therefore, accounts for aortic regurgitant volume plus effective forward flow. This is important since it is total transvalvular flow during systole that should be used for the calculation of aortic valve area.

Investigators have recently utilized the principle that the volume of systolic flow through the left ventricular outflow tract (LVOT) must equal the volume of systolic flow through the stenotic aortic valve (AV). This is based on the continuity principle (Figure 5). Since LV total output equals the product of the cross-sectional area (CSA) through which flow proceeds and the systolic flow velocity integral (FVI), the following simple equations can be derived:

(1) $$\mathrm{FLOW}_{LVOT} = \mathrm{FLOW}_{AV} \qquad \text{Since flow} = (\mathrm{CSA})(\mathrm{FVI}),$$

(2) $$(\mathrm{CSA})_{LVOT}\,(\mathrm{FVI})_{LVOT} = [\mathrm{AVA}]\,(\mathrm{FVI})_{AV} \text{ with rearrangement}$$

(3) $$\mathrm{AVA} = (\mathrm{CSA})_{LVOT}\left[\frac{\mathrm{FVI}_{LVOT}}{\mathrm{FVI}_{AV}}\right]$$

Multiple reports have validated the use of echo-Doppler techniques to measure aortic valve area by the continuity principle [16,26–30]. In one particularly well-conducted study, Zoghbi et al. [27] used Doppler derived flow from the LVOT to compare noninvasively derived AVA with catheterization calculated

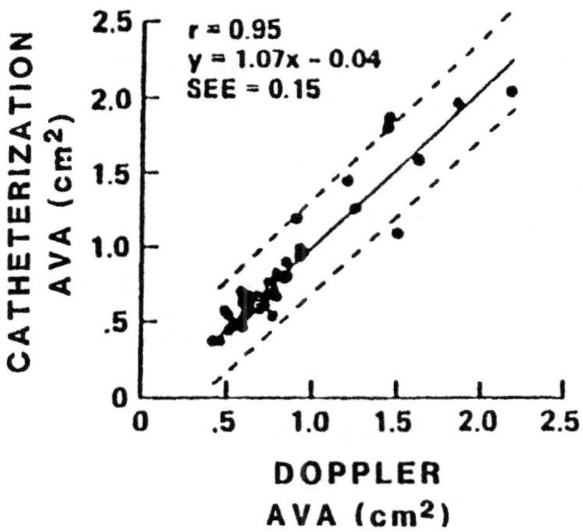

Figure 6. Correlation between aortic valve areas determined at cardiac catheterization and Doppler-derived aortic valve areas determined using the left ventricular outflow tract diameter method in 39 adults (Reprinted from WA Zoghbi et al. [27]).

estimates. For the 39 patients studied, the correlation coefficient was 0.95, with a standard error of 0.15 cm^2 (Figure 6).

5. *Color flow Doppler to assess severity of associated lesions.* In patients with aortic stenosis, color flow Doppler is useful to assess the relative magnitude of associated aortic and/or mitral regurgitation as well as the direction of forward blood flow through the stenotic valve. This latter information helps to determine if the angle between the direction of blood flow and incident ultrasound beam is appropriately small. Assessment of the severity of associated aortic regurgitation is particularly important when considering a patient as a possible candidate for aortic balloon valvuloplasty.

III. MITRAL STENOSIS

A. *Clinical assessment*

The most common symptom of mitral stenosis is dyspnea. In general, exercise is well tolerated when the area of the mitral valve orifice is narrowed to 2.5 cm^2. With narrowing to between 1.5 and 2.5 cm^2, moderately severe exercise may precipitate dyspnea. Further reduction in orifice area will be associated with progressive disability. Usually when the mitral orifice is diminished to a critical area of 1 cm^2, even mild exercise causes dyspnea. Because of accommodations in patients' life styles from active to sedentary modes with progression of the disease, symptoms are often difficult to quantify and do not always reflect the severity of the anatomic narrowing of the mitral valve orifice. Other objective evidence of the severity of mitral stenosis is thus essential for the proper management of patients with this condition. Traditionally, decisions regarding surgical interventions have been based on estimations of the mitral valve area using the Gorlin equation in conjunction with the presence of symptoms. But with the advent of echo and Doppler techniques our ability to noninvasively assess and quantify mitral stenosis has changed dramatically.

B. *Invasive assessment*

The Gorlin equation for the mitral valve [18] states that

$$\text{Mitral valve area} = \frac{\text{Cardiac output / Diastolic filling period}}{(\text{Constant})\,(\sqrt{\text{Mean diastolic gradient}})}$$

$$\text{Mean diastolic gradient} = \left[\frac{\text{Cardiac output / Diastolic filling period}}{(\text{Constant})\,(\text{Mitral valve area})}\right]^2$$

Given a fixed mitral valve area, the formula shows how variations in cardiac output and diastolic filling time (heart rate) affect the mean transmitral pressure gradient. Conditions that increase cardiac output or shorten the diastolic filling period (e.g., exercise, pregnancy, tachyarrythmias, excitement, fever) will raise the mean mitral valve gradient, thereby significantly elevating left atrial pressure leading to pulmonary capillary engorgement and dyspnea. Unfortunately, the Gorlin equation, currently the standard against which all new indices are measured, does not always provide an accurate approximation of the mitral valve area [31]. This is understandable considering the assumptions inherent in this formula. First, it assumes steady flow through an idealized fixed orifice, not through a rheumatically deformed, funnel-shaped mitral valve and submitral apparatus. Second, the calculation of mitral valve area using Gorlin's hydraulic formula depends heavily on the accurate estimation of cardiac output, yet the currently used clinical techniques for determining cardiac output (thermodilution and Fick principle) have their own inherent sources of imprecision. Third, the valve orifice area is not constant and appears to be flow dependent, especially at low flow rates [32,33]. Fourth, in the presence of mitral regurgitation the Gorlin equation underestimates mitral valve area since thermodilution or Fick techniques measure only the antegrade fraction of transmitral flow, thereby neglecting the regurgitant flow that recrosses the mitral valve. Furthermore, the constants employed in this formula were derived from valve areas obtained by blind digital palpation during operations. Finally, in most catheterization laboratories, pulmonary capillary wedge pressure is used as a substitute for left atrial or pulmonary venous pressures. Wedge pressure recordings in patients with mitral stenosis are often dampened (when compared to direct left atrial pressure recordings), thereby yielding higher mean diastolic gradients – which lead to erroneous valve area calculations [34].

C. *Noninvasive assessment*

1. *Ultrasound imaging.* Since 1956 when Edler first reported the ultrasonic features of mitral stenosis, echocardiography has been used extensively in the detection of rheumatic mitral stenosis as well as in the determination of etiologies of various other forms of mitral valve disease [35]. The first M-mode echo abnormality to be recognized in mitral stenosis was the marked reduction in the diastolic EF slope of the anterior mitral valve leaflet. Diagnosis was further refined by Duchak et al. who first described the abnormal anterior motion of the posterior mitral leaflet during diastole [36]. Two-dimensional echocardiography has considerably refined the assessment of rheumatic mitral valve disease by offering a tomographic visualization of the entire mitral valve apparatus in conjunction with real-time cross-sectional imaging of the mitral valve orifice [37]. Moreover, two-dimensional echo imaging is useful for estimating the severity of narrowing of the entire LV inflow tract. The suitability for mitral commissurotomy (closed, open or percutaneous) versus valve replacement can often be assessed using two-dimensional echo techniques [38]. Recently, transesophageal echo (TEE) has been shown to be useful for selecting patients amenable for mitral valve repair rather than replacement [39]. In addition TEE is a useful screening procedure for left atrial thrombus in a patient being considered as a possible candidate for mitral balloon valvuloplasty.

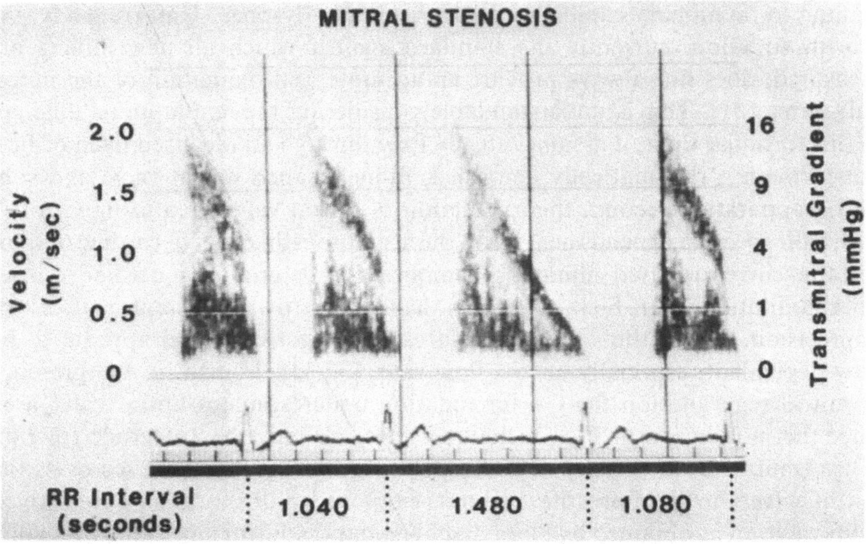

Figure 7. Continuous wave Doppler recording from a patient with mitral stenosis. The cardiac rhythm is atrial fibrillation. Late diastolic velocities are useful in calculating the end-diastolic gradient. Long RR intervals are associated with lower end-diastolic gradients while shorter RR intervals are associated with higher end-diastolic gradients. Despite different RR intervals the slope of the diastolic descent of the mitral valve velocity profile is the same, resulting in almost identical t½ values.

2. *Doppler estimation of transvalvular pressure gradients.* The Doppler flow profile of a stenosed mitral valve, unlike the normal valve, demonstrates a maximum diastolic velocity greater than 1 m/sec, slow deceleration of blood velocity after initial diastolic filling, and increased late diastolic velocity. In the presence of atrial fibrillation the late diastolic flow augmentation caused by atrial contraction is absent (see Figure 7). As the severity of mitral stenosis progresses, peak flow velocity increases with reduced flow deceleration over the remainder of diastole. The peak velocities present at any time during diastole can be used to estimate the corresponding instantaneous pressure gradients across the valve using the modified Bernoulli equation [40,41]. Mean diastolic gradients obtained during cardiac catheterization correlate well with those obtained by Doppler study [11,41].

In patients with mitral stenosis, late diastolic velocities are useful in calculating the end-diastolic gradient. As noted in Figure 7, the gradient is flow and heart rate dependent: long RR intervals are associated with low end-diastolic gradients while short RR intervals are associated with high end-diastolic gradients. In patients with mitral stenosis and atrial fibrillation, Doppler echocardiography can be used to determine the ventricular rate associated with the lowest late diastolic transmitral gradient in association with preserved cardiac output. Additionally, pharmacological interventions intended to control ventricular rates during exercise in patients with atrial fibrillation can be monitored.

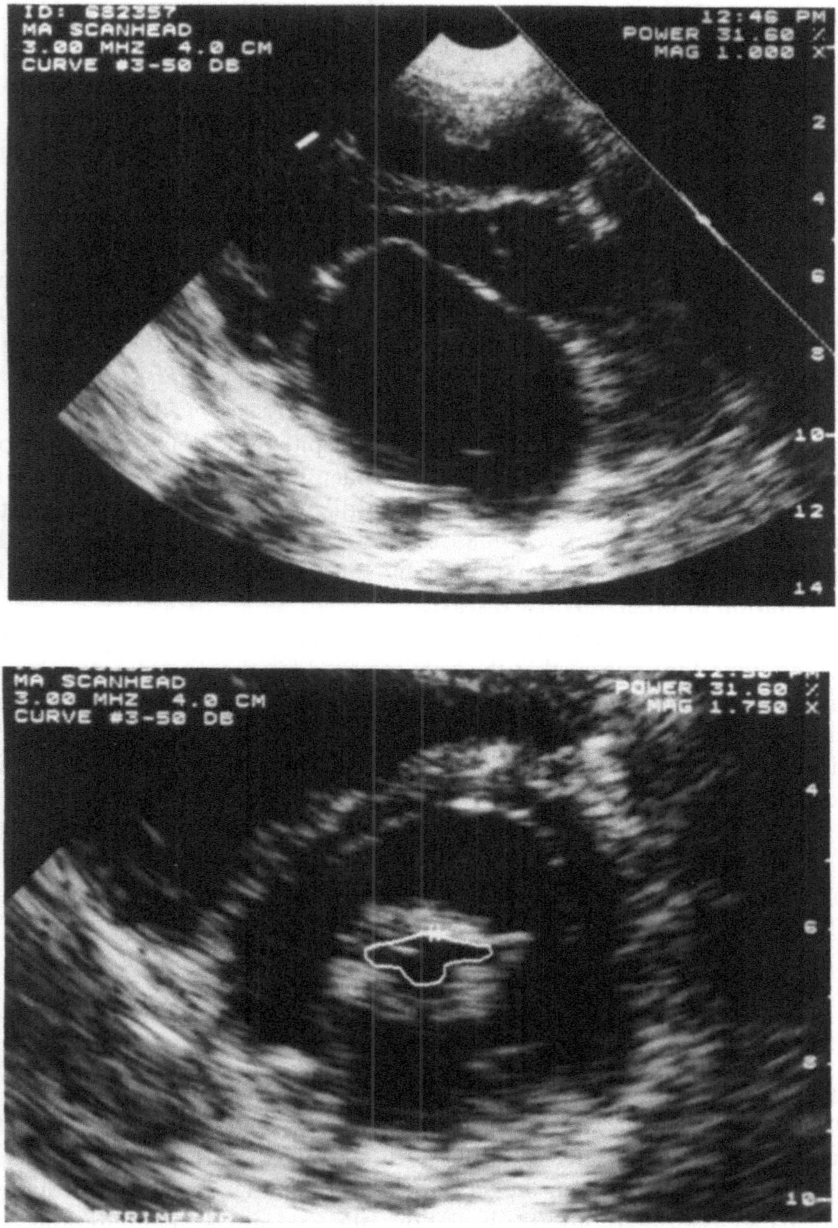

Figure 8. *Upper panel*: Early diastolic frame from a two-dimensional echocardiogram of a stenotic mitral valve. Note doming of the anterior mitral valve leaflet and enlargement of the left atrium. *Lower panel*: The short axis examination provides the opportunity for two-dimensional measurement of the mitral valve area. Planimetry resulted in a mitral valve area of 0.75 cm^2.

3. *Estimation of mitral valve area.* (a) *Two-dimensional echocardiography.* The mitral orifice size is best evaluated from the parasternal short-axis view [37,42]. Ideally, the plane of imaging should be parallel to the plane of the mitral valve orifice. Several tomographic cuts of the funnel-shaped mitral valve apparatus should be obtained in order to insure that the smallest diastolic mitral orifice is identified. By freezing this diastolic image and tracing its inner border at the black and white interface, the mitral valve orifice size can be determined (Figure 8). Certain factors may, however, limit the accuracy of this measurement. First, high-quality short-axis parasternal views of the mitral valve may be obtained in all but 15% of patients with mitral stenosis. In addition, dropout of lateral echos as well as the appropriateness of gain and reject settings may also negatively influence the accuracy of the planimetry. Planimetry does not appear to be accurate post commissurotomy due to the extensive leaflet distortion created by this procedure [43]. The separation of the fractured or incised commissures is frequently not well visualized and often excluded from the planimetered area. Despite these limitations, previous studies comparing measurements by two-dimensional echocardiography with those by the Gorlin equation derived from cardiac catheterization have reported correlation coefficients of $r = 0.83$ to 0.95 [37,41,43–45]. Importantly, this correlation appears to be unaffected by the presence of associated mitral regurgitation or other valvular disease.

(b) *Doppler echocardiography.* The Doppler pressure half-time [$P_{(t½)}$] method is based upon the concept that the time required for the diastolic mitral valve gradient to drop to half its initial peak value reflects the severity of the mitral stenosis [46]. With smaller valve areas, progressive increases in the pressure half-time occur. Hatle et al. noninvasively determined the pressure half-time and defined it as the time required for the early maximal diastolic velocity to fall to a value equal to the maximal velocity divided by the square root of two [40,47]. An estimate of mitral valve area is obtained by dividing an empirically derived number (220 msec/cm^2) by the pressure half-time in milliseconds:

$$\mathrm{MVA} = \frac{220}{P_{(t½)}}.$$

Figure 9 illustrates how the mitral pressure half-time is calculated. This approach is particularly suitable for patients in whom the two-dimensional examination is technically inadequate or mitral commissurotomy has been performed. It has also been shown to be useful in patients with mitral stenosis who have associated atrial fibrillation and/or mitral regurgitation [48]. Grayburn et al. demonstrated the lack of influence of aortic regurgitation on the pressure half-time assessment of mitral stenosis [49]; however, some investigators have shown that aortic regurgitation may shorten the pressure half-time leading to a Doppler overestimation of valve area. The discordance between studies emanates from differences in the LV end-diastolic pressure

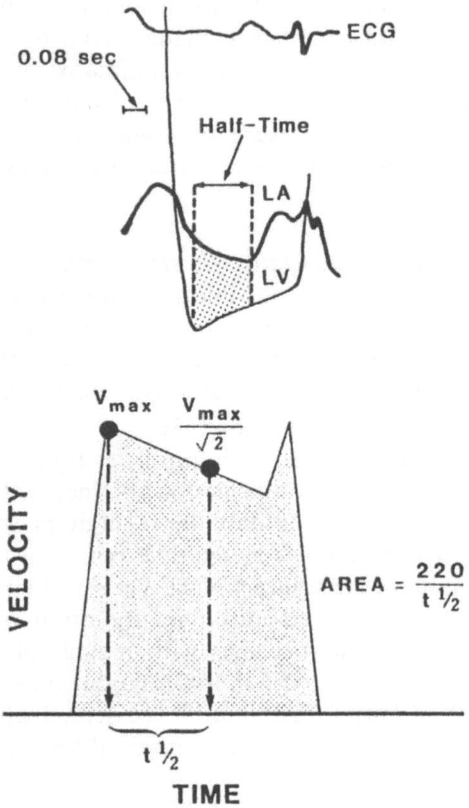

Figure 9. Illustration of the Doppler pressure half-time method for estimating mitral valve area. The transmitral diastolic velocities when used in the modified Bernoulli equation allow accurate estimates of instantaneous left atrial to left ventricular pressure gradients (shaded area). The pressure half-time is defined as the time required for the gradient to drop to half its initial peak value. Mitral valve area (cm^2) is calculated as 220 divided by the t½.

response to aortic insufficiency, which in turn is dependent mainly upon LV compliance. Recently, the ability of the pressure half-time formula to predict mitral valve areas has been validated for both native and prosthetic valves and compared to simultaneous catheterization and 2-D cross-sectional data yielding high correlation coefficients ($r \geqslant 0.90$) [41,43,48,49].

The pressure half-time method has several potential limitations. First, it requires operator experience. Failure to align the interrogating Doppler signal with the stenotic jet may result in underestimation of the mean mitral gradient and pressure half-time. Second, the mitral pressure half-time not only varies inversely with mitral valve area but also directly with left atrial and left ventricular compliance and proportionally to the square root of the initial transmitral gradient [50,51]. These findings explain why pressure half-time works as an accurate predictor of mitral valve area in the majority of clinical situations (i.e., pressure and compliance changes tend to offset each other). Conversely, the pressure half-time is a poor estimator of mitral valve area in those situations where anatomic distortion or physiologic derangement has independently changed either pressure or compliance. Examples of such situations include percutaneous balloon mitral valvuloplasty and acute myocardial ischemia [52].

4. *Color flow Doppler to assess associated mitral regurgitation.* With the addition of color flow mapping, it is now possible in mitral stenosis to identify jet shape and angulation as well as improve the rapidity and accuracy of pulsed and continuous-wave Doppler sampling. Moreover, with this technique, the LA-to-LV jet through the stenotic mitral valve can be distinguished more easily from coexisting aortic regurgitation [53].

Mitral stenosis is often associated with mitral regurgitation. By combining Doppler techniques with structural information obtained with two-dimensional echo imaging, it is possible to quantitate the regurgitant volume [54]. Color Doppler can rapidly visualize flows at multiple points in an imaging plane, thereby allowing mapping of the regurgitant jet. The sensitivity of color Doppler with angiographically documented mitral regurgitation ranges in different studies from 86–100% while the specificity with angiographically documented competent mitral valves is 100% [55,56]. Information concerning the presence as well as the severity of mitral regurgitation is essential when deciding upon the type of medical or surgical intervention planned for a patient with mitral stenosis.

Recently, the feasibility of percutaneous balloon dilation of stenotic mitral valves has been established. Echo-Doppler techniques are very important in the appropriate selection of candidates in whom balloon dilation might have a successful result. Severe calcification of the commissures, rigid valve leaflets and subvalvular disease are associated with smaller increases in mitral valve area when compared to patients with pliable, minimally calcified leaflets with no mitral regurgitation [57] (Figure 10). Cardiac ultrasound techniques including transesophageal echocardiography, have also been used to successfully monitor the delivery of valvular dilation catheters across the interatrial septum as well as detect and quantify residual shunts created by atrial septostomy. Using Doppler techniques, it has become evident that new or increased mitral regurgitation occurs in over one-third of patients post valvuloplasty [57].

IV. DOPPLER ESTIMATION OF RIGHT VENTRICULAR AND PULMONARY ARTERY PRESSURES

Moderate to severe mitral stenosis is usually associated with either passive or reactive pulmonary artery hypertension. In most patients, this results in

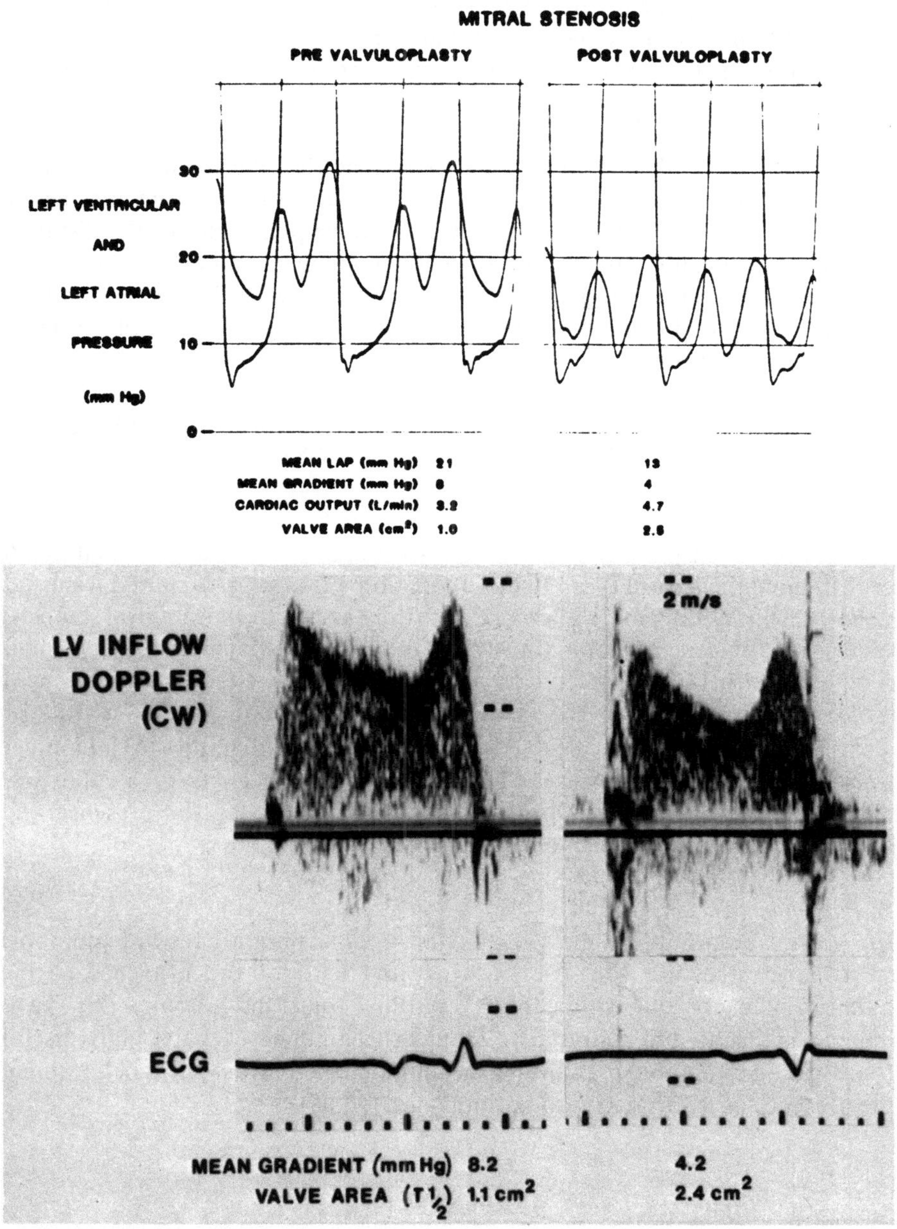

Figure 10. *Upper panel*: Left ventricular and atrial pressures recorded in the cardiac catheterization laboratory before and after mitral valvuloplasty using the double balloon technique. The mean diastolic gradient decreased from 8 mmHg to 4 mmHg with balloon dilation in assocation with a 47% increase in cardiac output and a marked increase in mitral valve area. *Lower panel*: Continuous wave Doppler recordings obtained before and after valvuloplasty in the same patient. Note that the mean gradient and valve areas obtained using Doppler techniques were almost identical to those obtained during cardiac catheterization.

some degree of RV dilation and functional tricuspid regurgitation [58]. Doppler echo, by estimating the RV to RA pressure drop (from the tricuspid regurgitant jet) and adding the measured or estimated right atrial pressure (RAP), can be used to predict the peak right ventricular systolic pressure (RVSP) [59,60]:

$$RVSP = RAP + 4(V_{max})^2$$

In the absence of valvular pulmonic stenosis, the RVSP provides an accurate estimate of peak PA pressure. The RAP can be estimated from the height of the jugular venous pulse above the sternal angle plus 5 cm for the distance from the right atrium to the sternal angle. Dividing this number by 1.3 converts the units to mmHg. Alternatively, an assumed RAP of between 5 and 15 mmHg can be used depending upon the size of the right atrium and severity of trecuspid regurgitation.

V. DOPPLER ESTIMATION OF TRANSVALVULAR PRESSURE GRADIENTS IN TRICUSPID STENOSIS AND PULMONIC STENOSIS

A. *Tricuspid stenosis*

The normal tricuspid valve has a cross-sectional area of approximately 10 cm^2. Rheumatic deformity is the most common etiology for acquired tricuspid stenosis. This lesion, which is almost uniformly associated with mitral stenosis, results in a mean diastolic transvalvular gradient which is usually small compared with that of the mitral valve. In general, a tricuspid valve area $\leqslant$ 1.5 cm^2 represents severe disease. Two-dimensional echo is useful for identifying thickened and calcified leaflets with restricted motion [61]. Doppler tracings can accurately measure instantaneous and mean transvalvular gradients [62,63]. Color flow Doppler is useful for assessing the presence and severity of associated tricuspid regurgitation.

B. *Pulmonic stenosis*

Congenital deformity of the valve is the most common cause of pulmonic stenosis. Obstruction can also occur at the level of the branches of the pulmonary artery and within the RV outflow tract (infundibular PS). Two-dimensional echo and quantitative Doppler techniques are particularly useful for assessing infundibular and valvular pulmonic stenosis as well as determining the presence of associated cardiac anomalies [64,65].

REFERENCES

1. Cross G, et al. (1972) Cardiovascular information from transcutaneous aortovelography. Proc 3rd Int Cont Med Physics 19.9 Gotenborg, Sweden
2. Colocousis JS, et al. (1977) Estimation of stroke volume changes by ultrasonic Doppler. *Circulation* 56:914
3. Magnin PA, et al. (1981) Combined Doppler and phased array echocardiographic estimation of cardiac output. *Circulation* 63:388

4. Huntsman LL, et al. (1983) Noninvasive Doppler determination of cardiac output in man: Clinical validation. *Circulation* 67:595
5. Neumann A, et al. (1988) Is it possible to obtain an accurate Doppler estimate of stroke volume in patients with decreased forward flow? *J Am Coll Cardiol* 11:121A
6. Holen J, et al. (1976) Determination of pressure gradient in mitral stenosis with a noninvasive ultrasound Doppler technique. *Acta Med Scand* 199:455
7. Folland ED, et al. (1984) Is peripheral arterial pressure a satisfactory substitute for ascending aortic pressure when measuring aortic valve gradients? *J Am Coll Cardiol* 4:1207
8. Carabello BA (1987) Advances in the hemodynamic assessment of stenotic cardiac valves. *J Am Coll Cardiol* 10:912
9. Hoffman T, et al. (1987) Determination of aortic valve orifice area in aortic valve stenosis by two-dimensional transesophageal echocardiography. *Am J Cardiol* 59:330
10. Hatle L, et al. (1980) Non-invasive assessment of aortic stenosis by Doppler ultrasound. *Br Heart J* 45:284
11. Stamm RB, et al. (1983) Quantification of pressure gradients across stenotic valves by Doppler ultrasound. *J Am Coll Cardiol* 2:207
12. Berger M, et al. (1984) Evaluation of aortic stenosis by continuous wave Doppler ultrasound. *J Am Coll Cardiol* 3:150
13. Williams GA, et al. (1985) Value of multiple echocardiographic views in the evaluation of aortic stenosis in adults by continuous wave Doppler. *Am J Cardiol* 55:445
14. Agatston AS, et al. (1985) Doppler diagnosis of aortic stenosis in patients over 60 years of age. *Am J Cardiol* 56:106
15. Currie PJ, et al. (1985) Doppler echocardiographic assessment of severity of calcific aortic stenosis: a simultaneous Doppler-catheter correlative study in 100 patients. *Circulation* 71:1162
16. Tierstein P, et al. (1986) Doppler echocardiographic measurement of aortic valve area in aortic stenosis: A noninvasive application of the Gorlin formula. *J Am Coll Cardiol* 8:1059
17. Borow KM, et al. (1987) Can the modified Bernoulli equation be used to accurately determine intraventricular pressures throughout systole in patients with valvular aortic stenosis? *J Am Coll Cardiol* 9:236A
18. Gorlin R, et al. (1951) Hydraulic formula for calculation of the area of the stenotic mitral valve, other cardiac valves, and central circulatory shunts I. *Am Heart J* 41:1
19. Goldberg SJ, et al. (1982) Evaluation of pulmonary and systemic blood flow by two-dimensional Doppler echocardiography using fast Fourier transform spectral analysis. *Am J Cardiol* 50:1394
20. Sanders SP, et al. (1983) Measurement of systemic and pulmonary blood flow and QP/QS ratio using Doppler and two-dimensional echocardiography. *Am J Cardiol* 51:952
21. Meijboom EJ, et al. (1987) A simplified mitral valve method for two-dimensional echo Doppler blood flow calculation. *Am Heart J* 113:335
22. Fisher DC, et al. (1983) The mitral valve orifice method for non-invasive two-dimensional echo-Doppler determination of cardiac output. *Circulation* 67:872
23. Lewis JF, et al. (1984) Pulsed Doppler echocardiographic determination of stroke volume and cardiac output: Clinical validation of two new methods using the apical window. *Circulation* 70:425
24. Minor WR (1982) *Hemodynamics*. Baltimore: Williams & Wilkins, p23.
25. Ihlene H, et al. (1984) Determination of cardiac output by Doppler echocardiography. *Br Heart J* 51:54
26. Skjaerpe T, et al. (1985) Non-invasive determination of valve area in patients with aortic stenosis by Doppler ultrasound and two-dimensional echocardiography. *Circulation* 72:810
27. Zoghbi WA, et al. (1986) Accurate non-invasive quantification of stenotic aortic valve area by Doppler echocardiography. *Circulation* 73:452
28. Richards KL, et al. (1986) Calculation of aortic valve area by Doppler echocardiography: a direct application of the continuity equation. *Circulation* 73:964
29. Otto CM, et al. (1986) Determination of the stenotic aortic valve area in adults using Doppler echocardiography. *J Am Coll Cardiol* 7:509

30. Neumann A, et al. (1989) Valve resistance in aortic stenosis: an alternative method for assessing the hemodynamic significance of flow obstruction. *J Am Coll Cardiol* 13:234A
31. Odemuyiwa O, et al. (1986) Assessing the severity of valve stenosis. *Br Heart J* 55:117
32. Rodrigo FA, et al. (1953) Estimation of valve area and 'valvular resistance.' *Am Heart J* 45:1
33. Ubago JL, et al. (1980) Hemodynamic factors that affect calculated orifice areas in the mitral Hancock xenograft valve. *Circulation* 61:388
34. Hosenpud J, et al. (1983) Overestimation of mitral valve gradients obtained by phasic pulmonary capillary wedge pressure. *Cath Cardiovasc Diag* 9:283
35. Edler I (1956) Ultrasound cardiogram in mitral valvular disease. *Acta Chir Scand* 111:230
36. Duchak JM Jr, et al. (1972) The posterior mitral valve echo and echocardiographic diagnosis of mitral stenosis. *Am J Cardiol* 29:628
37. Nichol PM, et al. (1977) Two-dimensional echocardiographic assessment of mitral stenosis. *Circulation* 55:120
38. Peller OG, et al. (1987) Role of Doppler and imaging echocardiography in selection of patients for cardiac valvular surgery. *Am Heart J* 114:1445
39. Marwick T, et al. (1989) Echo evaluation of immediate and late failed mitral valve repair. *J Am Coll Cardiol* 13:114A
40. Hatle L, et al. (1978) Noninvasive assessment of pressure drop in mitral stenosis by Doppler ultrasound. *Br Heart J* 40:131
41. David D, et al. (1989) Can the modified Bernoulli equation accurately estimate instantaneous transmitral pressure gradients in patients with cardiac pathology? *J Am Coll Cardiol* 13:234A
42. Mehlman DJ (1986) Doppler and two-dimensional echocardiographic assessment of mitral stenosis. *Echocardiography* 3:109
43. Smith MD, et al. (1986) Comparative acuracy of two-dimensional echocardiography and Doppler pressure half-time methods in assessing severity of mitral stenosis in patients with and without prior commissurotomy. *Circulation* 73:100
44. Nichol PM, et al. (1977) Two-dimensional echocardiographic assessment of mitral stenosis. *Circulation* 55:120
45. Yamamoto T (1983) Two-dimensional echocardiographic assessment of mitral stenosis: Preoperative detection of organic change in the mitral valve apparatus. *J Cardiovasc Ultrasound* 2:273
46. Libanoff AJ, et al. (1968) Atrioventricular pressure half-time. Measure of mitral valve orifice area. *Circulation* 38:144
47. Hatle L (1979) Noninvasive assessment of atrioventricular pressure half-time by Doppler ultrasound. *Circulation* 60:1096
48. Bryg RJ, et al. (1986) Effect of atrial fibrillation and mitral regurgitation on calculated mitral valve area in mitral stenosis. *Am J Cardiol* 57:634
49. Grayburn PA ,et al. (1987) Effect of aortic regurgitation on the assessment of mitral valve orifice area by Doppler pressure half-time in mitral stenosis. *Am J Cardiol* 60:322
50. Karp K, et al. (1989) Reassessment of valve area determinations in mitral stenosis by the pressure half-time method: Impact of left ventricular stiffness and peak diastolic pressure difference. *J Am Coll Cardiol* 13:594
51. Flachskampf FA, et al. (1989) Ventricular and atrial compliance changes affect pressure half time: experimental evidence. *J Am Coll Cardiol* 13:234A
52. Wilkins GT, et al. (1987) Failure of the Doppler pressure half-time to accurately demonstrate change in mitral valve area following percutaneous mitral valvotomy. *J Am Coll Cardiol* 9:218A
53. Panadian NG, et al. (1987) Color Doppler flow imaging in valvular stenosis. *Echocardiography* 4:515
54. Rokey R, et al. (1986) Determination of regurgitant fraction in isolated mitral or aortic regurgitation by pulsed Doppler two-dimensional echocardiography. *J Am Coll Cardiol* 7:1273
55. Miyatake K, et al. (1986) Semiquantitative gradings of severity of mitral regurgitation of real-time two-dimensional Doppler flow imaging technique. *J Am Coll Cardiol* 7:82

56. Helmcke F, et al. (1987) Color Doppler assessment of mitral regurgitation using orthogonal planes. *Circulation* 75:175
57. Reid CL, et al. (1987) Mechanisms of increase in mitral valve area and influence of anatomic features in double-balloon, catheter balloon valvuloplasty in adults with rheumatic mitral stenosis: A Doppler and two-dimensional echocardiographic study. *Circulation* 76:628
58. Miyatake K, et al. (1982) Evaluation of tricuspid regurgitation by pulsed Doppler and two-dimensional echocardiography. *Circulation* 66:777
59. Berger M, et al. (1985) Quantitative assessment of pulmonary hypertension in patients with tricuspid regurgitation using continuous wave Doppler ultrasound. *J Am Coll Cardiol* 6:359
60. Currie PJ (1985) Continuous wave Doppler determination of right ventricular pressure: a simultaneous Doppler-catheterization study in 127 patients. *J Am Coll Cardiol* 6:750
61. Hubbard WN, et al. (1987) Acquired abnormalities of the tricuspid valve – an ultrasonographic study. *Int J Cardiol* 14:311
62. Dennig K, et al. (1986) Doppler echocardiographic assessment of tricuspid stenosis. *Herz* 11:332
63. Parris TM, et al. (1987) Doppler echocardiographic findings in rheumatic tricuspid stenosis. *Am J Cardiol* 60:1414
64. Johnson Gl, et al. (1984) Accuracy of combined two-dimensional echocardiography and continuous wave recordings in the estimation of pressure gradient in right ventricular outlet obstruction. *J Am Coll Cardiol* 3:1013
65. Goldberg SJ, et al. (1986) Can the technique of Doppler estimate of pulmonary stenosis gradient be simplified? *Am Heart J* 111:709.

3. Proper timing of valve replacement in aortic stenosis

BLASE A. CARABELLO

INTRODUCTION

If prosthetic valves were perfect and could be inserted without operative mortality, the timing of surgery for aortic stenosis would be a simple matter. One could simply replace the valve prophylactically in anyone who had significant stenosis. Unfortunately, insertion of prosthetic valves carries a 5–10% operative risk. Following succesful surgery, one is still faced with the subsequent complications of thromboembolism, primary valve failure, and endocarditis. Because of these potential complications, valve replacement should be delayed as long as possible. On the other hand, excessive delay may lead to irreversible left ventricular dysfunction or sudden death. Thus the goal in the timing of replacement of the aortic valve for aortic stenosis is to avoid excessive years with a prosthesis in place but also to replace the valve prior to the occurrence of serious complications. The following is a review of clinical data which are useful in helping to decide when it is either too early or too late to perform aortic valve replacement for aortic stenosis.

WHEN IS IT *TOO EARLY* TO REPLACE THE VALVE FOR AORTIC STENOSIS?

The answer to the question posed above is best derived from the natural history of the disease. Figure 1 shows the survivorship of patients with aortic stenosis. In this data compiled in 1968 by Ross & Braunwald, it is evident that survivorship in patients with aortic stenosis is excellent until the onset of symptoms. Once symptoms occur, survivorship is greatly reduced in unoperated patients. One can expect approximately 50% of patients who develop angina to be dead within five years of the onset of that symptom unless valve replacement is performed. In the case of syncope the expected mortality is 50% within three years. If congestive heart failure develops the expectant mortality is 50% within one to two years. Although 20% of patients with aortic stenosis die suddenly, only 25% of that 20% (5%) die suddenly

E. Andries & R. Stroobandt (eds.), Hemodynamics in Daily Practice, 43–52.

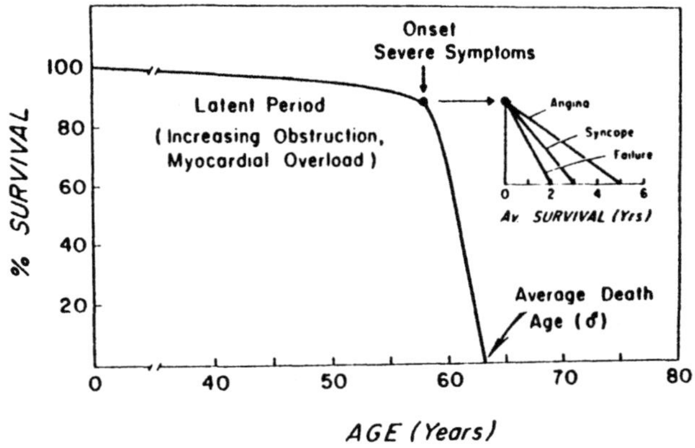

Figure 1. The natural history of aortic stenosis. The figure shows a long latent period (asymptomatic period) during which survivorship is nearly normal. With the onset of symptoms, the curve abruptly changes and mortality is profoundly increased. Reproduced by permission of the American Heart Association, Inc. (from Ross & Braunwald [1], Figure 1).

without the onset of symptoms [1]. Since operative mortality is at least 5%, there is little to be gained by surgery, from a risk-benefit standpoint, prior to the onset of symptoms. The data above compiled in the 1960s have recently been confirmed in a study by Kelly et al. [2]. In this study 51 asymptomatic patients with aortic stenosis who had a gradient of at least 50 mmHg were followed for a mean duration of 17 months. In that period of time only two of the 51 patients (4%) died and each had become symptomatic prior to death. Further confirmation of the natural history of aortic stenosis comes from the Mayo Clinic in a study by Pellikka et al. who followed 114 patients with asymptomatic aortic stenosis who had a gradient $\geqslant$ 64 mmHg for 20 months [3]. During that time period only three patients (<3%) died and each had become symptomatic for at least three months prior to death. Thus the data seem clear in giving an answer to the question posed above: It is too early to operate prior to the onset of symptoms because there is little to be gained by aortic valve replacement in asymptomatic patients.

One could ask the question whether with more modern medical therapy one should now delay surgery till after the symptoms have been present for some period of time. A recent study from the Mayo clinic by O'Keefe et al. demonstrates that currently mortality for patients with *symptomatic* aortic stenosis is till 44% at one year, 63% at two years, and 75% three years after the onset of symptoms [4]. Thus while one should delay surgery until symptoms develop, on the other hand, immediate surgery is required once symptoms do develop. The expected results of surgery are demonstrated in Figure 2 [5]. Survivorship for 125 patients with symptomatic aortic stenosis who underwent aortic valve replacement was 85% at five years but only 20% for patients with symptomatic aortic stenosis who refused surgery.

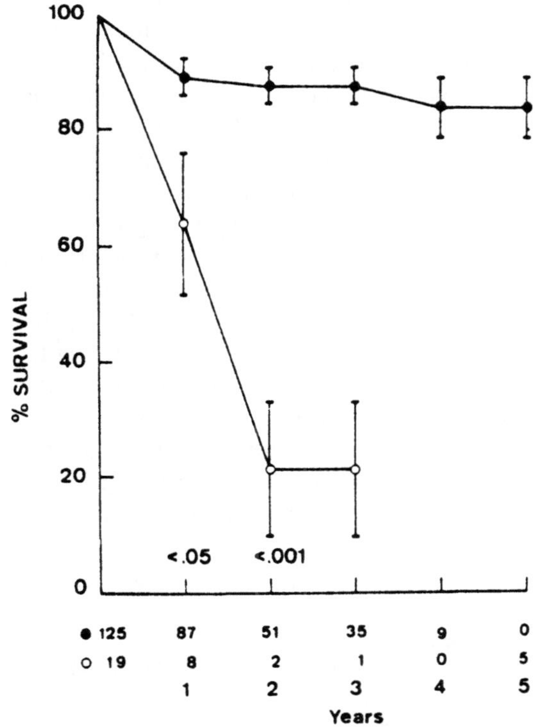

Figure 2. Survivorship of operated versus unoperated patients with symptomatic aortic stenosis. Survivorship in operated patients (●) was far superior to that of unoperated patients (○). Patients in both groups were similar with regard to severity of disease. Reproduced by permission of the American Heart Association, Inc. (from Schwarz et al. [5] Figure 1, left-hand panel) $\chi^2 = 23{,}5$; $p < 0.0001$.

WHEN IS IT *TOO LATE* TO OPERATE ON THE PATIENT WITH SEVERE AORTIC STENOSIS?

Although surgery is recommended as soon as symptoms occur, some patients neglect their symptoms until the symptoms are far advanced. It could be asked about patients with far-advanced disease: Is it now too late to operate?

Patients with aortic stenosis who have congestive heart failure and severe depression of left ventricular ejection performance still usually benefit from aortic valve replacement [6–8]. Even moribund patients may improve dramatically following aortic valve replacement. This distinction of dramatic acute improvement in ventricular performance following surgery which aortic stenosis shares with few other heart diseases stems from the pathophysiologic mechanisms responsible for congestive heart failure in this disease. The causes for reduction in systolic performance in aortic stenosis include afterload mismatch and contractile dysfunction [7,9–11]. Afterload mismatch defines a situation where ventricular ejection performance is reduced because load on the ventricle (created by the small outflow orifice) is greatly increased. In the situation of pure afterload mismatch, contractile function is normal yet ejection fraction is severely reduced because the ventricle (with normal contractile function) can not produce the force necessary to overcome the extraordinary amount of afterload present. The second mechanism by which left ventricular ejection performance can be reduced is that contractile function (muscle strength) itself has deteriorated [7,11]. In a group of 66 patients with aortic stenosis examined by Huber et al., 19 had normal afterload and normal left ventricular performance [11]. Of the 57 patients with abnormal function, an element of afterload mismatch was present in 48 (85%). It is the presence of afterload mismatch in the large majority of patients with aortic stenosis and congestive heart failure that contributes to the excellent surgical results in these patients. Surgical relief of the aortic valve obstruction acutely reduces afterload (Figure 3) [12]. This in turn results in an immediate postoperative increase in ejection performance (Figure 4), translating into a relatively low perioperative mortality for such ill patients and improvement in clinical status.

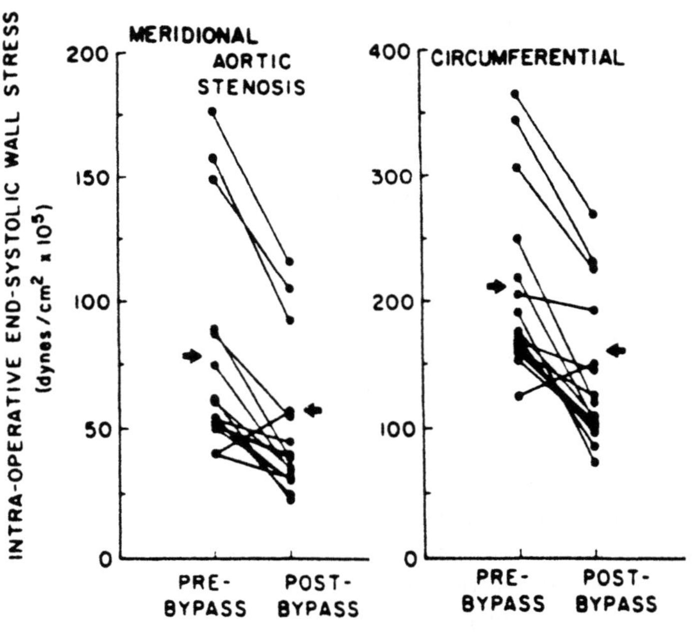

Figure 3. Wall stress (afterload) before and after aortic valve replacement (bypass). Both meridional and circumferential stress, indicators of left ventricular afterload, are significantly decreased immediately following surgery. Reproduced by permission of the American Heart Association, Inc. (from St. John Sutton et al. [12] Figure 2)
$p < 0.01$.

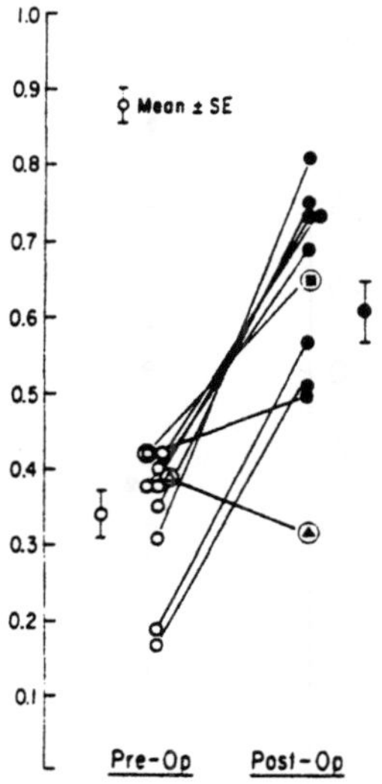

Figure 4. Ejection fraction before aortic valve replacement (Pre-op) and after aortic valve replacement (Post-op). Nearly all subjects with depressed preoperative ejection fraction had a striking improvement in ejection fraction following surgery. Reproduced by permission of the American Heart Association, Inc. (from Smith et al. [8] Figure 5, left-hand panel).
$p < 0.001$.
(■) = Peri-op: M1 and late CHB.
(▲) = Post-op: perivalvular aortic incompetence.

While the majority of patients with severe left ventricular dysfunction due to aortic stenosis improve after valve replacement, there is still a small group which still has a poor result. Carabello et al. found that patients with aortic stenosis, congestive heart failure, and poor ejection performance who had low transvalvular gradients (<30 mmHg) had a high operative mortality (Figure 5) [7]. This was recently confirmed by Smucker et al. [13]. The same is true for patients undergoing transluminal valvuloplasty [14]. Intuitively, this is not surprising. It is the patients with the lowest transvalvular gradients who experience the least afterload reduction since only a small reduction in left ventricular systolic pressure is accomplished by surgical relief of the aortic valve obstruction. Further, it is probably the patients with the worst contractile function who also have the lowest gradients. To summarize: If reduced ejection performance is primarily due to afterload mismatch, the outcome of aortic valve replacement is good because surgery acutely reverses the afterload excess and improves ejection performance and clinical condition. Conversely, if preoperative reduction in ejection performance is primarily due to contractile dysfunction in the absence of afterload mismatch, surgery does little acutely to improve ejection performance and hemodynamic state. This lack of acute improvement produces a high perioperative mortality and little immediate clinical improvement.

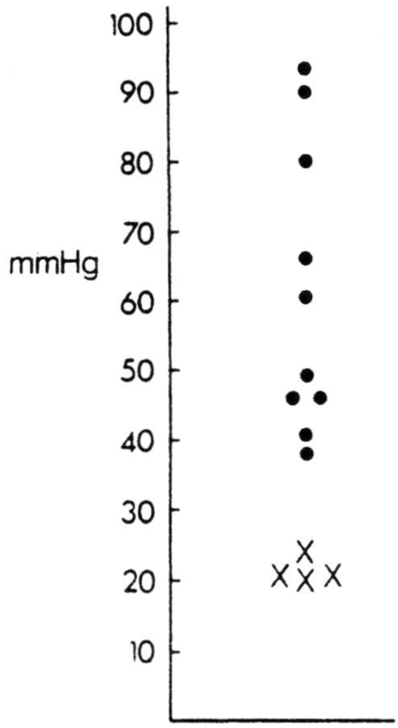

Figure 5. Relationship of transvalvular gradient to operative results in aortic stenosis. Patients with a *low* transvalvular gradient (×) died or remained severely symptomatic following aortic valve replacement while patients with *higher* transvalvular gradients (•) had an excellent outcome. Reproduced by permission of the American Heart Association, Inc. (from Carabello et al. [7] Figure 3).

A second reason (besides a lack of reversible afterload mismatch) for patients with low transvalvular gradients doing poorly at surgery is that some patients with small transvalvular gradients have 'pseudo aortic stenosis' rather than true aortic stenosis. I define a 'pseudo aortic stenosis' as a mildly stenotic aortic valve operating in conjunction with a coincidentally myopathic left ventricle. In the case of 'pseudo aortic stenosis' the valve disease did not cause the cardiomyopathy to begin with, thus its correction does not improve the patients condition. However, in 'pseudo aortic stenosis' the low cardiac output together with the low gradient still yields a small, even 'critical', valve area when the area is calculated by the Gorlin equation [15]. The orifice size may be calculated to be small because of one of two reasons. First, the myopathic ventricle may be unable to open the mildly stenotic valve to its full orifice area producing an orifice area which is in fact reduced. In support of this hypothesis Richards and his colleagues were able to demonstrate during surgery that a balloon placed in the stenotic aortic valve and inflated to pressures in the range of those generated by the left ventricle could open the valve substantially more at higher pressures than at lower pressures [16]. This finding suggests that the orifica area in aortic stenosis is not in fact fixed but can vary according to the force of ventricular contraction. In the instance of a

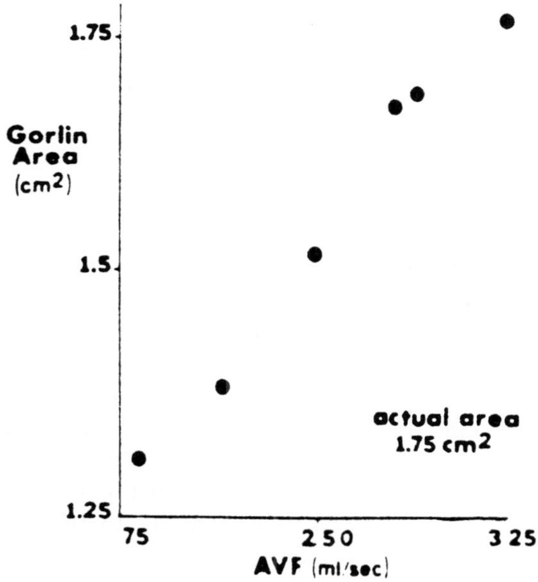

Figure 6. Effect of flow on Gorlin formula calculated area. This figure demonstrates that as aortic valve flow increased, calculated Gorlin formula area increased despite the fact that the actual valve area was fixed at 1.75 cm^2. Reproduced by permission of the American Heart Association, Inc. (from Cannon et al. [17] Figure 5).

weak contraction, the aortic orifice is small but the small orifice size is due more to the weak ventricle than to pathology in the valve. Thus there is 'pseudo aortic stenosis'. A second cause of 'pseudo aortic stenosis' are limitations inherent in the Gorlin formula used to calculate the valve area. In a recent study by Cannon and colleagues [17] valves of known and fixed orifice area were placed in a pulsatile flow chamber where flow and transvalvular pressure gradients could be measured accurately. As shown in Figure 6, calculated valve area increased directly with flow even though actual valve area was fixed. Since valve area, flow, and gradient were all known, Cannon et al. were able to recalculate the constant in the Gorlin equation. They found that the constant was not a constant at all but rather varied directly and closely ($r = 0.95$) with the square root of the mean valve gradient. Since the constant was proportional to the square root of the mean valve gradient, correction for the constant (k) is made by multiplying it by the square root of the mean valve gradient. When this new term $k \approx \sqrt{MVG}$ is introduced into the original Gorlin equation:

$$\text{Valve area} = \frac{\text{flow}}{44.3\sqrt{\text{MVG}}}$$

where MVG = mean valve gradient, it produces a new equation:

$$\text{Valve area} = \frac{\text{flow}}{44.3\ \sqrt{\text{MVG}}\cdot(\sqrt{\text{MVG}}\cdot \text{k})}$$

or

$$\text{Valve area} = \frac{\text{flow}}{44.3\ \cdot \text{MVG}\cdot \text{k}}$$

since multiplying a square root by a square root results in removal of the square root sign from the equation. It is probably this potential limitation in the original formula which makes calculated valve area potentially flow dependent. Thus in the patient with a cardiac output of 3 l/min and a mean valve gradient of 20 mmHg, the calculated valve area will likely be in the critical range at 0.7 cm^2. However, in such patients, if cardiac output were increased by exercise [18], or by inotropic agents [19], it would increase flow proportionally more than gradient yielding a higher valve area.

The above data suggests the following answer to the question posed at the beginning of this section: It is almost never too late to operate on patients with severe aortic stenosis and congestive heart failure since most patients, even those with severely reduced ejection fraction benefit from surgery. However, there is a small subgroup of patients with a low gradient and low output which may not benefit. In such patients it is probably advisable that during heart catheterization cardiac output be increased artificially by infusion of a positive inotropic agent such as dobutamine or by exercise. If an increase in cardiac output causes a large increase in aortic valve area, such patients probably have 'pseudo aortic stenosis' and a concomitant but independent cardiomyopathy. These patients are unlikely to benefit from surgery. On the other hand, if increasing cardiac output causes a substantial increase in gradient so that the valve area remains close to the critical range, then surgery can be offered to such patients with the understanding that they are still at high risk.

SUMMARY

Asymptomatic patients with aortic stenosis, even those with high transvalvular gradients, have an excellent prognosis without surgery. Since the onset of symptoms heralds an abrupt worsening of prognosis, asymptomatic patients should be followed carefully and operated upon immediately when symptoms develop.

Patients with aortic stenosis who have congestive heart failure, even those with severe reduction in ejection fraction, usually have an excellent response to surgery as long as they have a mean transvalvular gradient of at least 40 mmHg. Almost all such patients should be operated providing there are no extenuating circumstances such as the coincidental presence of other serious illnesses. Conversely, patients with a transvalvular gradient < 40 mmHg are less likely to benefit from surgery. Such patients should be stressed during catheterization to determine the valve area at a higher cardiac output. If the valve area stays within the critical range and gradient increases substantially, aortic valve replacement should still be contemplated.

REFERENCES

1. Ross J Jr, Braunwald E (1968) Aortic stenosis. *Circulation* 38 (Suppl V): V–61–67
2. Kelly TA, Rothbart RM, Cooper CM, Kaiser DL, Smucker ML, Gibson RS (1988) Comparison of outcome of asymptomatic to symptomatic patients older than 20 years of age with valvular aortic stenosis. *Am J Cardiol* 61:123–130
3. Pellikka PA, Bailey KR, Nishimura RA, Taylor CL, Taijk AJ (1989) The natural history of adults with asymptomatic, severe aortic stenosis. *J Am Coll Cardiol* 13:147A (abstract)
4. O'Keefe JH Jr, Vlietstra RE, Holmes DR Jr, Bailey KR (1987) Natural history of candidates for balloon valvuloplasty. *J Am Coll Cardiol* 9:195A (abstract)
5. Schwarz F, Baumann P, Manthey J, Hoffmann M, Schuler G, Mehmel HC, Schmitz W, Kübler W (1982) The effect of aortic valve replacement on survival. *Circulation* 66:1105–1110
6. Croke RP, Pifarre R, Sullivan H, Gunnar R, Loeb H (1977) Reversal of advanced left ventricular dysfunction following aortic valve replacement for aortic stenosis. *Ann Thorac Surg* 24:38–43
7. Carabello BA, Green LH, Grossman W, Cohn LH, Koster JK, Collins JJ Jr (1980) Hemodynamic determinants of prognosis of aortic valve replacement in critical aortic stenosis and advanced congestive heart failure. *Circulation* 62:42–48
8. Smith N, McAnulty JH, Rahimtoola SH (1978) Severe aortic stenosis with impaired left ventricular function and clinical heart failure: results of valve replacement. *Circulation* 58:255–264
9. Ross J Jr (1976) Afterload mismatch and preload reserve: a conceptual framework for the analysis of ventricular function. *Prog Cardiovasc Dis* 18:255–264
10. Gunther S. Grossman W (1979) Determinants of ventricular function in pressure-overload hypertrophy in man. *Circulation* 59:679–688
11. Huber D, Grimm J, Koch R, Krayenbuehl HR (1981) Determinants of ejection performance in aortic stenosis. *Circulation* 64:126–134
12. St. John Sutton M, Plappert T, Spiegel A, Raichlen J, Douglas P, Reichek N, Edmunds L (1987) Early postoperative changes in left ventricular chamber size, architecture, and function in aortic stenosis and aortic regurgitation and their relation to intraoperative changes in afterload: a prospective two-dimensional echocardiographic study. *Circulation* 76:77–89
13. Smucker ML, Manning SB, Stuckey TD, Tyson DL, Nygaard TW, Kron IL (1989) Preoperative left ventricular wall stress, ejection fraction, and aortic valve gradient as prognostic indicators in aortic valve stenosis. *Cathet Cardiovasc Diag* 17:133–143
14. Reddy PS, Uretsky BF, Trento A, Gallis-Davis K (1989) Is balloon valvuloplasty beneficial in patients with calculated critical aortic stenosis but low ejection fraction and pressure gradient. *J Am Coll Cardiol* 13:156A (abstract)
15. Gorlin R, Gorlin SG (1951) Hydraulic formula for calculation of area of stenotic mitral valve, other cardiac values, and central circulatory shunts, I. *Am Heart J* 41:1–29
16. Richards KL, Hart TT, Cannon SR, Lujan MS, Crawford MH, Harman PK, Grover FL, Trinkle JK (1986) Confirmation of variable orifice native valves in adults with severe aortic stenosis. *Circulation* 74 (Suppl II): II–314 (abstract)

17. Cannon SR, Richards KL, Crawford M (1985) Hydraulic estimation of stenotic orifice area: a correction of the Gorlin formula. *Circulation* 71:1170–1178
18. Bache RJ, Wang Y, Jorgensen CR (1971) Hemodynamic effects of exercise in isolated valvular aortic stenosis. *Circulation* 44:1003–1013
19. Wyman RM, Diver DJ, Lorell BH (1988) The effects of increasing inotropy and transvalvular flow on Gorlin formula aortic valve area calculations in aortic stenosis. *Circulation* 78 (Suppl II): II–124 (abstract)

4. Optimal timing of surgery for volume overload hypertrophy in mitral and aortic regurgitation

KENNETH M. BOROW

I. INTRODUCTION

Despite numerous clinical studies, the proper timing of corrective surgery in many patients with chronic aortic or mitral regurgitation remains a controversial issue. However, most investigators agree that it is the magnitude of left ventricular (LV) contractile abnormality in a given patient that subsequently determines clinical course. Ideally, patients should undergo surgery late enough in the natural history of their disease to justify the surgical risk yet before irreversible damage to the ventricular contractile mechanism or pulmonary vasculature has occurred. A long-standing problem has been the differentiation of myocardial contractility from overall LV performance. This is evident in most of the clinical studies of preoperative and postoperative LV function in chronic volume overload states in which highly load-dependent indices (e.g., ejection fraction, shortening fraction, LV volumes or dimensions) have been used [1, 2]. It is important to realize that overall LV performance reflects the net effect of preload, afterload and contractility [3]. These component parts interact to determine the magnitude of ventricular wall thickness and mass, the size of the left ventricle and the extent of ventricular fiber shortening during systole. Superimposed upon these conditions is the marked interdependence of systolic and diastolic events in the cardiac cycle. Because of all of these factors, the presence or absence of clinical symptoms does not necessarily correlate with the magnitude of pathophysiologic derangements. Indeed, because of 'successful' compensatory mechanisms, patients with aortic or mitral regurgitation can remain asymptomatic for years despite depression in LV contractile state.

Recently, it has become evident that improved preoperative care, surgical procedures and myocardial preservation techniques have made it necessary to reassess the data upon which we base our current decisions regarding the optimal timing for valve replacement. This chapter will give a brief overview of the pathophysiology of chronic aortic and mitral regurgitation as well as the advantages and limitations of various physiologic indices used previously

E. Andries & R. Stroobandt (eds.), Hemodynamics in Daily Practice, 53–76.

to determine optimal timing of valve replacement in these patients. Finally, a series of guidelines will be offered based upon the most important recent studies of operative mortality and long-term survival in patients with chronic aortic and mitral regurgitation.

II. PATHOPHYSIOLOGY

A. *Chronic aortic regurgitation*

This is characterized by progressive LV dilation secondary to the chronic LV volume overload that results from aortic valve incompetence. Severe AR may be associated with normal effective forward flow and normal overall LV performance even though the regurgitant fraction (i.e., regurgitant volume/total LV output) may exceed 0.75. In AR, the large total LV output is ejected into the relatively high pressure proximal aorta requiring marked elevations in LV work. The major compensatory mechanism enabling this to occur is augmentation of ventricular preload (i.e., force or load acting to stretch LV fibers at end-diastole) [4, 5]. With time, the LV passive diastolic pressure-volume relation is displaced rightward (i.e., improved chamber compliance) such that any end-diastolic volume is associated with a lower end-diastolic pressure than would be recorded in a normal subject [6]. This results in lowering

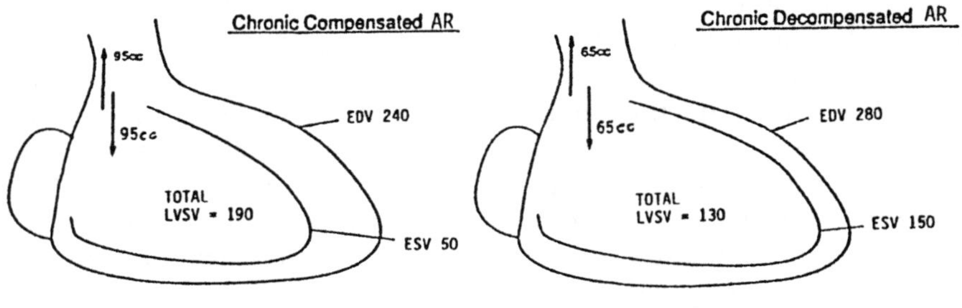

	Preload EDS (kd/cm²)	Afterload ESS (kd/cm²)	CS	EF	RF	FSV (CC)
NL	16	90	N	68	0	95
CCAR	40	110	N	0.79	0.50	95
CDAR	50	150	χ	0.46	0.50	65

Figure 1. Representative myocardial hemodynamics noted in patients with chronic compensated aortic regurgitation (CCAR) and chronic decompensated aortic regurgitation (CDAR). LVSV = left ventricular stroke volume; EDV = end-diastolic volume; ESV = end-systolic volume; NL = normal; EDS = end-diastolic stress; ESS = end-systolic stress; CS = contractile state; EF = ejection fraction; RF = regurgitant fraction; FSV = forward stroke volume.

of pulmonary venous pressures and increased ability to tolerate large LV diastolic volumes prior to the onset of symptoms of congestive heart failure.

In order to more fully understand the physiologic responses of the left ventricle to a chronic volume overload, it is necessary to differentiate changes in overall cardiac performance secondary to alterations in contractility from those due to abnormal loading conditions. Ventricular preload and afterload are measures of the forces or load acting on the myocardial fibers. In the clinical setting, these forces are best quantified as wall stress which relates ventricular pressure and size to wall thickness [6]. Chronic AR results in LV dilation leading to increased left ventricular peak systolic wall stress. This is thought to act as an important stimulus for replication of sarcomeres in series, elongation of fibers and an increase in end-diastolic and early systolic wall thickness thereby lowering peak systolic wall stress back towards the normal range [5]. Through these changes, the ratio of LV end-diastolic wall thickness to cavity radius (h/r) is maintained within the normal range until LV decompensation occurs [12]. At that time, any further increase in ventricular size can no longer be compensated for by increased wall mass resulting in a decreased h/r ratio. Despite these physiologic responses, wall stress at end-diastole, a measure of LV preload, remains somewhat elevated (Figure 1). Importantly, it is currently thought that the wall stress at end-systole rather than the wall stress throughout the course of LV ejection is the afterload that determines the overall extent of myocardial fiber shortening [13, 14]. As such, it is the end-systolic wall stress that establishes the size of the ventricle at end-ejection and is a major determinant of LV stroke volume [14]. Recent studies have shown that patients with chronic AR have elevated end-systolic wall stress providing a potential setting for afterload mismatch [15–17]. In this setting, operative relief of the AR with restoration of normal LV afterload can result in postoperative improvement of overall LV performance despite the amelioration of the preload augmented state.

B. *Chronic mitral regurgitation*

The pathophysiology of the LV volume overload associated with chronic mitral valve incompetence is somewhat similar to that described for chronic aortic regurgitation. However, several very important physiologic differences occur. Unlike AR where the left ventricle ejects its entire output into a high impedance circuit, the ventricle with MR decompresses into both the high impedance systemic circulation and the low impedance left atrium. This occurs predominantly during 'isometric' contraction and the early portion of LV ejection [18]. A clinically important compensatory mechanism that occurs in chronic MR is increased LV and LA compliance despite the volume overload present in both of these chambers [19, 20]. This permits accommodation of the large regurgitant volumes at relatively low pressures thereby reducing pulmonary venous pressure and pulmonary vascular congestion.

During the compensated phase of chronic MR, left ventricular peak, mean and end-systolic wall stresses remain normal (Figure 2) [16, 17, 21]. In such

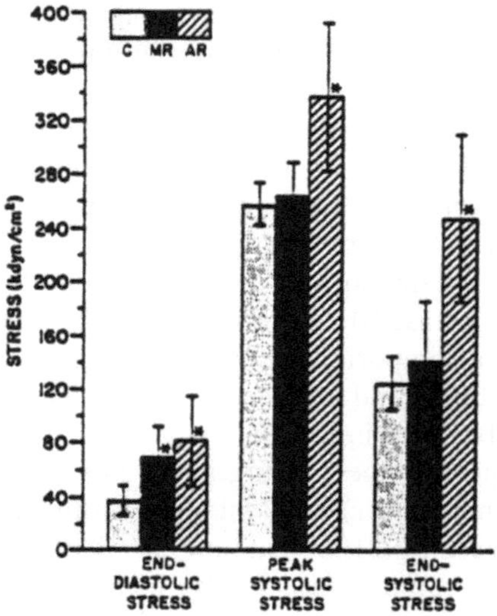

Figure 2. Comparison of preload measured as end-diastolic circumferential wall stress and afterload measured as peak or end-systolic wall stress in patients with aortic regurgitation (AR), mitral regurgitation (MR) and control subjects (C).
Values are mean ± standard deviation. The symbol * indicates a significant ($p \leqslant 0.05$) difference from the control group. (From Wisenbaugh et al. [16])

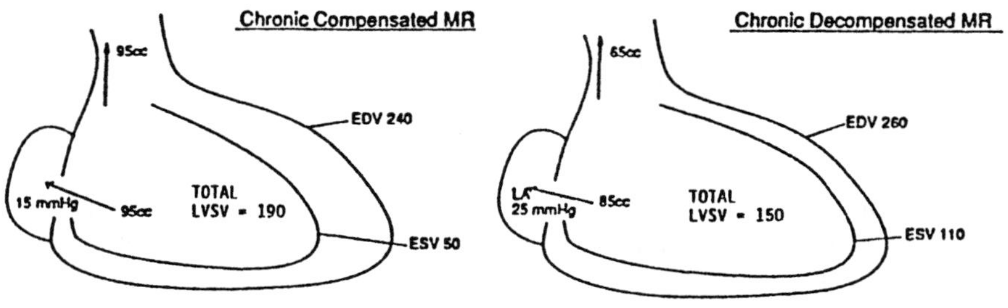

	Preload EDS (kd/cm²)	Afterload ESS (kd/cm²)	CS	EF	RF	FSV (CC)
NL	16	90	N	68	0	95
CCMR	40	90	N	0.79	0.50	95
CDMR	50	120	χ	0.58	0.57	65

Figure 3. Representative myocardial hemodynamics noted in patients with chronic compensated mitral regurgitation (CCMR) and chronic decompensated mitral regurgitation (CDMR).
LA = left atrium. All other abbreviations as in Figure 1. (Adapted from Carabello [2])

patients, overall LV performance (e.g., ejection fraction) is often normal or high reflecting predominantly increased preload rather than marked alterations in LV afterload (i.e., actual fiber load during systole). With time, however, the LV contractile mechanism (i.e., force generating capability of the individual myocardial fibers) becomes damaged. This decompensated phase of the disease is characterized by decreased end-diastolic wall thickness to radius (h/r) ratio as well as increased peak, mean and end-systolic wall stress [15]. The result of augmented LV afterload superimposed upon decreased contractile state is depression in overall LV performance and worsening symptoms of congestive heart failure (Figure 3) [17, 22].

III. ADVANTAGES AND LIMITATIONS OF VARIOUS PHYSIOLOGIC INDICES USED TO DETERMINE OPTIMAL TIMING OF VALVE SURGERY

From the preceding discussion, it is evident that the presence or absence of symptoms alone does not allow determination of the optimal timing of valve surgery in chronic AR or MR. Accordingly, indices based on the severity of valvular regurgitation, LV chamber size and performance and ventricular loading conditions have been evaluated as predictors of surgical outcome.

A. *Regurgitant volume and regurgitant fraction*

Regurgitant volume (RV) and fraction (RF) have been used to estimate severity of chronic AR and MR. They can be determined invasively as well as noninvasively. The ability to assess severity of regurgitation by Doppler (pulsed, continuous and color flow) and radionuclide techniques makes RV and RF determinations feasible in the outpatient setting [23–26]. However, severity of AR and MR is affected by multiple physiologic factors [27–29] including (1) regurgitant orifice size [AR and MR], (2) aortic impedance [AR and MR], (3) LV diastolic pressure and chamber compliance [AR and MR], (4) length of diastole [AR], and (5) LA chamber compliance [MR]. For example, in chronic AR, increased heart rate reduces regurgitant volume and regurgitant fraction per beat without necessarily significantly altering the effect of the LV volume overload on ventricular contractile state. Similarly, in MR, peripheral vasodilators such as nitroprusside and captopril can reduce regurgitant fraction while increasing forward cardiac output without altering LV contractility. Not unexpectantly, since regurgitant volume and regurgitant fraction do not measure LV contractility or intrinsic myofibrillar function, they are poor predictors of surgical outcome for valve replacement in chronic AR and MR.

B. *LV end-diastolic pressure, volume and dimension*

The physiologic response to chronic moderate to severe aortic or mitral regurgitation is ventricular dilation at end-diastole associated with a increase in left ventricle wall mass. This helps maintain normal end-diastolic wall thickness to chamber dimension ratio [4, 12]. End-diastolic wall stress (the product of end-diastolic pressure and dimension divided by wall thickness) is the best measure of the load acting to stretch left ventricular fibers at end-diastole (preload) [6]. However, in the clinical setting, LV end-diastolic pressure, volume or dimension have generally been used rather than end-diastolic wall stress as an estimate of true end-diastolic fiber load. In patients with chronic AR or MR, end-diastolic fiber load is affected by alterations in (1) chamber stiffness (2) myocardial contractility (3) intravascular blood volume and its distribution (4) atrial contribution to left ventricular filling (5) right ventricular-left ventricular interaction (6) intrapericardial and intrathoracic pressures and (7) systemic venous capacitance. These confounding variables mask the status of left ventricular contractility and, again, it is not surprising that the end-diastolic indices of LV performance in isolation are relatively insensitive predictors of postoperative clinical course [7, 9, 10].

C. *LV ejection phase indices*

1. *Rest data.* Overall left ventricular performance, as measured by ejection fraction (EF) or percent fractional shortening (% ΔD), reflects the interdependence of preload, afterload, heart rate and contractile state [3]. In chronic aortic and mitral regurgitation, left ventricular end-diastolic fiber load are significantly increased, as are end-diastolic volume and stroke volume. This preload augmentation helps maintain left ventricular ejection fraction within the normal range even if myocardial contractility is depressed. The inability to distinguish between changes in contractile state and altered myocardial load is an important limitation of all ejection phase indices of ventricular performance [3]. Superimposed on this problem is the effect of the interaction between systolic and diastolic events in the cardiac cycle. For example, in a patient with moderate to severe aortic regurgitation, preload, and subsequently ejection fraction, will vary depending on heart rate despite constancy of left ventricular contractile state [26, 27]. Nevertheless, several authors have reported reasonably good correlations between EF or %ΔD and risk of death or persistent LV dysfunction after valve replacement for chronic AR or MR [8, 9, 11, 30]. However, this appears to be true only at the extremes of overall LV performance.

2. *Exercise response.* The left ventricular ejection fraction (LVEF) response to exercise has been used for almost a decade as a measure of ventricular functional reserve in patients with chronic aortic or mitral regurgitation [27, 31–33]. Indeed, it has been suggested that failure to augment LVEF during exercise may be an early harbinger of myocardial dysfunction [32–34]. Despite its widespread use and popularity, the (LVEF) response to exercise appears to have limited predictive value as a marker for postoperative course in chronic LV volume overload lesions [31, 35]. This reflects the inability of the technique to distinguish between ejection fraction changes due to altered loading

conditions and those due to left ventricular contractile abnormalities. This limitation is further compounded by the complexity of acute circulatory events that occur with dynamic exercise [3]. These include: (1) peripheral vasodilation in exercising muscles (2) increases in sympathetic tone to the heart (3) release of catecholamines from the adrenal medulla (4) alterations in systemic venous capacitance leading to maintenance of venous return and ventricular preload and (5) augmentation of heart rate thereby resulting in a marked decrease in the length of the diastolic portion of the cardiac cycle. Derangements of any one of these mechanisms can result in failure to increase ejection fraction without implicating a depression in myocardial contractility [36].

In addition, the criteria for the 'normal' ejection fraction response to exercise have been defined in subjects without ventricular volume overload or valvular regurgitation. It is conceptually inappropriate to expect a highly load-dependent ejection phase index such as ejection fraction to respond to dynamic exercise in a similar manner in normal subjects and in patients with chronically altered left ventricular loading conditions. This is well illustrated in patients with aortic regurgitation, in whom exercise-induced tachycardia markedly reduces the duration of diastole, which reduces the duration and absolute value of the aortic regurgitant volume per beat [27, 37]. The ventricle, which is volume overloaded before exercise, becomes relatively 'preload deficient' during exercise. The preload augmented LVEF present at rest frequently falls with exercise, reflecting an acute change in ventricular loading conditions rather than depressed contractile reserve. This helps to explain the very high incidence of abnormal ejection fraction response to exercise seen in nearly all studies of aortic regurgitation regardless of the age, functional class or rest ejection fraction of the patient group. In a similar manner, the normal decrease in systemic vascular resistance and aortic impedance that occur with exercise can result in maintained overall LV performance in patients with MR despite the presence of a significant myopathic state. Thus, the multiplicity of factors operating simultaneously in the exercising patient with chronic aortic or mitral regurgitation results in too many discordantly changing variables to allow the ejection fraction response to be clinically reliable as a measure of ventricular contractile reserve.

D. *LV end-systolic indices*

1. *Volume or dimension.* The left ventricular fiber length at end-systole closely reflects the contractile performance of the myocardium because it is virtually independent of preload and varies with afterload. End-systolic volume (dimension) has therefore become an attractive index for assessing LV contractility in patients with chronic aortic or mitral regurgitation [7–10, 30] Clinical studies that have used LV end-systolic chamber size have assumed that alterations in end-systolic volume (dimension) reflected changes in LV contractility associated with chronic volume overload rather than derangements in LV afterload [7–10]. This assumption represents a potentially significant limitation

of these indices since if a contractile abnormality is present, poor postoperative outcome would be expected. However, if a systolic load mismatch is present, relief of the LV volume overload may allow a more favorable outcome than would be predicted by analysis of end-systolic volume (dimension) alone [15, 24]. This issue can be addressed only if, in addition to left ventricular preload, one considers afterload as a confounding variable.

2. *Pressure-volume relation.* In an attempt to incorporate afterload into the analysis of left ventricular performance, some investigators have turned to the end-systolic pressure-volume relation. The slope of this relation, which is usually determined using a pharmacologic challenge, is relatively independent of preload, incorporates afterload and is a sensitive measure of contractility. Several clinical investigators have substituted peak systolic pressure for end-systolic pressure to simplify determination of the end-systolic pressure-volume slope [33, 38]. However, the substitution of peak systolic for end-systolic pressure assumes that the relation between these two pressures is always constant. This is not the case when one considers the effects of pharmacologic interventions or dynamic exercise on such important hemodynamic variables as: (1) the timing and rate of left ventricular peak ejection (2) the volume of aortic regurgitant flow and (3) the velocity as well as the amplitude of reflected waves from the periphery. The further simplification of using the peak systolic pressure/end-systolic volume ratio as a contractility index is even less physiologically justified. This ratio, which is highly afterload dependent, assumes that the end-systolic pressure-volume relationship generated from a single point lies on a regression line that always passes through the origin of the pressure and volume axes. This is rarely the case for true LV end-systolic pressure-volume regression lines. Finally, the end-systolic pressure-volume relation resembles a force-length relation [3]. However, in an abnormally shaped, hypertrophied ventricle (as seen in chronic or mitral regurgitation), wall stress is a more appropriate measure of fiber load or force [3, 15]. This has the advantage of taking ventricular dimensions, shape, wall thickness and pressure into account when quantifying left ventricular forces acting on the myocardium. It also allows more appopriate comparisons between ventricles of different sizes and wall thicknesses.

3. *Stress-volume and stress-shortening (velocity) relations.* Left ventricular afterload can be thought of as the force opposing fiber shortening. It is the wall stress at end-systole rather than the wall stress during the course of ventricular ejection that most closely determines the extent and mean velocity of left ventricle fiber shortening for a given contractile state [13, 14]. As such, it is the end-systolic wall stress that determines end-systolic volume and dimension in patients with chronic aortic or mitral regurgitation. Most of the studies in patients with AR or MR that have incorporated wall stress measurements have related end-systolic wall stress to load-dependent ejection phase indices (e.g., ejection fraction and percent fractional shortening).

Although this approach eliminates problems with afterload, it does not address the effect of preload augmentation on overall left ventricular performance. Carabello and coworkers have suggested that the single point ratio between end-systolic wall stress and end-systolic volume is an easily obtained, load-independent index of left ventricular contractility that circumvents this problem [30]. However, it is now known that this simple ratio changes directly with alterations in left ventricular afterload, and is therefore of limited clinical utility as a measure of contractile state [39, 40]. This problem could potentially be overcome if the end-systolic wall stress-volume relation were determined over a wide range of afterload conditions induced with a pharmacologic intervention. In this manner, afterload could be incorporated directly into the analysis of the data. A promising contractility index that has not yet been studied in patients with chronic aortic or mitral regurgitation is the relation between end-systolic wall stress and the rate-corrected velocity of left ventricular fiber shortening [41]. This index, which can be determined using totally noninvasive techniques, is preload and heart rate independent and incorporates afterload. It has been successfully used to distinguish load alterations from contractile abnormalities in patients with chronic left ventricular pressure overload (e.g., valvular aortic stenosis and coarctation of the aorta), chronic volume overload (e.g., renal failure with arteriovenous fistula for hemodialysis) and dilated cardiomyopathy [41–44].

IV. IMPORTANT RECENT PHYSIOLOGIC STUDIES IN CHRONIC AORTIC AND MITRAL REGURGITATION

Because of the inherent limitations of existing clinical indices of left ventricular contractility and reserve, no single test can precisely identify those patients with chronic AR or MR who will die or develop severe, irreversible LV dysfunction after valve surgery (Table 1). However, over the past decade, important investigations of pre- and post-operative cardiovascular hemodynamics have allowed development of a multifactorial physiologically based framework for the 'optimal' timing of valve surgery in these lesions. The following summarizes a number of the recent clinical studies that have contributed significantly to these guidelines. Since the size of the study population, operative dates, duration of follow-up and techniques employed for pre- and post-operative data acquisition vary widely from investigation to investigation, these points will be specifically addressed.

A. *Aortic regurgitation*

1. *KM Borow et al.: End-systolic volume as a predictor of postoperative left ventricular performance in volume overload from valvular regurgitation* (1980) [7].
   Study population: 20 patients with chronic AR; no CAD. Operative dates: 1971–1979. Duration of follow-up: 2.3 years (mean).

Table 1. Physiologic framework for assessing preoperative predictors of surgical outcome in chronic aortic regurgitation or mitral regurgitation.

	Preload	Afterload	Heart Rate	Contractility
Severity of AR or MR				
Regurgitant volume	+	+	+	0
Regurgitant fraction	+	+	+	0
End-diastolic indexes				
Volume (dimension)	+	+	+	+/0
Pressure	+	+	+	+/0
Ejection phase indexes				
Rest data	+	+	+	+
Exercise response	+	+	+	+
End-systolic indexes				
Volume (dimension)	0	+	+/0	+
Pressure-volume slope	0	0	+/0	+
Wall stress/volume ratio	0	+	0	+
Wall stress-EF relation	+	0	+	+
Wall stress-Vcf_c relation	0	0	0	+

AR= aortic regurgitation; MR = mitral regurgitation; HR = heart rate; Vcf_c = rate-corrected velocity of fiber shortening; + = dependent; 0 = independent.

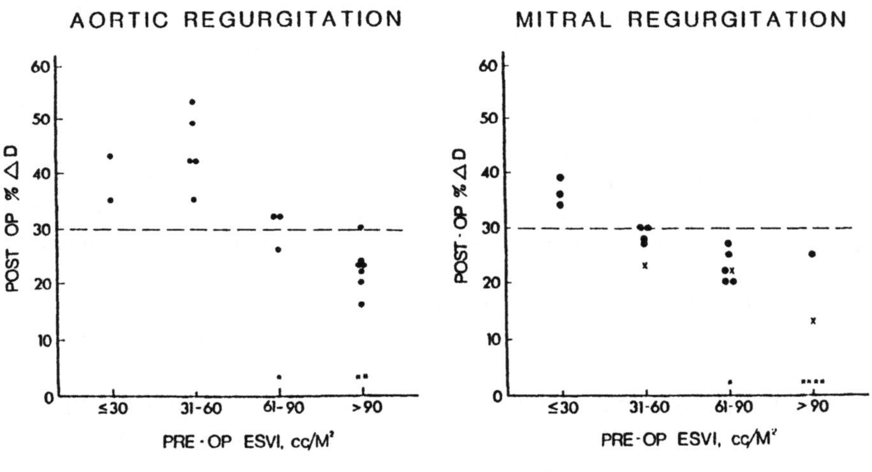

Figure 4. The relationship between postoperative left ventricular function (percent dimension change = % ΔD) and preoperative end-systolic volume index (ESVI) in patients with aortic regurgitation (•), mitral regurgitation (•) or combined mitral aortic regurgitation (×). Patients are grouped according to the degree of enlargement in end-systolic volume index (on the horizontal axis). Patients who died perioperatively from heart failure are demarcated by an asterisk at the bottom of the appropriate preoperative end-systolic volume index group. Normal left ventricular function is marked by the area above the horizontal dashed line at % ΔD = 30. (Adapted from Borow et al. [7])

This was the first study of LV volume overload from chronic valvular regurgitation to use an end-systolic index as its major predictor of subsequent course. Preoperative LV end-systolic volume index (ESVI) was determined by contrast ventriculography and compared to postoperative LV performance as measured by echocardiographic percent fractional shortening (%ΔD). As seen in Figure 4, preoperative ESVI correlated well with postoperative %ΔD ($r = 0.77$); much poorer correlations existed for preoperative LV ejection fraction ($r = 0.49$) and end-diastolic volume index ($r = 0.66$). Preoperative ESVI also predicted patients at high risk for postoperative cardiac death. Both preoperative ejection fraction and end-diastolic volume were less precise predictors of surgical outcome.

Conclusion: A preoperative ESVI $\geqslant 90$ ml/m^2 in patients with chronic AR accurately predicted late mortality as well as persistent LV dysfunction postoperatively.

2. *WL Henry et al.: Observations on the optimum time for operative intervention for aortic regurgitation* (1980) [8].
   Study population: 49 patients with isolated AR; 20% with associated CAD.
   Operative dates: 1972–1977. Duration of follow-up: 3.5 years (mean).

Forty-nine patients with moderate to severe AR were studied prospectively by echocardiography. Preoperatively, LV dilatation was present in all patients with overall LV performance significantly reduced (%ΔD $\leqslant$ 25) in 14/49 patients (29%). Postoperatively, LV end-diastolic dimensions significantly decreased with little additional change noted after the third postoperative week. Nine of 17 patients (53%) with a preoperative left ventricular end-systolic dimension greater than 55 mm either died at operation (2 patients) or died late postoperatively of congestive heart failure (7 patients). Eleven of 13 patients (85%) who had both a preoperative left ventricular end-systolic dimension greater than 55 mm and a left ventricular fractional shortening below 25% either died at operation (2 patients) or died late postoperatively of congestive heart failure (7 patients) or had moderate or severe residual systolic dysfunction postoperatively (2 patients). In contrast, of the 32 patients with left ventricular end-systolic dimension of 55 mm or less, only one (3%) died late postoperatively of congestive heart failure (Figure 5).

Conclusion: Aortic valve replacement should be performed in patients with AR immediately before or shortly after the LV end-systolic minor axis dimension exceeds 55 mm regardless of symptomatic status. This is especially true if %ΔD $\leqslant$ 25.

3. *MR Zile et al.: Left ventricular stress-dimension-shortening relations before and after correction of chronic aortic and mitral regurgitation* (1985) [17].
   Study population: 32 patients with AR; 11% with CAD. Operative dates: 1975–1980. Duration of follow-up: 1 year (mean).

Echocardiographic data were used to assess LV stress-dimension-shortening relations in 32 patients with chronic AR and normal subjects. All AR patients

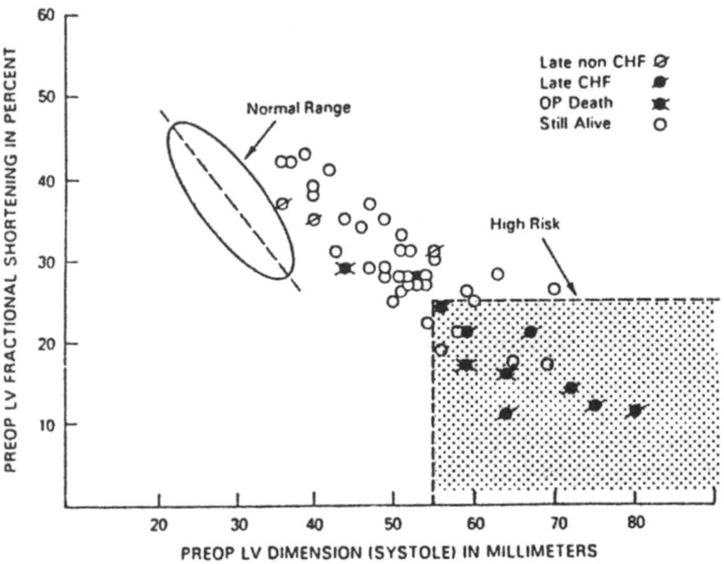

Figure 5. Aortic regurgitation. Plot of preoperative left ventricular (LV) fractional shortening (vertical axis) vs preoperative LV end-systolic dimension (horizontal axis). The elliptically shaped area indicates the 95% confidence region for normal subjects. The high-risk area (stippled) is the region in which the left ventricular end-systolic dimension is $\geqslant$ 55 mm and the fractional shortening is $\leqslant$ 25%. Operative (OP) deaths, late deaths from congestive heart failure (CHF) and late deaths not related to congestive heart failure (non-CHF) are indicated. (From Henry et al. [8])

had LV dilatation preoperatively. Patients were subsequently divided according to postoperative LV end-diastolic dimension (Group A $\leqslant 3.3\ cm/m^2$; Group B $\geqslant 3.3\ cm/m^2$). Preoperatively, patients in Group A had increased peak systolic stress but normal end-systolic stress and %ΔD; the patients in Group B had increased peak and end-systolic stresses and depressed %ΔD. One year after aortic valve replacement, the patients in Group A had normal systolic wall stresses and normal %ΔD whereas those in Group B had persistently elevated wall stresses and a decrease in shortening.

Conclusions: In some patients with postoperative LV dysfunction, persistent elevations of systolic wall stress may be an important contributing factor to the decrease in overall ventricular performance (i.e., afterload excess or mismatch) without necessarily implying the presence of depressed contractile state.

4. *K Taniguchi et al.: Preoperative LV function: minimal requirements for successful late results of valve replacement for aortic regurgitation* (1987) [9]. Study population: 62 patients with AR; no CAD. Operative dates: 1978–1985. Duration of follow-up: 3.8 years (mean).

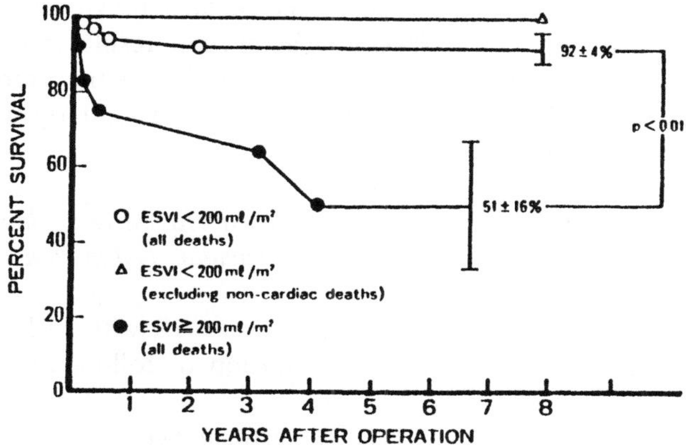

Figure 6. Postoperative survival in 48 patients with preoperative left ventricular end-systolic volume index (ESVI) $\leqslant$ 200 ml/m^2 versus the 12 patients with a preoperative ESVI $\geqslant$ 200 ml/m^2. (From Taniguchi et al. [9])

Postoperative survival and left ventricular function were studied in 62 patients who underwent aortic valve replacement for isolated chronic aortic regurgitation. There were three in-hospital and six late deaths. Five (56%) of the 9 postoperative deaths were of cardiac-related causes. The preoperative variables of age, functional class, cardiothoracic ratio, left ventricular end-diastolic pressure, end-diastolic and end-systolic volume indices and ejection fraction were subjected to stepwise multiple discrimination analysis. As seen in Figure 6, the most important indicator for postoperative cardiac death was the preoperative ESVI ($p \leqslant 0.001$). The 6.5 year survival rate was 92 ± 4% for patients with an end-systolic volume index $\leqslant$ 200 ml/m^2 compared with 51 ± 16% for those whose index was $\geqslant$ 200 ml/m^2. All 5 patients who died of cardiac-related causes had an end-systolic volume index $\geqslant$ 200 ml/m^2 and an ejection fraction $\leqslant$ 0.35 preoperatively. None of the 48 patients with an end-systolic volume index $\leqslant$ 200ml/m^2 died of cardiac-related causes. Twenty-three of the 48 patients with an end-systolic volume index $\leqslant$ 200 ml/m^2 (Group 1) and 6 of the 12 patients with a higher index (Group 2) underwent repeat catheterization 26 months postoperatively. Preoperative afterload, assessed by end-systolic wall stress, was elevated in both groups, but decreased postoperatively, becoming identical to the afterload in 20 normal control subjects. Despite correction of the disadvantageous LV afterload conditions with aortic valve replacement, the ejection fraction in Group 2 patients (preoperative end-systolic volume index $\geqslant$ 200 ml/m^2) failed to return to normal, indicating that associated irreversible myocardial dysfunction was primarily responsible for the reduced ejection fraction in these patients.

Conclusions: Owing to improved myocardial preservation and surgical techniques, patients currently undergoing aortic valve replacement for chronic AR display better restoration of LV performance then previously reported (e.g., Borow et al. [7], Henry et al. [8]). Satisfactory late results in both long-term survival and reversal of LV dysfunction occur when the preoperative LV end-systolic volume index is ⩽ 200 ml/m^2. This is particularly true when preoperative LV ejection fraction is ⩾ 0.35.

5. *BA Carabello et al.: Predictors of outcome for aortic valve replacement in patients with aortic regurgitation and left ventricular dysfunction: a change in the measuring stick* (1987) [10].
   Study population: 14 patients with chronic severe AR with LVEF ⩽ 0.55; no CAD. Operative dates: 1980–1987. Duration of follow-up: 1.9 years (mean).

Fourteen patients with decreased overall LV performance (EF = 0.45 ± 0.02) in association with chronic severe AR were studied by echocardiographic and invasive techniques prior to valve replacement. Follow-up was performed using radionuclide angiographic assessment of resting LV ejection fraction. The patients had 82 (58%) of a possible 140 predictors of negative outcome preoperatively. Twelve of the 14 patients had a decrease in symptoms and an increase in ejection fraction into the normal range after operation (average postoperative ejection fraction 0.59 ± 0.04). There was a significant correlation between postoperative LVEF and eight of the tested preoperative predictors. Preoperative end-systolic dimension correlated best (r = –0.91) with postoperative ejection fraction (Figure 7). An end-systolic dimension of 60 mm correlated with a postoperative LVEF of 0.55. Preoperative LV percent fractional shortening correlated moderately well (r = 0.71) with postop LVEF such that a preop %ΔD of 0.21 would be expected to give a postop LVEF of 0.55.

Conclusions: Preoperative LV function is an important determinant of outcome of aortic valve replacement for aortic regurgitation. However, current

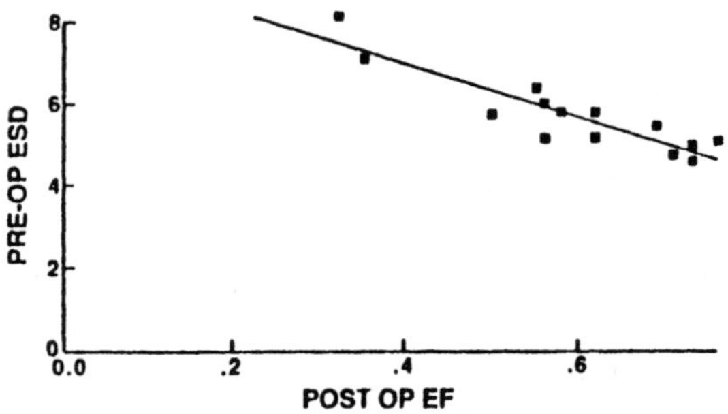

Figure 7. Preoperative echocardiographic end-systolic dimension (PRE-OP ESD) demonstrated a good negative correlation with postoperative ejection fraction (POST-OP EF) in patients with chronic aortic regurgitation. (From Carabello et al. [10])

medical and surgical techniques permit a better prognosis in the presence of reduced ventricular function than was previously considered possible. It appears that patients with preoperative LV end-systolic dimensions as large as 60 mm or preoperative %ΔD as low as 0.21 can still have normal overall LV performance after valve replacement.

6. *ES Monrad et al.: Time course of regression of left ventricular hypertrohy after aortic valve replacement* (1988) [45].
   Study Population: 10 patients with predominant AR and 11 control subjects. Operative dates: 1974–1982. Duration of follow-up: Study 1 = 1.6 years (mean); Study 2 = 8.1 years (mean)

Ten patients with predominant AR were studied preoperatively, after an intermediate period (Study 1) and late (Study 2) after aortic valve replacement. Results were compared with those in 11 control patients. Preoperative LV end-diastolic volume index (EDVI), which was more than twice normal in the AR patients, fell significantly by Study 1 but was still greater than normal (Figure 8). By Study 2, no difference in LVEDVI was present between the groups. At the preoperative study, LV muscle mass index was 250% higher than normal for the AR patients. At the intermediate postop study, LV muscle mass index had decreased but remained greater than in the control subjects. By the time of late postop study, there was only a trend ($p \leqslant 0.06$) to a higher LV muscle mass index in those patients with prior AR. Thus, the regression of LV hypertrophy was characterized by a reduction in wall mass that was less than the reduction in chamber size. The ventricle was remodeled from a predominantly spherical shape to a more ellipsoidal geometry.

Conclusions: In patients with chronic AR who undergo successful valve replacement, the remodeling of LV volume, mass and shape is a process that may proceed long after correction of the primary valvular abnormality.

7. *RO Bonow et al.: Long-term serial changes in left ventricular function and reversal of ventricular dilation after valve replacement for chronic aortic regurgitation* (1988) [11].
   Study Population: 61 patients with severe AR. Operative dates: 1976–1983. Duration of follow-up: Study 1 = 0.6 years (mean); Study 2 = 5.0 years (mean).

Patients were studied by echocardiography and radionuclide angiography preoperatively, 6–8 months after and 3–7 years after aortic valve replacement. Between preoperative and early postoperative studies, left ventricular end-diastolic dimension decreased from 75 ± 6 to 56 ± 9 mm ($p \leqslant 0.001$), peak systolic wall stress decreased from 247 ± 50 to 163 ± 42 kdynes/cm^2 ($p \leqslant 0.001$), and ejection fraction increased from 43 ± 9% to 51 ± 16% ($p \leqslant 0.001$). Between early and late postoperative studies, diastolic dimension and peak systolic wall stress did not change, but ejection fraction increased further (to 56 ± 19%, $p \leqslant 0.001$). The increase in ejection fraction correlated with the

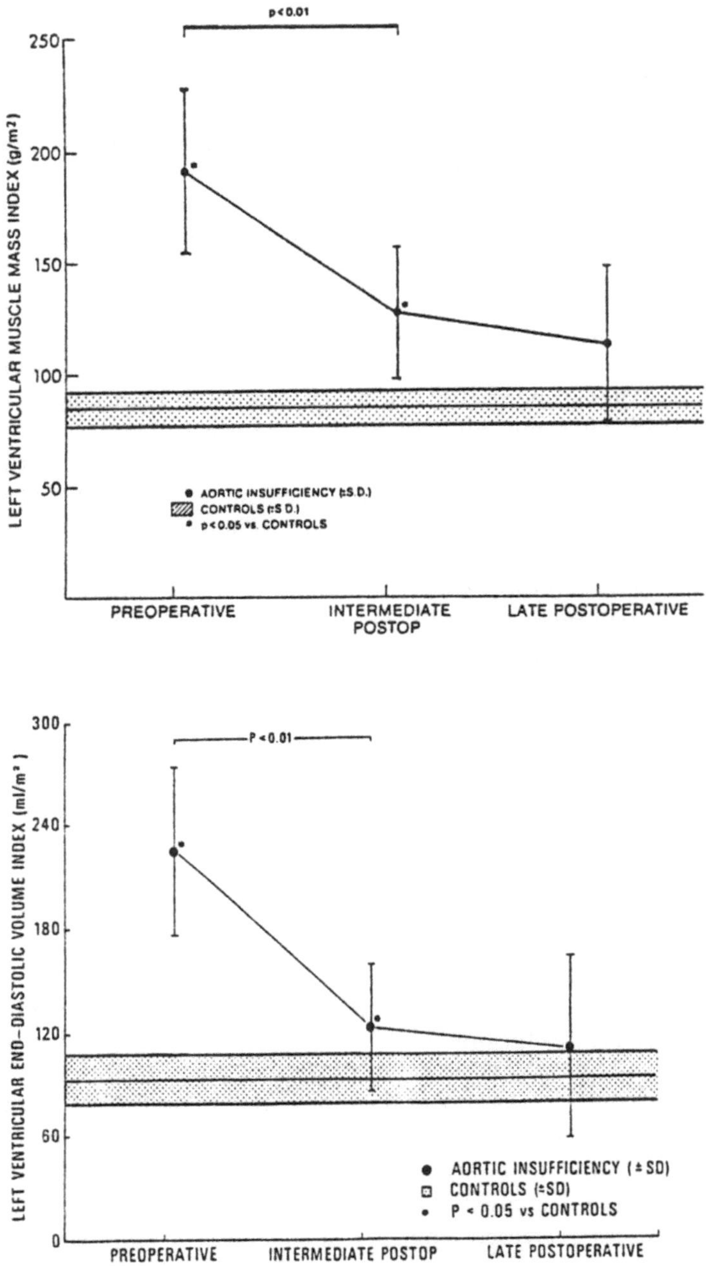

Figure 8. Serial changes in left ventricular muscle mass index and end-diastolic volume index comparing preoperative, intermediate postoperative and late postoperative data. (Modified from Monrad et al. [45])

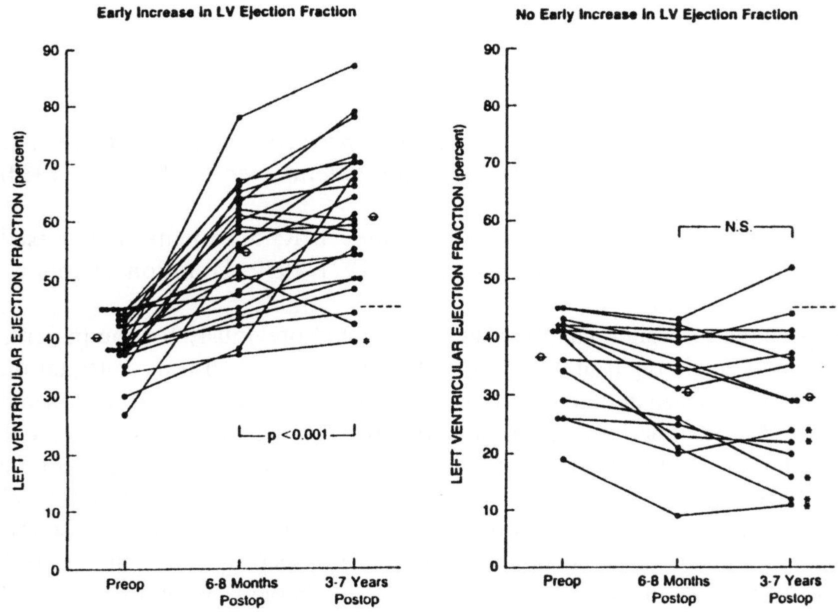

Figure 9. Plots of serial changes in left ventricular (LV) ejection fraction in patients with subnormal preoperative ejection fractions. Patients are subdivided on the basis of an early increase in ejection fraction within 6–8 months after operation (*left panel*) and no such early increase in ejection fraction (*right panel*).
*Patients who died from chronic congestive heart failure after the late postoperative study. (From Bonow et al. [11])

magnitude of reduction in end-dialostic dimension between preoperative and early postoperative studies (r = 0.63), between early and late postoperative studies (r = 0.54), and between preoperative and late postoperative studies (r = 0.69). Late increases in ejection fraction usually represented the continuation of an initial increase occurring early after operation (Figure 9). Among the 83 consecutive patients undergoing aortic valve replacement for AR during the timeframe of this study, 15 of the 16 postoperative deaths occurred in patients with preoperative LV dysfunction and impaired exercise tolerance or with preoperative systolic dysfunction of unknown duration. Such patients had a higher risk of irreversible LV dysfunction and death after operation than did patients with preserved exercise tolerance and only a brief duration of preoperative systolic dysfunction.

Conclusions: Short-term and long-term improvement in left ventricular function after operation is related to the early reduction in left ventricular dilation arising from correction of left ventricular volume overload. Moreover, late improvement in ejection fraction occurs commonly in patients with an early increase in ejection fraction after valve replacement but is unlikely to occur in patients with no change in ejection fraction during the first 6 months after operation.

B. *Mitral regurgitation*

1. *KM Borow al.: End-systolic volume as a predictor of postoperative left ventricular performance in volume overload from valvular regurgitation* (1980) [7].
   Study population: 16 patients with chronic MR; 5 patients with mixed MR and AR; no CAD. Operative dates: 1971–1979. Duration of follow-up: 2.3 years (mean).

The experimental design was the same as outlined previously for the patients with isolated aortic regurgitation. All of the patients with mitral regurgitation who had any increase in their end-systolic volume index in excess of the normal range ($\geqslant$ 31 cc/m^2) had abnormal postoperative left ventricular function. The degree of such dysfunction was related to the severity of the preoperative ESVI enlargement (Figure 4). Patients with mitral regurgitation and an ESVI $\geqslant$ 90 cc/m^2 fared poorly with operation, with four of five dying postoperatively. Overall, the correlation coefficient between preoperative LV end-systolic volume index and postoperative %ΔD was 0.73. Patients were also grouped according to their preoperative LV ejection fraction: Group I, normal ejection fraction ($\geqslant$ 0.55); Group II, mildly to moderatly depressed ejection fraction (0.40 to 0.54); Group III, markedly depressed ejection fraction ($\leqslant$ 0.40). No useful relationship could be discerned between preoperative ejection fraction and postoperative per cent dimension change. Cardiac deaths occurred in all groups, including the group with normal preoperative ejection fractions. The correlation coefficient between preoperative LVEF and postoperative %ΔD was 0.62. Finally, patients were grouped according to LV end-diastolic volume index. Preoperative end-diastolic volume index separated patients with normal postoperative function from those with abnormal postoperative function, in that all patients with an end-diastolic volume index that was abnormally elevated had a reduced percent dimension change postoperatively. However, the degree of preoperative LV enlargement did not correlate well with the extent of postoperative impairment in left ventricular function ($r = 0.56$). When compared with the patients with AR, these patients with MR appeared to be less able to tolerate increases in LV end-systolic volume index.

Conclusion: Preoperative LV end-systolic volume index can predict patients with MR at high risk for preoperative cardiac mortality or for residual postoperative impairement of overall LV performance.

2. *MR Zile et al.: Left ventricular stress-dimension-shortening relations before and after correction of chronic aortic and mitral regurgitation* (1985) [17].
   Study population: 20 patients with MR; 15% with CAD. Operative dates: 1975–1981. Duration of follow-up: 1 year (mean).

Data were acquired as noted previously for the patients with aortic regurgitation. Patients were divided according to postoperative LV end-diastolic dimension (Group A $\leqslant$ 3.3 cm/m^2; Group B $\geqslant$ 3.3 cm/m^2). Preoperatively, patients in Group A (n = 16) had only modest elevations of peak stress, while end-systolic stress and fractional shortening were normal; in patients in Group B (n = 4) the peak stress was similar to that seen in Group A, but end-systolic stress was increased and shortening was depressed. This suggests that at least some component of the decreased overall LV performance noted preoperatively in the Group B patients could be accounted for by disadvantageous LV afterload conditions. One year after mitral valve replacement, patients in Group A had no change in end-systolic stress, but peak stress fell and shortening decreased; patients in Group B had persistently abnormal stress-shortening relations.

Conclusions: Afterload excess and LV contractile abnormalities are relatively common 1 year post mitral valve replacement for chronic MR.

3. *B Carabello et al.: Hemodynamic predictors of outcome in patients undergoing valve replacement* (1986) [30].
   Study population: 13 patients with chronic MR; no CAD. Operative dates: 1980–1985. Duration of follow-up: 1.5 years (mean).

Thirteen patients with mitral regurgitation were studied invasively prior to

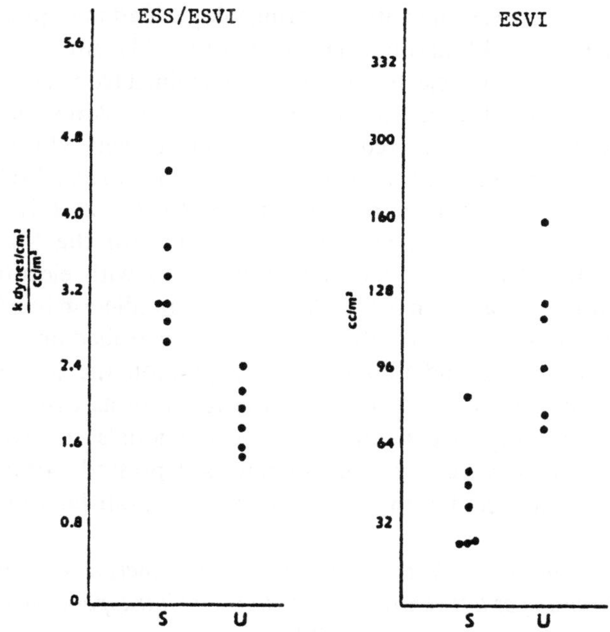

Figure 10. Predictors of outcome in patients undergoing valve replacement. Abbreviations: ESS = end-systolic stress; ESVI = end-systolic volume index; S = satisfactory outcome; U = unsatisfactory outcome. (Modified from Carabello et al. [30])

surgery. Twelve preoperative predictors of postoperative clinical status were determined. Outcome was considered satisfactory if the patient was *NYHA Class I* or *II* post valve replacement and unsatisfactory if the patient died of a cardiac cause or remained *NYHA Class III* or *IV*. Seven of 13 (54%) patients had satisfactory outcomes. The LV endsystolic stress-volume index ratio (ESS/ESVI) was the only independent predictor of outcome. Patients with ESS/ESVI $\leqslant 2.6$ had a poor surgical result (Figure 10). A left ventricular end-systolic volume index $\geqslant 70$ cc/m^2 also tended to be predictive of outcome.

Conclusions: It is likely that these indices detect patients with MR who have preperative LV dysfunction that persists postoperatively and results in poor clinical outcome. Of note, a recent study by Corin and associates has questioned the clinical utility of the ESS/ESVI ratio in patients with mitral regurgitation [40].

4. *T Wisenbaugh: Does normal pump function belie muscle dysfunction in patients with chronic severe mitral regurgitation?* (1988) [22].
   Study population: 27 patients with chronic severe MR and 23 normal subjects. Operative dates: 1983–1987. Duration of follow-up: 1.6 years (mean).

Left ventricular cineangiography and micromanometry were performed simultaneously in 27 patients with chronic severe mitral regurgitation (MR group) and in 23 normal subjects. Stress and volume were computed frame by frame. Measurements were repeated after pharmacologic load manipulation in subsets of MR patients (n = 10) and normal subjects (n = 11). An inverse relationship (r = -0.90) between EF_c (ejection fraction determined from a common preload) and afterload was observed for the normal group. Afterload, estimated as end-systolic stress, was not reduced in the group with chronic MR (204 ± 70 kdynes/cm^2 vs 192 ± 54 kdynes/cm^2 for the normals). Preload estimated as end-diastolic stress was increased in the MR (71 ± 29 kdynes/cm^2) vs the normal group (49 ± 19 kdynes/cm^2; $p \leqslant 0.01$). For the MR group, 10 of 14 with ejection fraction $\leqslant 0.60$ and four of 13 with ejection fractions $\geqslant 0.60$ had muscle dysfunction (i.e., below the 95% prediction band of the normal EF_c–σ_{es} relationship). Mitral valve surgery was performed on 19 of the patients with MR. All survived and all but one were symptomatically improved.

Conclusions: Left ventricular contractile function as assessed by the EF_c-afterload relationship is frequently normal in individuals with MR when ejection fraction is normal. When ejection fraction is depressed, contractile function is frequently depressed, but this does not preclude a satisfactory surgical result.

5. *ME Goldman et al.: Mitral valvuloplasty is superior to valve replacement for preservation of left ventricular function – an intraoperative two-dimensional echocardiographic study* (1987) [46].
   Study population: 18 patients with isolated severe MR; no CAD. Operative dates: Intraoperative study without long-term follow-up (n = 10 for repair; n = 8 for replacement).

Eighteen patients with pure, severe mitral regurgitation were studied by intraoperative two-dimensional echocardiography immediately before and immediately after the operative procedure. No patient had any residual mitral regurgitation. Preoperative hemodynamics were similar for both groups. However, the patients with valve repair postoperatively had a lower pulmonary capillary wedge pressure than did the patients with valve replacement ($p \leqslant 0.04$). Although intraoperative echocardiographic ejection fraction fell significantly after mitral valve replacement (0.64 ± 0.11 to 0.40 ± 0.09; $p \leqslant 0.0001$), it was maintained after valve repair (0.44 ± 0.20 to 0.49 ± 0.16; p = NS) [Figure 11]. Additionally, regional wall motion abnormalities in the anterior and posterior septum were detected immediately after the procedure by intraoperative echocardiography in the patients with valve replacement, but not in those with repair.

Conclusions: By preserving the chordal attachments to the papillary muscles, mitral valve repair helps preserve overall LV performance, enabling the ventricle to overcome loading changes caused by elimination of mitral valve competence. Mitral valve repair has the additional advantage of leaving the patient with a native mitral valve instead of a prosthesis, thereby obviating complications of prosthetic heart valves. It appears that whenever possible, mitral valve repair is preferable to valve replacement.

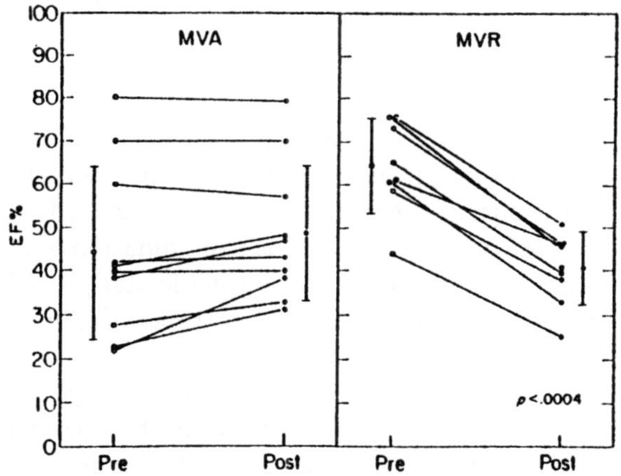

Figure 11. Comparison of pre-procedure (Pre) and post-procedure (Post) ejection fraction (EF) measured by intraoperative two-dimensional echocardiography in patients undergoing mitral valve repair or anuloplasty (MVA) or mitral valve replacement (MVR). (From Goldman et al. [46])

V. GUIDELINES FOR OPTIMAL TIMING OF OPERATIVE INTERVENTION

These guidelines are based on the operative mortality and long-term survival data presented in the preceding section. Because of the 'real world' difficulties encountered in sending asymptomatic or minimally symptomatic patients to valve surgery, the specific recommendations are divided according to the severity of symptoms in conjunction with more quantitative criteria based on left ventricular size, performance and loading conditions. It must be emphasized that surgery should be performed prior to the onset of irreversible LV contractile abnormalities.

A. *Chronic AR: operative indications*

1. In the patient with *significant AR and limiting symptoms*, one should consider AVR to decrease symptoms and prolong life. If preoperative LV systolic performance is normal to moderately impaired, ventricular size and function usually improve after valve replacement. If preoperative LV performance is significantly impaired (LVEF $\leqslant$ 0.35 or %ΔD $\leqslant$ 0.25), the risk of irreversible LV contractile abnormality postoperatively is markedly increased. This is especially true if LVESVI $\geqslant$ 200 cc/m^2.
2. In the patient with *significant AR and minimal or no symptoms*, use of combined LV size and performance parameters is important in decision making. If normal to moderately increased LV end-systolic size [ESD $\leqslant$ 55mm (26 mm/m^2) or ESVI $\leqslant$ 90 cc/m^2] in association with LVEF $\geqslant$ 0.40 or %ΔD $\geqslant$ 25% are present, serial evaluation is important. Regardless of the results, these patients are at risk for progression of LV dilatation and development of irreversible LV dysfunction. Aortic valve replacement is indicated if short term follow-up studies show deterioration of LV performance. If LV end-systolic size is markedly increased [ESD $>$ 60 mm (29 mm/m^2) or ESVI $>$ 150 cc/m^2], especially if LVEF $<$ 0.35–0.40 or %ΔD $<$ 0.25, AVR should be performed.

B. *Chronic MR: operative indications*

1. In the patient with *significant MR and limiting symptoms*, decreased myocardial performance may progress rapidly. Surgery is indicated if LVEF $\geqslant$ 0.40 in which case surgical mortality is low. However, LV performance will frequently decrease postoperatively due to elimination of the LV volume overload and unmasking of depressed contractile state. If LVEF $\leqslant$ 0.40, the incidence of operative mortality and postoperative congestive heart failure may be unacceptably high.
2. In the patient with *significant MR and minimal or no symptoms*, one should consider operation to preserve LV contractility in the presence of an ESVI $\geqslant$ 60 cc/m^2 or ESD $\geqslant$ 50 mm (26 mm/m^2), a left ventricular EF $\leqslant$ 0.55 or % ΔD $\leqslant$ 28%, and possibly an ESS/ESVI ratio less than 2.6.
3. As a general principle, whenever possible a reconstructive procedure rather than mitral valve replacement should be performed.

REFERENCES

1. Borow KM (1987) Surgical outcome in chronic aortic regurgitation: a physiologic framework for assessing preoperative predictors. *J Am Coll Cardiol* 10:1165
2. Carabello BA (1988) Mitral regurgitation: basic pathophysiological principles and proper timing of mitral valve replacement. *Mod Concept Cardiovasc Dis* 57:53
3. Borow KM (1988) Clinical assessment of contractility in the symmetrically contracting left ventricle. *Mod Concepts Cardiovasc Dis* 57:29
4. Gaasch WH (1979) Left ventricular radius to wall thickness ratio. *Am J Cardiol* 43:1189
5. Grossman W (1980) Cardiac hypertrophy: useful adaptation or pathologic process. *Am J Med* 69:576
6. Grossman W, et al. (1975) Wall stress and patterns of hypertrophy in the human left ventricle. *J Clin Invest* 56:56
7. Borow KM, et al. (1980) End-systolic volume as a predictor of postoperative left ventricular performance in volume overload from valvular regurgitation. *Am J Med* 68:655
8. Henry WL, et al. (1980) Observations on the optimum time for operative intervention for aortic regurgitation. *Circulation* 61:471
9. Taniguchi K, et al. (1987) Preoperative left ventricular function: minimal requirements for successful late results of valve replacement for aortic regurgitation. *J Am Coll Cardiol* 10:510
10. Carabello B, et al. (1987) Predictors of outcome for aortic valve replacement in patients with aortic regurgitation and left ventricular dysfunction: a change in the measuring stick. *J Am Coll Cardiol* 10:991
11. Bonow RO, et al. (1988) Long-term serial changes in LV function and reversal of ventricular dialation after valve replacement for chronic aortic regurgitation. *Circulation* 78:1108
12. Gaasch WH, et al. (1983) Chronic aortic regurgitation: prognostic value of left ventricular end-systolic dimension and end-diastolic radius/thickness ratio. *J Am Coll Cardiol* 1:775
13. Weber KT, et al. (1982) The contractile behavior of the heart and its functional coupling to the circulation. *Prog Cardiovasc Dis* 24:375
14. Borow KM, et al. (1982) Left ventricular end-systolic stress-shortening and stress-length relations in humans: normal values and sensitivity to inotropic state. *Am J Cardiol* 50:1301
15. Ross J Jr (1985) Afterload mismatch in aortic and mitral valve disease: implications for surgical therapy. *J Am Coll Cardiol* 5:811
16. Wisenbaugh T, et al. (1984) Differences in myocardial performance and load between patients with similar amounts of chronic aortic versus chronic mitral regurgitation. *J Am Coll Cardiol* 3:916
17. Zile MR, et al. (1985) Left ventricular stress-dimension-shortening relations before and after correction of chronic aortic and mitral regurgitation. *Am J Cardiol* 56:99
18. Eckberg DL, et al. (1900) Mechanics of left ventricular contraction in chronic severe mitral regurgitation. *Circulation* 47:1252
19. Braunwald E, et al. (1963) The syndrome of severe mitral regurgitation with normal left atrial pressure. *Circulation* 27:29
20. Wong CYH, et al. (1981) Systolic and diastolic properties of the human left ventricle during valve replacement for chronic mitral regurgitation. *Am J Cardiol* 47:40
21. Corin WJ, et al. (1987) The relationship of afterload to ejection performance in chronic mitral regurgitation. *Circulation* 76:59
22. Wisenbaugh T (1988) Does normal pump function belie muscle dysfunction in patients with chronic severe mitral regurgitation? *Circulation* 77:515
23. Grayburn PA, et al. (1987) Quantitative assessment of the hemodynamic consequences of aortic regurgitation by means of continuous wave Doppler recordings. *J Am Coll Cardiol* 10:135
24. Goldberg SJ, et al. (1986) Quantitative assessment by Doppler echocardiography of pulmonary and aortic regurgitation. *Am J Cardiol* 56:131
25. Bolger AF, et al. (1988) Quantifying valvular regurgitation: limitations and inherent assump-

tions of Doppler techniques. *Circulation* 78:1316
26. Firth BG, et al. (1982) Effect of increasing heart rate in patients with aortic regurgitation: Effect of incremental atrial pacing on scintigraphic, hemodynamic, and thermodilution measurements. *Am J Cardiol* 49:1860
27. Gerson MC, et al. (1984) Effects of dynamic and isometric exercise on the radionuclide determined regurgitation fraction in aortic insufficiency. *J Am Coll Cardiol* 3:98
28. Meyer T, et al. (1987) Echocardiographic and hemodynamic correlates of diastolic closure of mitral valve and diastolic opening of aortic valve in severe aortic regurgitation. *Am J Cardiol* 59:1144
29. Judge TP, et al. (1971) Quantitative hemodynamic effects of heart rate in aortic regurgitation. *Circulation* 44:355
30. Carabello BA, et al. (1986) Hemodynamic predictors of outcome in patients undergoing valve replacement. *Circulation* 74:1309
31. Gee DS, et al. (1985) Prognostic significance of exercise-induced left ventricular dysfunction in chronic aortic regurgitation. *Am J Cardiol* 56:605
32. Borer JS, et al. (1978) Exercise-induced left ventricular dysfunction in symptomatic and asymptomatic patients with aortic regurgitation: assessment with radionuclide cineangiography. *Am J Cardiol* 42:351
33. Iskandrian AS, et al. (1986) Radionuclide angiographic evaluation of left ventricular performance at rest and during exersice in patients with aortic regurgitation. *Am Heart J* 111:1143
34. Massie BM, et al. (1985) Ejection fraction response to supine exercise in asymptomatic aortic regurgitation: relation to simultaneous hemodynamic measurements. *J Am Coll Cardiol* 5:847
35. Bonow RO, et al. (1985) Survival and functional results after valve replacement for aortic regurgitation from 1976 to 1983: impact of preoperative left ventricular function. *Circulation* 72:1244
36. Borow KM, et al (1990) Myocardial mechanics in young adult patients with diabetes Mellitus: effects of altered load, inotropic state and dynamic exercise. *J Am Coll Cardiol* 15:1508
37. Boucher CA, et al. (1983) Exercise testing in asymptomatic or minimally symptomatic aortic regurgitation: relationships of left ventricular ejection fraction to left ventricular filling pressure during exercise. *Circulation* 67:1091
38. Iskandrian AS, et al. (1985) LV pressure-volume relationship in aortic regurgitation. *Am Heart J* 110:1026
39. Wisenbaugh T, et al. (1985) The superiority of maximum fiber elastance over maximum stress-volume ratio as an index of contractile state. *Circulation* 72:648
40. Corin WJ, et al. (1987) Inability of the end-systolic stress/end-systolic volume index ratio to predict postoperative outcome in chronic mitral regurgitation. *J Am Coll Cardiol* 9:85A
41. Colan SD, et al. (1984) Left ventricular end-systolic wall stress-velocity of fiber shortening relation: a load-independent index of myocardial contractility. *J Am Coll Cardiol* 4:715
42. Borow KM, Colan SD, Neumann A (1985) Altered left ventricular mechanics in valvular aortic stenosis and coarctation of the aorta: effects on systolic performance and late outcome. *Circulation* 72:515
43. Lang RM, et al. (1988) Effects of varying serum ionized calcium concentration on left ventricular contractility in humans. *Ann Int Med* 108:524
44. Borow KM, et al. (1988) Physiologic mechanisms governing hemodynamic responses to positive inotropic therapy in dilated cardiomyopathy. *Circulation* 77:625
45. Monrad ES, et al. (1988) Time course of regression of left ventricular hypertrophy after aortic valve replacement. *Circulation* 77:1345
46. Goldman ME, et al. (1987) Mitral valvuloplasty is superior to valve replacement for preservation of left ventricular function. An intraoperative two-dimensional echocardiographic study. *J Am Coll Cardiol* 10:568

5. Acute effects of myocardial ischemia on left ventricular function

How to differentiate myocardial infarction, stunned myocardium, and hibernating myocardium

GUY R. HEYNDRICKX

Diagnosis and treatment of myocardial infarction were based untill recently upon the concept that in almost all instances myocardial ischemia was thought to be caused by an unbalance between myocardial oxygen demand and oxygen delivery in the presence of a fixed, atherosclerotic lesion of a major epicardial coronary artery. A slow but steadily progression of a stenosis led invariably to total coronary artery occlusion, with myocardial infarction and necrosis inescapably as the end result.

In recent years we have witnessed important changes in our understanding of the pathophysiology of myocardial ischemia and the once static concept of ischemic heart disease has evolved into a complex dynamic system, introducing at the same time new concepts into our clinical practice, such as stunned myocardium, and hibernating myocardium [1–4].

This chapter will review some of the salient features relating to myocardial ischemia which bears some importance for the practicing cardiologist.

1. MYOCARDIAL ISCHEMIA

Adequate oxygen delivery to support high energy phosphate production by the oxidative phosphorylations in the mitochondria, is of paramount importance to sustain normal myocardial function. When the amount of oxygen delivered to the myocardium is insufficient, myocardial infarction may temporarily run on high energy phosphates produced by anaerobic glycolysis with accumulation of lactate as end product. With decreasing O_2 supply, energy production is decreased while catabolites accumulate, thereby inhibiting cellular functions, including contractility, transport systems and synthetic function. At this point the cellular damage is still reversible. With prolonged oxygen deficiency, irreversible damage occurs to some critical subcellular organelles. Coagulation necrosis ensues with secondary inflammatory response, removal of the dead myocytes and replacement by scar tissue resulting in non-functional myocardial segments [1].

E. Andries & R. Stroobandt (eds.), Hemodynamics in Daily Practice, 77–90.

2. REPERFUSION

If reperfusion occurs either spontaneously, by relieving coronary spasm, dislodgment of platelet plug or thrombus or through experimental or clinical thrombolysis or mechanical recanalisation, the fate of the myocardium will depend upon the extent of reperfusion as well as on the state of the myocardium at the time of reperfusion (Figure 1). Reperfusion can occur at different points in time:

a) When myocytes have been irreversibly damaged, restoration of blood flow does not achieve cellular recovery but rather results in an explosive cell swelling of myocytes due to massive calcium overload and disruption of myofibrillar apparatus evidenced as contraction band necrosis. Concomitant microvascular injury results in heterogenous reperfusion with zones of no reflow leading to sustained regional ischemia.

b) When reperfusion occurs at the time when myocytes injury is still in a reversible phase, evolution towards necrosis is aborted and cell death prevented with recovery of all cellular, ultrastructural, metabolic and contractile function. This recovery is however not immediate but takes time, leaving the reperfused myocardium, so to speak recovering from K.O. This situation is referred to as 'stunned myocardium' [2–4].

c) In some instances minimal perfusion is preserved either through preex-

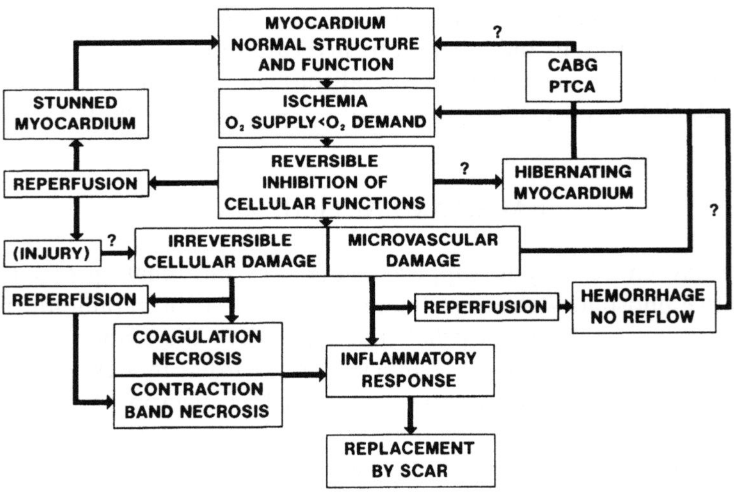

Figure 1. Dynamics of myocardial ischemia. Myocardial infarction is the end result of a dynamic process whereby myocardial cells undergo necrosis. During this time frame reperfusion may avert the evolution towards necrosis. Reperfused myocardium displays temporarily postischemic dysfunction, i.e., stunned myocardium, but is able to recover completely. Chronic ischemic myocardium may undergo adaptive metabolic changes, whereby prolonged survival of myocytes are made possible (hibernating myocardium).

isting collaterals or through minimal antegrade perfusion leading to a chronic stage of myocardial ischemia , resulting in chronic regional LV dysfunction. How stable a condition this is, is however unknown.

d) Occasionally, the myocardium may undergo adaptive changes in order to cope with reduced perfusion in order to stay alive. This hibernating response of the heart may be viewed as an act of selfpreservation [5–7]. Reperfusion injury is a popular concept and is thought to occur at the time of reperfusion whereby reversibly injured myocytes are killed by restoration of blood flow. If this hypothesis is correct, some ischemic myocytes that die despite reperfusion might be salvaged if reperfusion conditions are appropriately modified. Oxygen free radicals have been incriminated as potential culprits. Their mechanism of action seems to involve lipid peroxidation at the cellular membrane, resulting in permeability changes with intracellular calcium overload [8,9].

3. RELATION BETWEEN MYOCARDIAL FLOW AND FUNCTION

The coronary circulation, in contrast to many other vascular beds, is primarily under metabolic control, i.e., myocardial perfusion rate varies directly with the rate of myocardial metabolism. This metabolic autoregulation is responsible for the close match between changes in oxygen consumption and myocardial flow. Since resting coronary vascular resistance is high, relative to the rate of tissue metabolism, coronary extraction of oxygen and other substrates is elevated. As a consequence of high basal resistance, coronary flow can increase several fold above resting value. This increment is called the coronary reserve.

In the presence of a stenosis of one of the epicardial vessels, resistance of epicardial vessels increases with severity of the stenosis, while the arteriolar resistance decreases, thereby maintaining myocardial flow at normal levels. Once vasodilation reserve is exhausted, further increase in stenosis leads to a decrease in flow. This occurs when a stenosis results in a diameter reduction of 70%.

As a result of coronary stenosis, a transstenotic pressure gradient develops resulting in a decrease in coronary driving pressure distal to the stenosis. Once the driving pressure reaches 40 mmHg, any further decrease in pressure is followed by a concomitant decrease in regional flow. The relationship between regional flow and function shows a rather linear relationship.

Translated into clinical practice: A stenosis may progress slowly until 70% diameter reduction is reached without affecting basal flow significantly distal to the stenosed artery [10].

4. STUNNED MYOCARDIUM

The acute effects of myocardial ischemia on regional mechanical function are now well established [11,12]. The sequence of events upon coronary artery

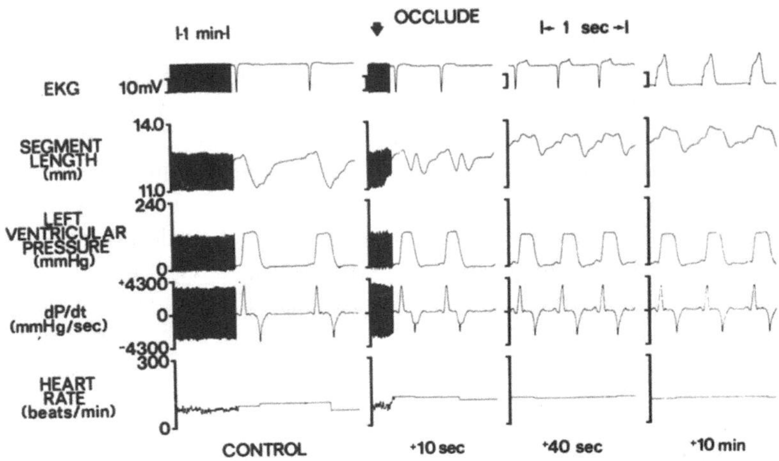

Figure 2. Tracings of intramyocardial ECG, segment length, left ventricular pressure, dP/dt and heart rate during control, during coronary occlusion at 10 sec, 40 sec and 10 min. Arrow indicates the time of occlusion. With the onset of ischemia there is an early systolic lengthening followed by late systolic shortening ('W') phenomenon). At 40 sec active shortening is abolished and replaced by systolic expansion. The peak rate of LV pressure decay (dP/dt) is reduced and delayed at 10 sec to return to preocclusion level when holosystolic expansion is complete. Note the late intramyocardial ECG changes. (From Heyndrickx et al. [20]). Reproduced with permission)

occlusion are shown in Figure 2. Regional contraction in the area subserved by the occluded artery is almost immediately altered with decrease in systolic segment shortening, followed by early relaxation and secondary shortening at the end of ejection.

This loss in contraction forces gradually progresses until systolic contraction is replaced by frank paradoxical motion. In contrast, regional ST segment elevation occurs only after contractile function has completely ceased. Pain is usually a late symptom. The alteration of global LV function will depend primarily on the percent LV mass involved in the ischemic process.

It is only recently that attention has been paid to the time course of recovery of function of ischemic myocardium upon reperfusion. From this observation the concept of stunned myocardium has evolved [2–4]. Stunned myocardium has been described as a temporary condition of postischemic LV dysfunction characterized by post-reperfusion depressed myocardial function in the zone which has been subject to an ischemic insult of which severity and duration did not result in permanent myocardial damage.

The time course of mechanical recovery has been well described and spans several days depending on the experimental conditions [2,13]. Reperfusion following a complete coronary artery occlusion with a duration of less than 20 minutes is followed by a well defined sequence of events:

a) The instantaneous reactive hyperemic response lasts several minutes and depends upon the duration of the ischemic insult. The presence and the degree of this hyperemic response is a good hallmark for the ultimate extent of functional recovery. Indeed, with longer episodes of coronary occlusion of more than 3 hours no reactive hyperemic response is observed presaging no recovery of regional function due to evolution towards infarction [14].

b) Full reperfusion is associated with almost immediate normalization of ECG changes despite persistent abnormal regional function, emphasizing different time course of recovery for different parameters of ischemia. This rapid normalization of ECG does not imply normalization of mechanical function.

c) Regional contractile function resumes as soon as perfusion is restored, despite an initial apparent hypercontractile response in part elicited by the reactive hyperemic response responsible for a temporary engorgement of blood in the ischemic segment resulting in an erectile phenomenon. When the reactive hyperemic response has subsided, the systolic function is depressed and does not return completely to preocclusion values until several hours or days after reperfusion (Figure 3). The degree of regional dysfunction ranges from – 70% to – 30% depending upon the experimental model used as well as the degree and duration of the ischemic insult [13].

d) Enzyme leakage from stunned myocardium has been documented in the absence of evidence of myocardial necrosis or permanent regional contractile deficit, suggesting that short episodes of myocardial ischemia, not long enough

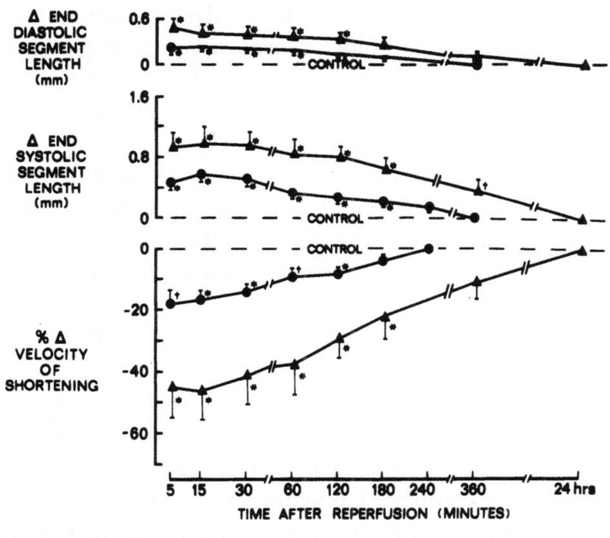

Figure 3. The prolonged recovery times for end-diastolic and end-systolic segment length and velocity of shortening after 5 min (●) and 15 min (▲) occlusions are compared. Recovery times from 5 to 24 hr after reperfusion are shown. Note that regional mechanical function remains depressed for more than 3 hr after a 15 min coronary artery occlusion. Significantly different from preocclusion control: * $p < 0.01$; + $p < 0.05$. (From Heyndrickx et al. [2]. Reproduced with permission)

to induce necrosis, are able to alter membrane permeability in a reversible way, whereby creatine kinase is permeating into the plasma. This is supported by the fact that adenosine triphosphate (ATP) and high energy phosphate-pool, necessary for membrane integrity remain also depressed for prolonged period of time after reperfusion. The currently accepted view that release of enzyme from ischemic myocardium reflects irreversible injury and necrosis may have to be revisited in the light of these observations [15].

e) Although the pathophysiological substrate of stunned myocardium is not yet completely understood, we know that stunned myocardium is associated with a decrease in high energy phosphate stores. In addition, the time course of refilling ATP stores and mechanical function are similar, however the cause and effect relationship has not been confirmed. Stunned myocardium is able to respond to sympathetic and other stimuli with increased contractility disclosing a potential inotropic reserve. In addition to the ischemic damage produced by the deprivation of oxygen and the accumulation of metabolites, there is evidence that reperfusion in itself can cause additional damage probably induced by acute increase in oxygen free radicals and/or cellular calcium overload [8, 9].

5. HIBERNATING MYOCARIUM

Rahimtoola in 1981 introduced the concept of hibernating myocardium referring to persistent severe regional myocardial dysfunction in the absence of clinical, electrocardiographic or biochemical signs of ongoing ischemia. He hypothesized that under some circumstances of reduced O_2 supply the myocardium may undergo adaptive changes to cope with reduced perfusion in order to prevent the occurrence of necrosis.

He framed this hypothesis on the observation that surgical myocardial revascularization results, in a number of patients, in striking improvement in left ventricular ejection fraction and regional wall motion [5, 6]. Although the concept is attractive, a distinct pathopysiological substrate has thus far not been identified.

The presence of persistent chronic regional dysfunction in the absence of ongoing ischemia can be explained in several ways.

a) akinetic segments could be composed of a mixture of infarcted tissue with some residual normal myocytes, which may be only moderately ischemic in the presence of adequate residual collateral flow and unable to contribute to active shortening of this segment. Upon revascularization, a small improvement in function of those remaining myocytes may explain overall improvement of regional function.

b) Prolonged hypokinesia may be due to an homogenously moderate reduction in function secondary to an uniformly reduction in flow. This situation, if prolonged, may result in small subendocardial necrosis in papillary muscle as shown in dogs to occur after 6 hours of steady state flow reduction, but with full reperfusion, prolonged depression with delayed recovery of contractile function is observed (stunned myocardium) [16]. It is however unknown how the myocardium will react to episodes of prolonged ischemia of more than six hours.

c) It is conceivable, but not yet proven, that in the phase of prolonged severe reduction in perfusion the majority of surviving myocytes are 'playing death' by some kind of metabolic adaptation towards anaerobic metabolism, whereby resetting of an ischemic treshold is proposed. This would allow myocytes to survive for a long time safeguarding the potential for full recovery. This situation could be viewed as chronic silent ischemia. One then could expect upon full reperfusion the reverse adaptation to higher O_2 supply to occur with a similar delay. The observation by Topol et al that revascularization of such segments results in almost immediate functional improvement, points towards chronic ongoing ischemia rather than hibernating myocardium [17].

6. MYOCARDIAL INFARCTION

If ischemia is severe enough and lasts long enough ($\geqslant$ 3hr), irreversible changes in cellular function occur, leading invariably to coagulation necrosis and scar formation. Since the subendocardium in humans is more susceptible to ischemic injury than the subepicardium, most human infarctions are most extensive in the subendocardial region.

While transmural progression of injury has been demonstrated in dogs going from the subendocardium towards the subepicardium, this wavefront injury has not been proven sofar in patients with myocardial infarction [1, 6]. The presence of collateral circulation, induced by repetitive short ischemic episodes throughout the course of progressive atherosclerosis, and the occurence of preconditioning of the myocardium to ischemia from repetitive episodes of ischemia delays adenosin triphosphate (ATP) depletion and the onset of myocardial ischemia .

7. DIAGNOSTIC APPLICATION OF POSITRON EMISSION TOMOGRAPHY

Recent advances in technology with the development of positron emission tomography (PET) offers a unique opportunity for studying noninvasively regional myocardial tissue perfusion and probing regional metabolism [18, 19]. Regional myocardial blood flow, glucose utilization, fatty acid metabolism and, more recently, oxygen consumption can now be evaluated noninvasively and can be quantified. Briefly, this imaging technique relies on the emission in diametrically opposed directions of two 511 KeV photons during positron annihilation which are detected by a ring of external detectors.

The tomographic reconstruction produces cross-sectional images reflecting a quantitative measurement of regional radioactivity. The physiologic tracers used with PET are compounds labeled with positron emitting isotopes of elements that are abundantly present in vivo such as carbon^{-11}, fluorine^{-18}, nitrogen^{-13} or oxygen^{-15}. Labeled substrates, substrate analogs and drugs can be synthetized in high specific activity without disturbing their biological properties. Combining these physiologic tracers with the quantitative capabilities of PET allows imaging of the distribution, uptake and turnover of tracers in the myocardium.

The myocardium is able to oxidize several substrates to meet its energy demands. The selection between the use of fuel of fatty acids, glucose, lactic acid, ketone bodies and amino acid depends largely upon the arterial concentration which in turn is regulated by the dietary state, physical activity and humoral balance.

The metabolic imaging with PET of stunned myocardium using tracers of glucose and fatty acid metabolism, as well as tracers probing the oxidative metabolism have yield important new information.

Figure 5 shows an example of a C-11 palmitate (CPA) study in stunned myocardium obtained 24 hours after reperfusion of a 1 hr coronary artery stenosis in a conscious dog, chronically instrumented for regional function measurements. Four representative images acquired 15 sec, 3 min, 9 min and 13 min after intravenous injection of CPA. The cross-sectional images were recorded at the same level where regional function was monitored. C-11 activity is colour-coded, the highest activity being in red, the lowest in dark blue. The images demonstrate the left ventricular blood pool early after injection, thereafter the rapid and homogeneous accumulation of CPA in all segments of left ventricular myocardium in septal, anterior, lateral and posterior wall segments indicating homogeneous myocardial blood flow. Finally the C-11 activity clears rapidly from the normal septal and anterior wall, but shows late stagnation in the posterior wall, stunned by one hour coronary artery stenosis.

Quantitative data are derived from these nuclear images. CPA tissue clearance curves are obtained from regions of interest both in stunned posterior zone and normal anterior zones (Figure 4). These time activity curves typically show two components, a first rapid decline followed by a more flatter part. Earlier studies have shown that the early phase of the curve is related to oxidation of fatty acids. Biexponential curve fitting allows to derive the halftime T½ of this early phase. Stunned myocardium displays typically an increase in early phase T½ compared to normal myocardium. This accounts for the stagnation of activity in the stunned zone on the images in Figure 5. Similarly, C-11 acetate clearance, a marker of oxidative metabolism at the mitochondrial level is typically delayed in stunned compared to normal myocardium.

In the clinical setting the advent of positron emission tomography has offered new possibilities to probe regional metabolism of various dyskinetic segments using the combination of a myocardial flow marker (ammonia) and a marker for regional metabolism (glucose).

In a number of patients, examined several days after acute symptoms of

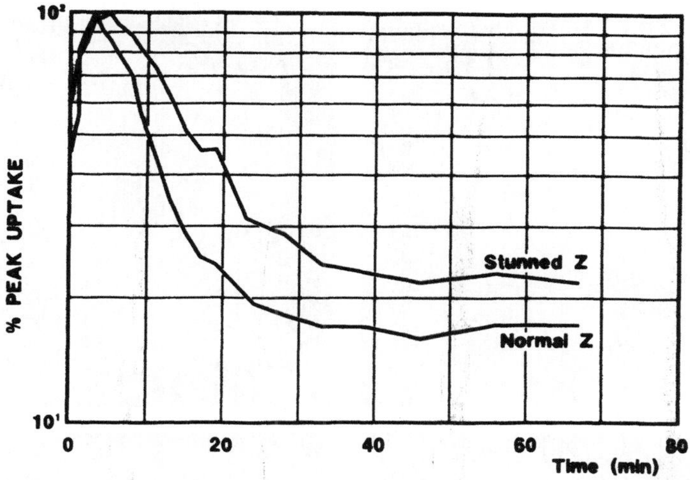

Figure 4. PET imaging with C-11 palmitate (CPA) in a dog 24 hr after a transient ischemic insult produced by a 1 hr circumflex coronary artery stenosis reducing transmural blood flow to 40% of control. Note the delayed clearance of activity from the lateral and posterior wall (arrows). The time of acquisition after intravenous CPA injection is indicated next each image. (For more detailed explanation see text)

myocardial infarction, exhibiting akinesia, PET scan has demonstrated two different patterns. In one group akinetic segments display a match between decrease or absence in regional blood flow and decrease or absence of regional metabolism, indicating myocardial necrosis with non-functional myocardium (Figure 6). Another group of patients with akinetic segments display a mismatch between regional blood flow and metabolism revealing segments with decreased or absent myocardial flow but preserved metabolism as evidenced by increased glucose uptake. Thus, myocardial viability in dyskinetic zones is characterized by a perfusion-metabolism mismatch (Figure 7).

Because impaired contractile function in segments of reduced flow may be interpreted as either infarcted segments, chronic ischemia or hibernating myocardium, PET scan may prove of importance in distinguishing between both conditions.

Analysis of wall motion abnormalities by echocardiography, LV cineangiogram or electrocardiography, nor the analysis of regional blood flow will adequately differentiate between necrosis and hibernating or chronic ischemic myocardium. The sensitivity of 201-Thallium scintigraphy for detecting myocardial viability in these conditions is rather low.

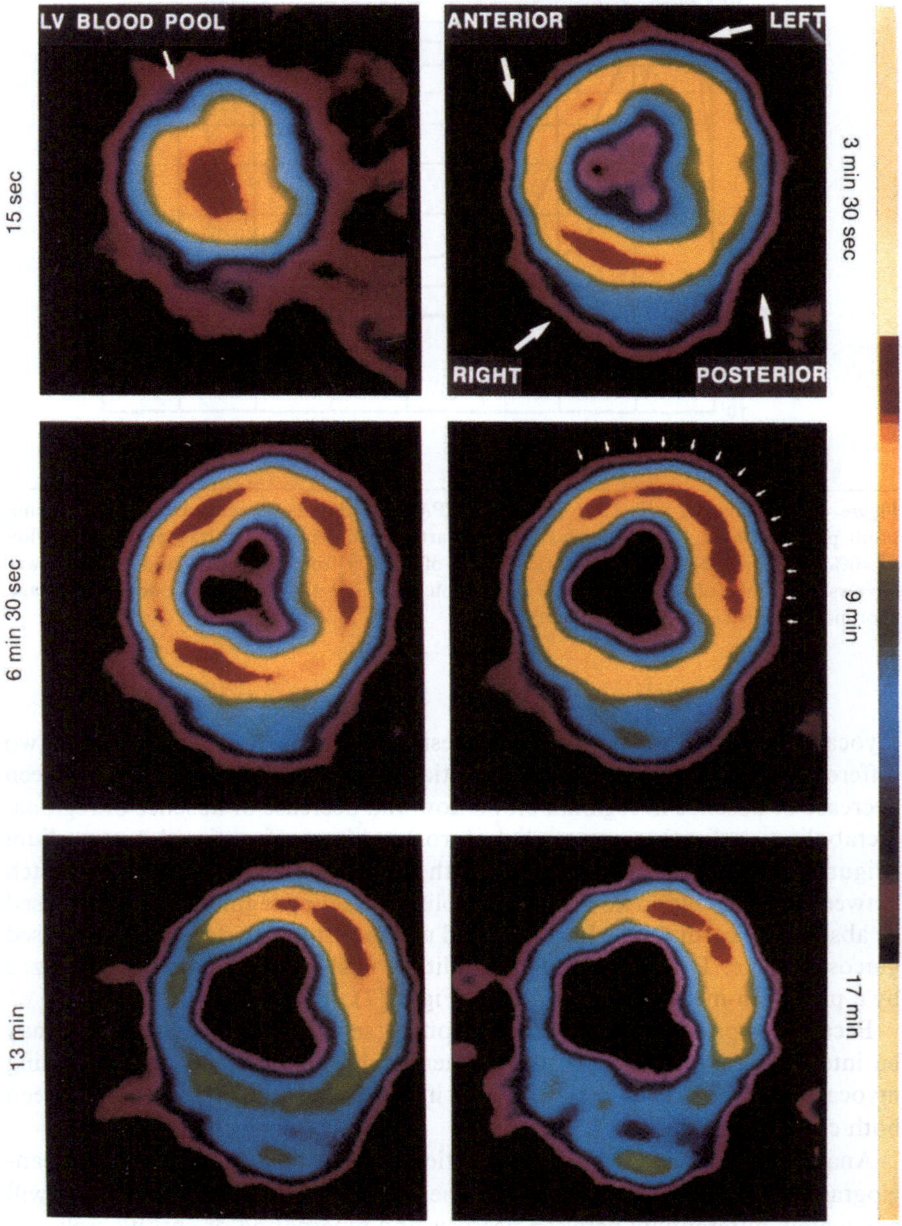

Figure 5. Time activity curve for uptake and clearance of C-11 palmitate (CPA), derived from region of interest in normal and stunned myocardium, 24 hr after an ischemic insult produced by a 1 hr severe coronary artery stenosis of the circumflex coronary artery in a dog followed by full reperfusion. As compared with the normal septal and anterior wall, clearance of C-11 activity is delayed in the stunned zones in posterior and lateral wall. The halftime of the early phase is increased from 4.2 min in the normal zone to 7.2 min in the stunned zone.

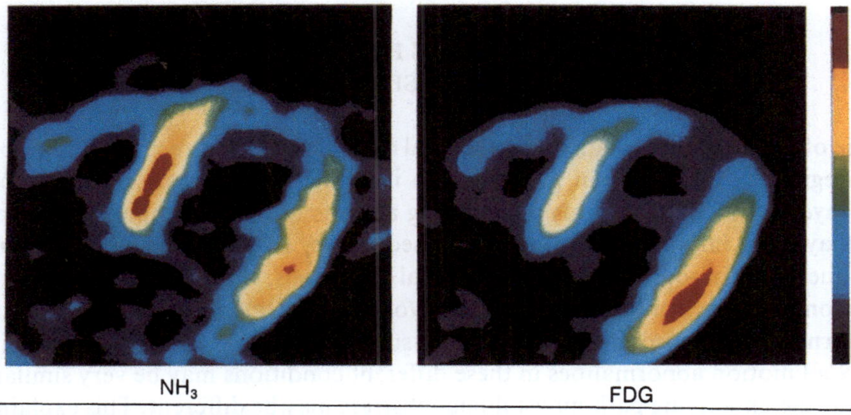

Figure 6. Positron emission tomogram of blood flow (*left panel*) and glucose metabolism (*right panel*) in a patient with coronary artery disease 60 days post anterior myocardial infarction treated with intravenous thrombolytic therapy. Blood flow (NH_3) in the anterior wall is markedly decreased which is consistent with total occlusion of the left anterior descending coronary artery. Uptake of ^{18}F 2-deoxyglucose (FDG) in the anterior segments is proportionally decreased. This pattern is an example of blood flow-metabolism match, indicative of myocardial necrosis.

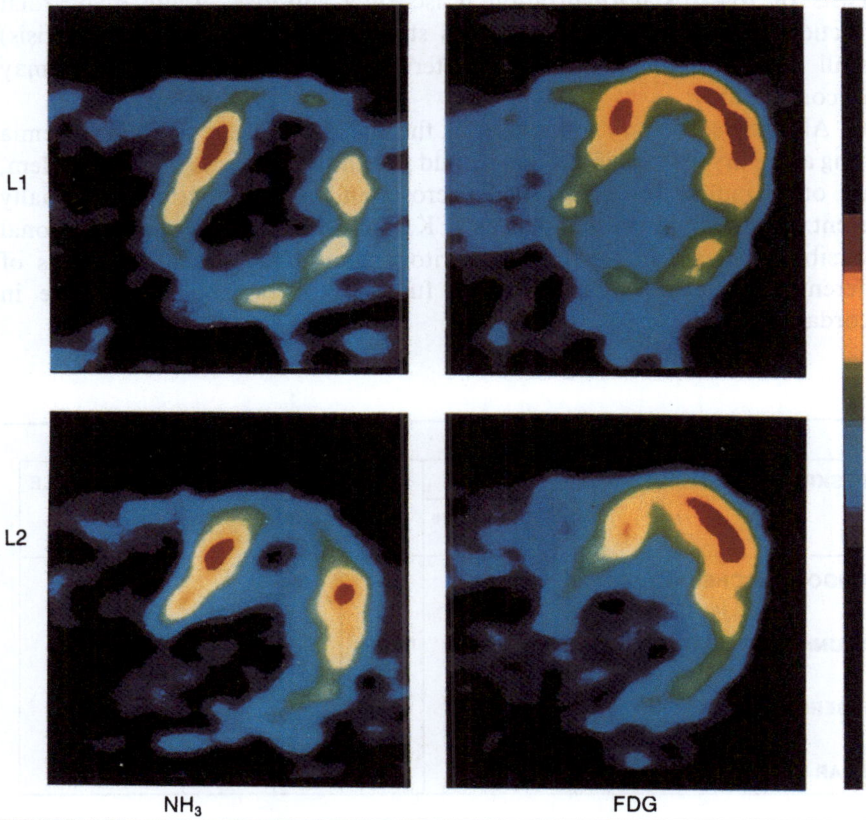

Figure 7. Positron emission tomograms in two planes of myocardial blood flow (*left panel*) and glucose metabolism (*right panel*) in a patient with coronary artery disease 60 days post anterior myocardial infarction treated with intravenous thrombolytic therapy. Blood flow (NH_3-ammonia) is markedly reduced in the anterior segments compatible with subtotal occlusion of left anterior descending coronary artery. Uptake of ^{18}F 2-deoxyglucose (FDG) differs from the distribution of ^{13}N-labeled ammonia, that is, it is increased in the anterior segments relative to blood flow. This pattern is an example of blood flow-metabolism mismatch indicative of viable myocardium in the anterior segments.

8. DIFFERENTIAL DIAGNOSIS FOR LEFT VENTRICULAR REGIONAL DYSFUNCTION

One of the diagnostic challenges in clinical cardiology is a correct interpretation of regional dysfunction in patients with ischemic heart disease. Recognition of myocardial viability in dysfunctioning areas is of clinical importance since it may have important therapeutic consequences. Regional dysfunction may be due to one of several pathophysiological conditions, alone or in combination: (a) ongoing ischemia, (b) stunned myocardium, (c) chronic ischemia or hibernating myocardium, and (d) scar tissue.

Wall motion abnormalities in these different conditions may be very similar, while the underlying pathophysiologic substrate may be different. This explains the differences observed in clinical features and potentially requires different treatment strategies (Figure 8).

a) Ongoing ischemia is characterized by an evolving pattern in clinical symptoms, ECG changes, heart enzymes and mechanical function. This evolving pattern may reveal evolution either towards necrosis if ischemia persists or towards normalization if ischemia subsides. Acute myocardial infarction, unstable angina, as well as stable angina (during anginal crisis) are all characterized by changing patterns, the time course of which may vary considerably.

b) Akinesia secondary to necrosis as the end result of myocardial ischemia during acute myocardial infarction should pose no difficult diagnostic problem, since other indices for myocardial necrosis and scar formation are usually present: Q-wave, increased plasma CK, etc. No evidence for additional reversible ischemia in the infarct territory should be present. Analysis of different parameters: ECG, regional function or metabolism will be in accordance.

DYSKINETIC SEGMENTS	EKG		FLOW	METABOLISM		CONTRACTILE RESERVE
	ST-T	Q-wave		fatty acids	glucose	
ONGOING ISCHEMIA	+	−	↓	↓	↓	+
STUNNED MYOCARDIUM	−	−	normal	↓	↑	+
HIBERNATING MYOCARDIUM	−	±	↓	?	↑	?
SCAR TISSUE	−	+	↓	↓	↓	−

Figure 8. Evaluation of myocardial viability in dyskinetic segments of the left ventricle in the early phase after acute coronary ischemic event.

c) Stunned myocardium reflected by regional motion abnormalities implies a previous but actually resolved ischemic episode. Myocardial blood flow in stunned zones is usually normal or slightly reduced. In the absence of signs indicative for myocardial necrosis, stunned myocardium is usually a retrospective diagnosis, since it implies full recovery of mechanical function upon reperfusion. Stunned myocardium retains the potential for inotropic stimulation. Searching for contractile reserve in akinetic segments (postextrasystolic potentiation, dobutamine infusion) may help differentiating scar tissue from stunned myocardium. Stunned myocardium is characterized by regional dysfunction in the phase of normal myocardium perfusion and decreased oxidative metabolism as well as decreased utilization of fatty acids. Both scar tissue and stunned areas may however, occur simultaneous when for instance thrombolytic therapy results in only partial myocardial salvage.

d) Chronic ischemia and/or hibernating myocardium may mimic myocardial necrosis. Several facts may, however, arouse suspicion for myocardial viability: (1) discrepancy between the extent of akinesia and the absence of extensive Q-wave on the standard ECG, and (2) additional episodes of transient ischemia (pain, ST-T changes). PET studies may add a new dimension as a noninvasive test for assessing muscle viability in dyskinetic segments by showing perfusion-metabolism mismatch. Further investigation will have to await until wide application of PET-scan can be advocated.

SUMMARY

Myocardial ischemia does not induce an all-or-none cell death. On the contrary, myocardial ischemia triggers a cascade of events, resulting in a dynamic process with several possible outcomes, depending on several autoregulatory mechanisms and medical interventions. The final result will depend upon the time frame when interventions are made and the particular situation of the myocardium at the time of these interventions. This results in distinctive pathophysiological entities such as stunned myocardium, chronic ischemia, hibernating myocardium or scar tissue. The clinical presentation of these syndromes may be confusing at times, but technological advances now offers new possibilities to differentiate between scar tissue, stunned myocardium and hibernating myocardium.

REFERENCES

1. Reimer KA Jennings RB (1986) Myocardial ischemia, hypoxia, and infarction, pp. 1133–1201, in *The Heart and the Cardiovascular System*, ed. by HA Fozzard et al. New York: Raven Press
2. Heyndrickx GR, Millard RW, McRitchie RJ, Maroko PR, Vatner SF (1975) Regional myocardial functional and electrocardiographic alterations after brief coronary artery occlusion in conscious dogs. *J Clin Invest* 56: 978–985

3. Heyndrickx GR, Baig H, Nellens P, Leusen I, Fishbein MC, Vatner SF (1978) Depression of regional blood flow and wall thickening after brief coronary occlusion. *Am J Physiol* 234: H 653–659
4. Braunwald E, Kloner RA (1982) The stunned myocardium: Prolonged, postischemic ventricular dysfunction. *Circulation* 66: 1146–1149
5. Rahimtoola SH (1985) A perspective on the three large multicenter randomized clinical trials of coronary bypass surgery for chronic stable angina. *Circulation* 8 (Suppl V): V 123–135
6. Rahimtoola SH (1989) The hibernating myocardium. *Am Heart J* 117: 211–221
7. Braunwald E, Rutherford JD (1986) Reversible ischemic left ventricular dysfunction: Evidence for 'hibernating myocardium'. *J Am Coll Cardiol* 8: 1467–1470
8. Weisfeldt M (1987) Reperfusion and reperfusion injury. *Clin Res* 35: 13–20
9. Bolli R (1988) Oxygen-derived free radicals and postischemic myocardial dysfunction ('Stunned myocardium'). *J Am Coll Cardiol* 12: 239–249
10. Olson RA, Bugni WJ (1986) Coronary circulation, pp 987–1037, in *The Heart and the Cardiovascular System*, ed. by HA Fozzard et al. New York: Raven Press
11. Tenant R, Wiggers LJ (1935) The effect of coronary occlusion on myocardial contraction. *Am J Physiol* 112: 351–361
12. Pagani M, Vatner SF, Baig H, Braunwald E (1978) Initial myocardial adjustment to brief periods of ischemia and reperfusion in conscious dogs. *Circ Res* 43: 83–92
13. Przyklenk K, Kloner RA (1989) What factors predict recovery of contractile function in the canine model of the stunned myocardium. *Am J Cardiol* 64: 18F–26F
14. Heyndrickx GR, Amano J, Patrick TA, Manders WT, Rogers GG, Rosendorff C, Vatner SF (1985) Effects of coronary artery reperfusion on regional myocardial blood flow and function in conscious baboons. *Circulation* 71: 1029–1037
15. Heyndrickx GR, Amano J, Kenna T, Fallon JT, Patrick TA, Manders WT, Rogers GG, Rosendorff C, Vatner SF (1985) Creatine Kinase release not associated with myocardial necrosis after short periods of coronary artery occlusion in conscious baboons. *J Am Coll Cardiol* 6: 1299–1303
16. Matsuzaki M, Gallagher K, Kemper WS, White F, Ross J Jr (1983) Sustained regional dysfunction produced by prolonged coronary stenosis: Gradual recovery after reperfusion. *Circulation* 68: 170–182
17. Topol EJ, Weiss JL, Guzman PA, Dorsey-Lima S, Blanck TJJ, Humphrey LS, Baumgartner WA, Flaherty JT, Reitz BA (1984) Immediate improvement of dysfunctional myocardial segments after coronary revascularization: Detection by intraoperative transoesophageal echocardiography. *J Am Coll Cardiol* 4: 1123–1134
18. Bergmann SR, Fox KAA, Geltman EM, Sobel BE (1985) Positron emission tomography of the heart. *Progr in Cardiovasc Dis* 28: 165–194
19. Schelbert HR, Buxton D (1988) Insights into coronary artery disease gained from metabolic imaging. *Circulation* 78: 496–505
20. Heyndrickx GR, et al. (1978) in: *Coronary Heart Disease. 3rd International Symposium*, ed. by Kaltenbach et al. Stuttgart: George Thieme Publishers

6. Effects of coronary reperfusion on left ventricular function and survival

Some remaining problems

FRANS VAN DE WERF

Although intravenous administration of thrombolytic agents has now become widely accepted as standard treatment for acute myocardial infarction, some important problems remain to be solved. First, the results of large placebo-controlled studies with different thrombolytic agents suggest that the clinical benefit (including the reduction of mortality) can hardly be explained by myocardial salvage and preservation of left ventricular function alone. Second, the effect of adjunctive treatment such as PTCA, β-blockers and scavengers of oxygen free radicals on left ventricular function and long-term clinical follow-up has not been conclusively studied. Third, the incidence and time course of infarct expansion and left ventricular remodeling after successful reperfusion and the possible effect of medical treatment (e.g., ACE-inhibitors, xamoterol, β-blockers...) thereon is largely unknown.

I. DISCREPANCIES BETWEEN THE EFFECTS OF REPERFUSION ON LEFT VENTRICULAR FUNCTION AND SURVIVAL

It is widely accepted that salvage of acutely ischemic but reversibly damaged myocardium is responsible for the preservation of left ventricular function and for the improved survival observed after thrombolytic treatment for acute myocardial infarction [1–17]. However, a number of recent observations seem to indicate that the relationship between coronary reperfusion and the reduction of left ventricular dysfunction, and their effect on the improvement of both early and late survival, is more complex than initially thought [18].

A first hint is the surprising observation that all placebo-controlled left ventricular function trials with intravenously administered thrombolytic agents have failed to show beneficial effects on *both* survival and global left ventricular function [5–8, 11, 13–17]. Indeed, a statistically significant beneficial effect on both endpoints has never been demonstrated so far – and thus will never be demonstrated in the future – in the *total* population of placebo-controlled trials with intravenous thrombolytic agents (Table 1). In the New Zealand

E. Andries & R. Stroobandt (eds.), Hemodynamics in Daily Practice, 91–100.

Table 1. Early mortality and global left ventricular function in placebo controlled trials with intravenous thrombolytic agents.

Reference	EF (%) Controls	EF (%) Active treament	Early mortality (%) Controls	Early mortality (%) Active treatment	Total numbers of patients in the trial
ISAM [5]	53.9	56.8 *	7.1	6.3 NS	1741
White et al. [6]	50.7	54.0 NS	12.5	3.7 *	219
Kennedy et al. [7]	50.7	54.3 NS+	9.6	6.3 NS	368
Guerci et al. [14]	46.4	53.2 *	7.6	5.6 NS	138
O'Rourke et al. [15]	54	61 *	5.6	5.4 NS	147
Australian [16]	51.7	57.7 *	4.2	9.6 NS	145
Van de Werf et al. [11]	48.5	50.7 *	5.7	2.8 NS++	721
Meinertz et al. [13]	54	53 NS	12.6	5.6 *	313
Bassand et al. [17]	47	53 *	5.0	6.3 NS	231

* Significantly different from control group; NS: not significantly different from controls; +: p = 0.056; ++: p = 0.53.

trial [6] with streptokinase in 219 patients, a significant improvement in global ejection fraction *and* survival was demonstrated in patients with a *first* myocardial infarction (n=172) but not in the total group of patients (n=219) in whom the difference in global ejection fraction between patients treated with streptokinase and controls was no longer statistically significant (p=0.09; not published, personal communication of H. White). In the European Cooperative Study Group trial in 721 patients [11], the difference in global ejection fraction between patients treated with tissue plasminogen activator and controls was small (2.2 absolute % points) but statistically significant (p=0.04). On the other hand the reduction in mortality at 14 days was large (51%) in this trial but only of borderline significance (p=0.053). In the Western Washington trial [7] with intravenous streptokinase only the difference in global ejection fraction was of borderline significance (p=0.056). In all other trials (see Table 1) either global ejection fraction or early survival was significantly improved. Moreover, in the Australian trial with rt-PA [16] and in the APSIM trial with APSAC [17] early mortality was higher in the thrombolysis group than in controls in spite of the significant 6% absolute difference in global ejection fraction observed in both studies.

In the Western Washington trial with intracoronary streptokinase [19] and in the TIMI-phase I trial with tissue plasminogen activator [20] improved long-term survival was demonstrated in the thrombolysis group without a significant effect on left ventricular function. Successful recanalization of the infarct-related coronary artery turned out to be the most important predictor of late survival in both trials [19, 20, 21].

The results of a recent randomized comparative trial with streptokinase and tissue plasminogen activator carried out in New Zealand in 271 patients [22] point in the same direction. Although global left ventricular ejection fraction was nearly identical in both treatment groups (satistically not significant) differences in early mortality rate were observed: 10 out of 136 patients died in the stroptokinase group (7.4%) compared with 5 out of 135 patients in the rt-PA group (3.7%). A similar trend was observed in the plasminogen activator Italian Multicentre study (PAIMS) [23]: hospital mortality was higher in streptokinase treated patients (8.2%, 7 out of 85) than in patients treated with tissue plasminogen activator (4.7%, 4 out of 86) whereas the difference in global ejection fraction (angiographically measured) was small (53% vs 55%).

Long-term follow-up in placebo-controlled trials with thrombolytic agents have shown that the beneficial effect of thrombolytic treatment on survival persists for at least 1 year [3, 9, 12, 24, 25]. If preservation of left ventricular contractile function is the only or at least the most important beneficial effect of successful coronary reperfusion one would expect divergent survival curves and a greater difference in survival rate at 1 year than at the time of hospital discharge.

The important and persistent mortality reduction observed in the ISIS-2 trial [9] in patients treated as late as 12 to 24 hours after the onset of symptoms – a time window far too late to allow substantial salvage of ischemic myocardium – also suggests that beneficial effects of reperfusion other than salvage of ischemic myocardium could be involved.

The observed discrepancies between the effects of coronary reperfusion on left ventricular function and survival do not detract from the importance of left ventricular dysfunction for long-term prognosis [26]. Nor should they weaken our efforts to treat patients very early during the course of an acute myocardial infarction, since, whatever the responsible mechanisms, the greatest clinical benefit is obtained in early treated patients. Mechanisms that could play a beneficial role in the acute stage of an evolving myocardial infarction, besides salvage of ischemic myocardium, are prevention of cardiac rupture and arrhythmia and, in a later stage, prevention or limitation of infarct expansion and left ventricular remodeling (*vide infra*).

An additional partial explanation for the observed discrepancies in effects could be the 'time of treatment paradox'. A detailed post hoc analysis of the data from the European Cooperative Study Group trial [11] revealed that in patients treated within 3 hours after the onset of symptoms the mortality reduction at 14 days was 82% (p=0.009) while global ejection fraction at 10 to 22 days in the surviving patients was nearly identical: 49.8% in controls vs 50.8% in the group treated with tissue plasminogen activator. Reversely, in patients treated after 3 hours, the 14 day mortality in the thrombolysis group was only slightly lower when compared to controls (4.5% vs. 5.0%) while in the surviving patients treated within this time window (3 to 5 hours after the onset of symptoms) global ejection fraction was significantly higher (4 absolute % points, $p \leqslant 0.01$) in the thrombolysis group (Table 2). Similarly,

Table 2. Paradoxical effects of thrombolytic treatment on early mortality and global left ventricular ejection fraction according to the time of treatment.

	< 3 hours		> 3 hours	
	Controls	rt-PA	Controls	rt-PA
Mortality (%) at 14 days	6.3 n = 207	1.1 * n = 179	5.0 n = 159	4.5 NS n = 176
EF (%) at 10–22 days	49.8 n = 165	50.8 n = 149	46.8 n = 121	50.7 * n = 138

Data from the European Cooperative Study Group rt-PA vs placebo trial [11].
* $p < 0.01$; NS: not significant different from controls.

in the Western Washington trial with intravenous streptokinase. [7, 8] the reduction in 14 day mortality in patients treated within 3 hours was 54% (from 11.3% in controls to 5.2% in the streptokinase group) with an improvement in ejection fraction of only 2% points (51% vs 49%) in a subgroup of surviving patients at 2 months. In patients treated between 3 and 6 hours after the onset of symptoms the 14 day mortality was identical in both treatment groups (7.5%) while global ejection fraction at 2 months was 5% points higher in the streptokinase group when compared to controls (50% vs 45%). In the ISAM study [5] where streptokinase was also used, the reductions in early mortality observed in thrombolysis patients were less pronounced and very similar in patients treated within 3 hours (from 6.5% to 5.2%) and in those treated between 3 and 6 hours (from 7.7% to 6.8%). Accordingly, the absolute differences in ejection fraction when compared with controls were also very similar in the 2 groups: 3.4% when treatment was started within 3 hours and 2.2% for treatment started within 3 to 6 hours after the onset of infarction. Thus, it can be argued that when an effective thrombolytic agent is administered very early in the course of an acute myocardial infarction some patients with a very poor left ventricular function will be saved. These patients would have died if no thrombolytic treatment would have been given or if thrombolytic treatment would have been started later (e.g., later than 3 hours after onset of symptoms). The (very) low ejection fractions of these early reperfused patients will mask the gain in ejection fraction obtained in other reperfused patients and therefore distort the comparison with surviving controls. The greater the reduction in early mortality obtained with a thrombolytic agent the more likely this 'paradoxical' phenomenon will play a part.

If recanalization of an infarct-related coronary artery in itself has beneficial effects by mechanisms other than salvaging ischemic myocardium and preserving left ventricular function, this could have very important consequences for the future of thrombolytic therapy. Among other things the following could be of particular significance: (1) thrombolytic agents with the highest reperfusion rate should be preferred since they would yield the greatest clinical benefit, (2) to prove the superiotity of a thrombolytic agent or the advantage of antithrombotic or other adjunctive treatment, trials that compare left ventricular function rather than mortality would be inappropriate [25], and (3) patients with an infarction of more than 6 hours should also be submitted to thrombolytic therapy.

II. LONG-TERM EFFECTS OF ADJUNCTIVE TREATMENT

It has been shown by the European Cooperative Study Group that in patients with an acute myocardial infarction treated with rt-PA, heparin and aspirin, immediate PTCA has no additional benefit on infarct size, left ventricular function and early survival [28]. Also in other studies performed in the United States [29, 30], invasive strategies including early coronarography and prophylactic PTCA did not result in a greater preservation of global left ventricular function. However, in the European Cooperative Trial [28] the remaining infarct-related residual stenosis at the time of hospital discharge was less severe in patients allocated to immediate PTCA (which had to be attempted on all lesions with a 50% or smaller diameter stenosis after reperfusion or on all occluded infarct vessels). Therefore, it can be argued that the reduction in diameter stenosis of the culprit lesion by immediate PTCA might have long-term beneficial effects. The one year follow-up of the European rt-PA/ PTCA trial is now available [31]. No difference in the incidence of new cardiac events between the 2 groups was observed between hospital discharge and one year follow-up. Mortality was 2.7% and 5.5% at 14 days and 1 year, respectively in conservatively treated patient as compared with 6.5% at 14 days and 9.6% at 1 year in the PTCA group. Very similarly, in the TIMI Phase II trial [30], reinfarction or death within 6 weeks occurred in a similar proportion of the patients allocated to the conservative or to the invasive strategy including coronary angiography and PTCA (to be performed on suitable lesions only). The results of these trials from both sides of the Atlantic therefore seem to advocate a conservative strategy after thrombolysis with coronary arteriography, eventually followed by mechanical therapy (PTCA or bypass surgery), being restricted to patients with clinical, electrocardiographic or scintigraphic signs of recurrent ischemia.

Early intravenous β-blockade has been shown to reduce early mortality in patients with an acute myocardial infarction not treated with thrombolytic agents [32, 33]. Moreover, in experimental animals acute intravenous administration of a β-blocker further reduced the amount of myocardial necrosis induced by reperfusion and accelerated the functional recovery of the reperfused infarction area [34]. In the already mentioned TIMI-phase II study [30], patients who were eligible for intravenous β-blockade were also randomly assigned to immediate (15 mg metoprolol intravenously) or to deferred (oral metoprolol started on day 6) β-blocker therapy. Global ejection fraction at rest and during exercise and mortality, both at discharge and at 6 weeks, were very similar in the 2 treatment groups. However, in patients allocated to immediate

β-blockade, recurrent ischemia and reinfarction occurred less frequently than in patients assigned to deferred oral β-blockade. Moreover, in patients treated within 2 hours after the onset of symptoms, the incidence of recurrent infarction or death was significantly lower in the immediate β-blocker group (5.0% vs 12.1%, $p \leqslant 0.01$). In low-risks patients, immediate intravenous β-blockade significantly reduced mortality at 6 weeks as compared with deferred β-blockade (0% vs 2.8%, p=0.007). These results could be partly explained by an 'antithrombotic' effect of metoprolol: in a recent study [35], metoprolol significantly reduced the plasma levels of the plasminogen activator inhibitor (PAI-1). This could result in a greater fibrinolytic effect of the thrombolytic agent used and/or in a lower incidence of rethrombosis afterwards. Doubtless, the favourable results of intravenous β-blockade in addition to thrombolysis of the TIMI-phase II trial warrant further detailed investigations, including long-term follow-up studies.

III. INFARCT EXPANSION AND LEFT VENTRICULAR REMODELING

Recently it has been shown that global remodeling of the left ventricle starts immediately after infarction and may continue for some months [36–40]. The result of this process is left ventricular dilatation and, eventually, heart failure. McKay et al. [40] have demonstrated this progressive remodeling process to include expansion of the infarcted areas and volume-overload hypertrophy of noninfarcted segments. These authors also hypothesized that increased diastolic wall stress is the trigger for these changes.

There are many theoretical possibillities to prevent or to limit left ventricular remodeling. One very important mechanism could be recanalization of the infarct vessel. Indeed, it is attractive to speculate that, apart from salvaging ischemic myocardium and limiting infarct size, reperfusion of an infarct-related vessel alters the viscoelastic properties of the (ischemic or necrotic) myocardium supplied by the coronary artery, thereby preventing or limiting further expansion of the infarction. The GISSI-I findings of smaller left ventricular volumes and less regional wall motion abnormalities in the presence of an identical ejection fraction at 6 months in a subset of patients treated with streptokinase as compared with conventionally treated patients, support this hypothesis [41]. The beneficial effects of thrombolytic therapy observed in patients treated late after the onset of symptoms in ISIS-2 [9] could also be partly explainded by this mechanism. However, in one small, detailed study in 36 patients with acute infarction, relatively late thrombolysis did not prevent subsequent development of delayed ventricular dilatation [42].

In view of the supposed mechanisms of diastolic dysfunction, interventions that reduce loading conditions might be beneficial. Pfeffer et al. have demonstrated that the early administration of captopril reduces geometric changes of the left ventricle after experimental infarction and that this blunting effect of remodeling was assiociated with improved survival at 1 year [36, 37]. These beneficial effects have been confirmed in patients [43].

Xamoterol (Corwin), a B_1-elective partial agonist with approximately 43% of the agonist activity of isoproterenol, has been shown to increase isovolumic rate, to reduce mean diastolic wall stress and left ventricular filling pressure, and to improve myocardial contractility [44]. This drug has been given to patients with anterior myocardial infarction and single-vessel disease. Beneficial effects on left ventricular diastolic geometry were observed in xamoterol treated patients as compared with controls [45].

Fishbein et al. [46] recently reported severe ventricular enlargement during long-term treatment with propranolol as compared to placebo in a rat model of myocardial infarction. From these potentially important data on might speculate that chronic β-blockade treatment after infarction could promote the processes leading to ventricular enlargement. Therefore, it would be very interesting to compare in a prospective randomized trial in post-infarction patients the effects of a classical β-blocker with those of xamoterol, which, as already mentioned, not only improves diastolic function but also has a moderate positive inotropic effect at rest, and, when the sympathetic tone is high, also attenuates the adrenergic reponse.

IV. CONCLUSION

It is obvious that intravenous thrombolytic therapy is a major breakthrough for the treatment of patients with an acute myocardial infarction. As explained, many questions remained to be answered. In view of the complexity of the remaining problems, the answers can only come form carefully performed randomized multicenter trials. It is to be hoped that the recently finished, ongoing or planned multicenter trials such as the GISSI-2 trial evaluating mortality *and* cardiac function, the International streptokinase versus tissue plasminogen activator Mortality Trial, the ISIS-3 trial, the TIMI-phase II trial, and the placebo-controlled trials with streptokinase (EMERA) and tissue plasminogen activator (LATE) in patients presenting late ($\geqslant$ 6 hours) after the onset of pain will throw an new light on the complex relationship between coronary thrombolysis, preservation of left ventricular function survival. The results are anxiously awaited.

REFERENCES

1. Kennedy JW, Ritchie JL, Davis KB, Fritz JK (1983) Western Washington randomized trial of intracoronary streptokinase in acute myocardial infarction. *N Engl J Med* 309: 1477–1482
2. Ritchie JL, Davis KB, Williams DL, Caldwell JH, Kennedy JW (1984) Global and regional left ventricular function and tomographic radionuclide perfusion: The Western Washington Intracoronary Streptokinase in Acute Myocardial infarction Trial. *Circulation* 70: 867–875
3. Simoons ML, Serruys PW, Van den Brand M, et al. (1985) Improved survival after early thrombolysis in acute myocardial infarction. *Lancet* 1985/2: 578–581

4. Gruppo Italiano per Lo Studio della Streptokinasi nell' infarcto Miocardico (GISSI) (1986) Effectiveness of intravenous thrombolytic treatment in acute myocardial infarction. *Lancet* 1986/1: 397–401
5. ISAM Study Group (1986) A prospective trial of intravenous streptokinase in acute myocardial infarction (ISAM). Mortality, morbidity and infarct size at 21 days. *N Engl J Med* 314: 1456–1471
6. White HD, Norris RM, Brown MA, et al. (1987) Effect of intravenous streptokinase on left ventricular function and early survival after acute myocardial infarction, *E Engl J Med* 317: 850–855
7. Kennedy JW, Martin CV, Davis KB, et al. (1988) The Western Washington Intravenous Streptokinase in acute Myocardial infarction randomized trial. *Circulation* 77: 345–352
8. Ritchie JL, Cerqueira M, Maynard C, Davis K, Kennedy JW (1988) Ventricular function and infarct size: the Western Washington Intravenous Streptokinase in myocardial infarction trial. *J Am Coll Cardiol* 11: 689–697
9. ISIS-2 Collaborative Group (1988) Randomized trial of intravenous streptokinase, oral aspirin, both, or neither among 17, 187 cases of suspected acute myocardial infarction: ISIS-2. *Lancet* 1988/2: 349–360
10. Wilcox RG, Olsson CB, Skene AM, von der Lippe G. Jensen G, Hampton JR (1988) Trial of tissue plasminogen activator for mortality reduction in acute myocardial infarction: Anglo-Scandinavian study of early thrombolysis 'ASSET'), *Lancet* 1988/2: 525–530
11. Van de Werf F, Arnold AER, (1988) Intravenous tissue plasminogen activator and size of infarct, left ventricular function, and survival in acute myocardial infarction. *Br Med J* 297: 1374–1379
12. The AIMS Trial Study Group (1988) Effect of intravenous APSAC on mortality after acute myocardial infarction: Preliminary report of a placebo-controlled clinical trial. *Lancet* 1988/1: 545–549
13. Meinertz T, Kasper W, Schumacher M, Just H, for the APSAC Multicenter Trial Group (1988) The German multicenter trial of anisoylated plasminogen streptokinase activator complex versus heparin for acute myocardial infarction. *Am J Cardiol* 62: 347–351
14. Guerci AD, Gerstenblith G, Brinke JA, et al. (1987) A randomized, placebo-controlled, double blind trial of intravenous plasminogen activator for acute myocardial infarction with subsequent randomization to elective coronary angioplasty. *N Engl J Med* 317: 1613–1618
15. O'Rourke M, Baron D, Keogh A, et al. (1988) Limitation of myocardial infarction by early infusion of recombinant tissue-type plasminogen activator. *Circulation* 77: 1311–1315
16. National Heart Foundation of Australia Coronary Thrombolysis Group (1988) Coronary Thrombolysis and myocardial salvage by tissue plasminogen activator given up to 4 hours after onset of myocardial infarction. *Lancet* 1988/1: 203–207
17. Bassand JP, Machecourt J, Cassagnes J et al. (1989) Multicenter trial of intravenous anisoylated plasminogen streptokinase activator complex (APSAC) in acute myocardial infarction: effects on infarct size and left ventricular function. *J Am Coll Cardiol* 13: 988–997
18. Van de Werf (1989) Discrepancies between the effect of coronary reperfusion on left ventricular function and survival. *Lancet* 1989/1: 1367–1369
19. Kennedy JW, Ritchie JL, Davis KB, Stadius ML, Maynard C, Fritz JK (1985) The Western Washington randomized trial of intracoronary streptokinase in acute myocardial infarction: A 12 month follow-up report. *N Engl J Med* 321: 1073–1078
20. Dalen JE, Gore JM, Braunwald E, et al. (1988) Six- and twelve-month follow-up of the phase I thrombolysis in myocardial infarction (TIMI) trial. *Am J Cardiol* 62: 179–185
21. Stadius ML, Davis K, Maynard C, Ritchie JL, Kennedy JW (1986) Risk stratification for 1 year survival based on characteristics identified in the early hours of acute myocardial infarction. *Circulation* 74: 703–711
22. White HD, Rivers JT, Norris RM, et al. (1988) Is rt-PA or streptokinase superior for preservation of left ventricular function after myocardial infarction? *Circulation* 78 (Suppl II): II–303 (abstract)
23. Magnani B et al (1989) Plasminogen activator Italian multicenter study (PAIMS): comparison

of intravenous recombinant single-chain human tissue-type plasminogen activator (rt-PA) with intravenous streptokinase in acute myocardial infarction. *J Am Coll Cardiol* 13: 19–26

24. Gruppo Italiano per lo Studio della Streptochinasi nell' Infarto miocardico (1987) Long-term effects of intravenous thrombolysis in acute myocardial infarction: Final report of the GISSI-study. *Lancet* 1987/2: 871–874
25. Van de Werf F, Arnold AER (1989) The European Cooperative rt-PA versus placebo trial: 1 year follow-up. *Circulation* 80 (Suppl. II): II–520 (Abstract)
26. White HD, Norris RM, Brown MA, Brandt PWT, Whitlock RML, Wild CJ (1987) Left ventricular end-systolic volume as the major determinant of survival after recovery from myocardial infarction. *Circulation* 76: 44–51
27. Norris RM, White HD (1988) Therapeutic trials in coronary thrombolysis should measure left ventricular function as primary end-point of treatment. *Lancet* 1988/1: 104–106
28. Simoons ML, Arnold AER, Betrice A et al (1988) Thrombolysis with tissue plaminogen activator in acute myocardial infarction: no additional benefit from immediate percutaneous coronary angiography. *Lancet* 1988/1: 197–203
29. Topol EJ, Califf RM, George BS et al. (1987) A randomized trial of immediate versus delayed elective angiography after intravenous tissue plasminogen activator in acute myocardial infarction. *N Engl J Med* 317: 581–588
30. TIMI Study Group (1989) Comparison of invasive and conservative strategies after treatment with intravenous tissue plasminogen activator in acute myocardial infarction. *N Engl J Med* 320: 618–627
31. Simoons ML, Arnold A (1989) One year follow-up of rt-PA without and with immediate PTCA. *Circulation* 80 (Suppl. II): II–520 (Abstract)
32. ISIS-I (1986) Randomized trial of intravenous atenolol among 16 027 cases of suspected acute myocardial infarction. *Lancet* 1986/2: 57–66
33. MIAMI Trial Research Group (1985) Metoprolol in acute myocardial infarction. A randomized placebo-controlled international trial. *Eur Heart J* 6: 199–226
34. Van de Werf F, Vanhaecke J, Jang IK, Flameng W, Collen D, De Geest H (1987) Reduction in infarction and enhanced recovery of systolic function after coronary thrombolysis with tissue-type plasminogen activator combined with B-adrenergic blockade with metoprolol. *Circulation* 75: 830–836
35. Teper-Nilsson AC, Dahlöf C, Haglund E, Hedman C, Olsson G, Ablad B (1989) Metoprolol reduces plasminogen activator inhibitor (PAI–1) in man (abstract, submitted to FASEB)
36. Roberts CS, Maclean D, Maroko P, Kloner RA (1984) Early and late remodeling of the left ventricle after acute myocardial infarction. *Am J Cardiol* 54: 407–410
37. Erlebacher JA, Weiss JL, Weisfeld ML, BulKley BH (1984) Early dilatation of the infarcted segment in acute transmural myocardial infarction: role of infarct expansion in acute left ventricular enlargement. *J Am Coll Cardiol* 4: 201–208
38. Pfeffer JM, Pfeffer MA, Braunwald E (1985) Influence of chronic captopril therapy on the infarcted left ventricle of the rat. *Circ Res* 57: 84–95
39. Pfeffer MA, Pfeffer JM, Steinbert C, Finn P (1985) Survival after an experimental infarction: beneficial effects of long-term therapy with captopril. *Circulation* 72: 406–413
40. McKay RG, Pfeffer MA, Pasternak RC et al. (1986) Left ventricular remodeling after myocardial infarction: a corollary to infarct expansion. *Circulation* 693–702
41. Marino P, Zanolla L, Golia G, Zardini P (1988) Effects of intravenous streptokinase on left ventricular modeling after myocardial infarction: the GISSI-trial. *Circulation* 78 (Suppl. II) II–275 (Abstract).
42. Warren SE, Royal HD, Markis JE, Grossman W, McKay RG (1988) Time course of left ventricular dilatation after myocardial infarction: influence of infarct-related artery and success of coronary thrombolysis. *J Am Coll of Cardiol* 11: 12–19
43. Pfeffer MA, Lamas GA, Vaughan DE, Parisi AF, Braunwald E (1988) Effects of captopril on progressive ventricular dilatation after anterior myocardial infarction. *New Engl J Med* 313: 80–86
44. Nuttall A, Snow HM (1982) The cardiovascular effects of ICI 118, 587: A B1-adrenoreceptor

partial agonist. *Br J Pharmacol* 77: 381–388
45. Pouleur H, van Eyll C, Hanet C, Cheron P, Charlier AA, Rousseau Mf (1988) Long-term effects of Xamoterol on left ventricular diastolic function and late remodeling: a study in patients with anterior infarction and singel-vessel disease. *Circulation* 77: 1081–1089
46. Fishbein MC, Lei LQ, Rubin SA (1988) Long-term propranolol administration alters myocyte and ventricular geometry in rat hearts with and without infarction. *Circulation* 78: 369–

7. Effects of revascularization on left ventricular function in the stunned and hibernating myocardium

W. FLAMENG

INTRODUCTION

The pathophysiological basis of postischemic heart failure is not fully understood and the underlying mechanisms may be manyfold. There is increasing evidence that at least three different conditions of ischemia-induced heart failure can be recognized and that they probably represent a sequence of stages of the same process. These conditions are: the akinetic state of the myocardium during acute ischemia, the postischemic myocardial dysfunction in the reperfusion phase (stunned myocardium [1]) and the chronically ischemic hypo-of akinetic myocardium (hibernating myocardium) [2]. All three conditions differ considerably in terms of subcellular pathophysiological abnormalities, biochemical alternations and ultrastructural changes.

Because differences between these types of contractile failure are fundamental, a given therapeutical intervention will not necessarily elicite the same responses.

A. ACUTE MYOCARDIAL ISCHEMIA

A rather common cause of pump failure is a loss of contractile function related to acute myocardial infarction. This type of contractile failure is well documented in the course of evolving infarction and is characterized by a complete akinesia of the portion of the left ventricle previously supplied by the blocked coronary artery. Pump failure occurs then when this segment represents a considerable part of the left ventricle. Hyperkinesia of the contralateral segment may compensate, to a certain degree, for the akinetic segment and can prevent global pump failure. Akinesia in the context of complete occlusion of a coronary artery however is an extreme situation: it can be preceded by different degrees of low flow ischemia leading to progressive impairment of regional contractility. Pump failure may result from extensive hypoperfusion in multiple coronary vessels producing diffuse hypokinesis of the left ventricle without evidence of infarction.

E. Andries & R. Stroobandt (eds.), Hemodynamics in Daily Practice, 101–112.

The basic mechanism of contractile failure due to acute ischemia is still unknown. Acute ischemic contractile failure occurs whithin seconds after cessation of coronary blood flow. Several mechanisms are involved in this process.

a) A first event in ischemia, which parallels in time (i.e., within seconds) with contractile failure is *a loss of cellular K^+*. This results in an increase in extracellular K^+ up to 15 mMol after 10 minutes. Such an early K^+ leak, although its mechanism is unknown, parallels also in time with the efflux of anions (mainly lactate and Pi) from the cell. Most probably a K^+ channel is activated when intracellular (ATP) falls below 1–2 mM. The accumulation of K^+ in the extracellular space leads to depolarization of the membrane and a small shortening of the action potential. This phenomenon in turn induces a rapid *decline in muscle tension.* However, because the loss of contractility after induction of ischemia is rapid and complete, potassium leakage cannot be the full answer for contractile failure.

b) Although the 'overall' cytoplasmic concentration of ATP does not change much in the first minutes of ischemia, the *change in free energy of ATP hydrolysis* changes rapidly and in parallel with changes in contractility. It was suggested by Kammermeier as the basic mechanism of ischemic contractile failure [3].

c) *Acidosis* during ischemia, by retention of lactate, reduces muscle tension by a competition between H^+ and Ca^{2+} for binding to troponin.

d) Due to the catabolism of high energy phosphates, mainly of creatine phosphate wich catabolises within a few minutes, *anorganic phosphate accumulation* is one of the earliest features in ischemia. Pi depresses tension production very significantly although it does not depress the ATP-ase activity at the myofibrils. Pi accumulation may play a significant role in the induction of acute contractile failure under ischemic conditions.

When coronary blood flow is not restored energy supply will become the limiting factor for the preservation of cellular integrity because mitochondrial oxydative phosphorylation is shut down immediately and anaeraobic ATP production will be inhibited by feed back inhibitory processes. Because Ca^{2+}, Na^+ and H^+ in the myocyte are present below the electrochemical equilibrium an active, i.e., energy consuming process is needed to pump these ions out of the cell. Efflux of sodium is mainly energy dependent (Na^+/K^+ ATPase, while sodium influx appears via fast sodium channels (voltage dependent) or Na^+–Ca^{2+} exchange or Na^+–H^+ exchange. Calcium is pumped out also actively by a Ca^{2+} ATPase system.

Under conditions of ischemia the Na^+/K^+ ATPase pump is deficient, which results in increased myoplasmic Na^+ concentration. This will, in turn, result in cell swelling and membrane disruption. It has, however, consequences on myoplasmic Ca^{2+} concentration: the Na^+–Ca^{2+} exchanger will extrude less Ca^{2+} than before and the active Ca^{2+} pump will be deficient because it is energy dependent. Therefore cytosolic Ca^{2+} will rise also because active pumping of Ca^{2+} in the sarcoplasmic reticulum (SR–Ca^{2+} pump) is decreased due to limited ATP. Total cell calcium at this moment is relatively unchanged.

Increased cytosolic Ca^{2+}, however, is potentially dangerous because it activates phospholipases, proteases and Ca^{2+} sensitive ATPases. This results in further breakdown of the adenylate pool and membrane and organel destruction.

The severity and incidence of cellular and subcellular damage to the myocardium during acute ischemia are closely related to the duration of the ischemic interval and the temperature of the heart. During the first 10–15 minutes of normothermic ischemia, the ultrastructural alterations are quite modest: besides some intracellular edema and the loss of osmiophillic granules in the mitochondria, subcellular structure remains intact. When ischemia persists, more pronounced lesions are found in the mitochondria: clearing of the mitochondrial matrix, rupture of the cristae and the appearance of flocculent densities. Finally electron dense, calcium containing granules observed in the mitochondria as a sign of irreversible damage of the cell. This feature is accompanied by rupture of the sarcolemma, oedema; abnormal arrangement of the sarcomeres and marginal clumping of chromatin in the nucleus.

The only possible treatment of contractile failure in acute ischemia is reperfusion. In regional ischemia reperfusion can be obtained either by coronary thrombolysis or emergency coronary bypass surgery.

In a recent study we could demonstrate that emergency coronary revascularisation can be a life-saving operation, limits infarct size and restores ventricular function, provided reperfusion was performed within 4 hours of the onset of symptoms [4].

The problem with reperfusion however is that when the ischemic myocardium is reperfused before this final stage of irreversible ischemic damage occurs, myocardial contractile *function does not recover* immediately [1]. This phenomenon of postischemic myocardial dysfunction in the presence of viable myocardial tissue is called myocardial 'stunning' [1].

B. MYOCARDIAL STUNNING

The basic mechanisms reponsible for the transiently reduced postischemic contractility (up to 7 days before complete recovery) are not fully elucidated.

At first glance, a loss of nucleotide-precursors (mainly adenosine and inosine) upon reperfusion is the most plausible cause of stunning. Indeed, the de novo-synthesis of ATP takes at least 72 hours [5].

In recent experiments however we could shown that, under conditions of short periods of ischemia (up to 10 minutes) myocardial ATP is catabolized to ADP and AMP without significant accumulation of adenosine and inosine. Reperfusion resulted in a rephosphorylation of nucleotides to ATP at near normal levels. Postischemic dysfunction however remained unaltered. The remaining possible mechanisms of myocardial stunning are a defect in:

a) *Energy producing processes.* A decreased oxidative phosphorylation in the mitochondria of the postischemic myocardium.

b) *Energy transport processes.* ATP cannot diffuse freely from its site of production (mitochondria) to its site of utilization (myofibrils). Energy is transferred via the creatine phosphate shuttle from production to utilization sites via two separate isoenzyme systems, the mitochondrial creatine kinase isoenzyme and the myofibrillar creatine kinase isoenzyme. Hypothetically, the loss or inactivation of, for example, the myofibrillar bound CK isoenzyme can be responsible for stunning and can even explain the 'overshoot' of postischemic tissue levels of creatine phosphate. Experimental evidence for this kind of mechanism was given recently [6].

c) *Energy utilizing processes.* Recent studies of Schaper et al. [7] on ATP turn-over and on the relation between energy metabolism and function after repeated short periods of ischemia provided evidence that ATP utilization in reperfused myocardium is reduced in the presence of a sufficient ATP supply. Moreover, postischemic contractile dysfunction can be reversed by inotropic stimulation indicating that even in the presence of reduced tissue levels, ATP turnover can be increased. The mechanism for the reduced ATP splitting by the sarcomeres is unclear: it may reside in the sarcomeres themselves or in disturbances of the electromechanical coupling.

Ito et al. [8] reported that an intracoronary infusion of calcium increased regional contractile function in stunned myocardium and suggested a defect at the level of the exitation-contraction coupling, probably involving calcium fluxes.

In a recent experimental study we could demonstrate that in case of 'pure stunning' the energetic state of the heart is intact in terms of high energy phosphate contents and mitochondrial function.

Therefore we conclude that *myocardial stunning is rather a problem of energy utilization than of energy production.*

We reported recently on our clinical experience of surgical reperfusion during evolving myocardial infarction and its effects on left ventricular function [4]. Although it is known from previous reports that emergency aortocoronary bypass surgery for evolving myocardial infarction (EMI) can be performed with acceptable mortality rates [9–12], still some controversy exists around the results of these studies [13–14]. One of the criticisms concerns a certain bias in selection of surgically treated patients. Indeed when prognosis is considered, patients developing a myocardial infarction must be classified into uncomplicated cases or 'low risk' patients and in complicated cases or 'high risk' patients. In medically treated cases one year mortality rate differs considerably between both groups and therefore also surgically treated patients should be divided into low and high risk groups before assessing results in terms of mortality rate. Reduction of mortality rate must be of course the first option in the search of treatment of acute myocardial infarction , but a further goal has to be limitation of infarct size and improvement of left ventricular function. Only when surgical therapy will be shown to be superior to medical therapy in this respect, it should become our treatment of choice. It is however known from experimental studies and also from recent reports on coronary thrombolysis [15–16], that the time interval between the onset of symptoms i.e., coronary occlusion and reperfusion is very critical for the achievement of true benefit in terms of reduction in infarct size and recovery of functions. Therefore we report here the results of very early surgical reperfusion, i.e., between 2 and 4 hours after the onset of symptoms. We assessed recovery of regional function using equilibrium gated blood pool scintigraphy, the incidence of residual infarction using electrocardiographic follow-up and histologic examination of intraoperatively obtained biopsy specimens, and infarct size using postoperative Thallium-201 scintigraphy.

Forthy eight consecutive patients with evolving myocardial infarction underwent coronary emergency aortocoronary bypass surgery. The patients were divided into a 'low risk' group and a 'high risk' group according to the preoperative status. The 'low risk' group comprised 26 patients in a hemodynamically stable condition, the 'high risk' group consisted of 22 patients which were in cardiogenic shock defined by a systolic blood pressure below 70mmHg (n=14) or by a low cardiac output state requiring cardiac massage (n=8). Clinical preoperative data are summarized in Table 1.

A transmural left ventricular biopsy was taken from the center of the area at risk before revascularization and another biopsy was obtained from the same area after 1 hour of reperfusion. The biopsy specimen were divided into a subepicardial and subendocardial part and after immersion fixation processed for light and electron microscopy as described before [17].

Morphologic assessment of the biopsy specimens taken before reperfusion in 18 patients showed ischemic damage in 17 subepicardial samples and no damage in one. After 1 hour of reperfusion nine subepicardial samples were normal (see Figure 1), five remained ischemic, and four were necrotic. This was in clear contrast to findings in the subendocardial samples: before reperfusion 13 samples were necrotic and five were ischemic. After reperfusion

Table 1. Pre-operative data in patients undergoing emergency aortocoronary bypass grafting.

	Low risk group	High risk group
Number of patients	26	22
Age (years – mean)	55	55
Sex (male/female)	23/3	18/4
Vessel disease (%) 1	58%	32%
2	31%	23%
3	11%	45%
No previous infarction	65%	68%
Incidence anterior infarction	58%	64%
Operative mortality	0%	18%
Mean coronary occlusion time (minutes – mean range)	172(105–108)	161(–360)
Number of graft/patient (mean and range)	2.2(1–5)	2.7(1–5)

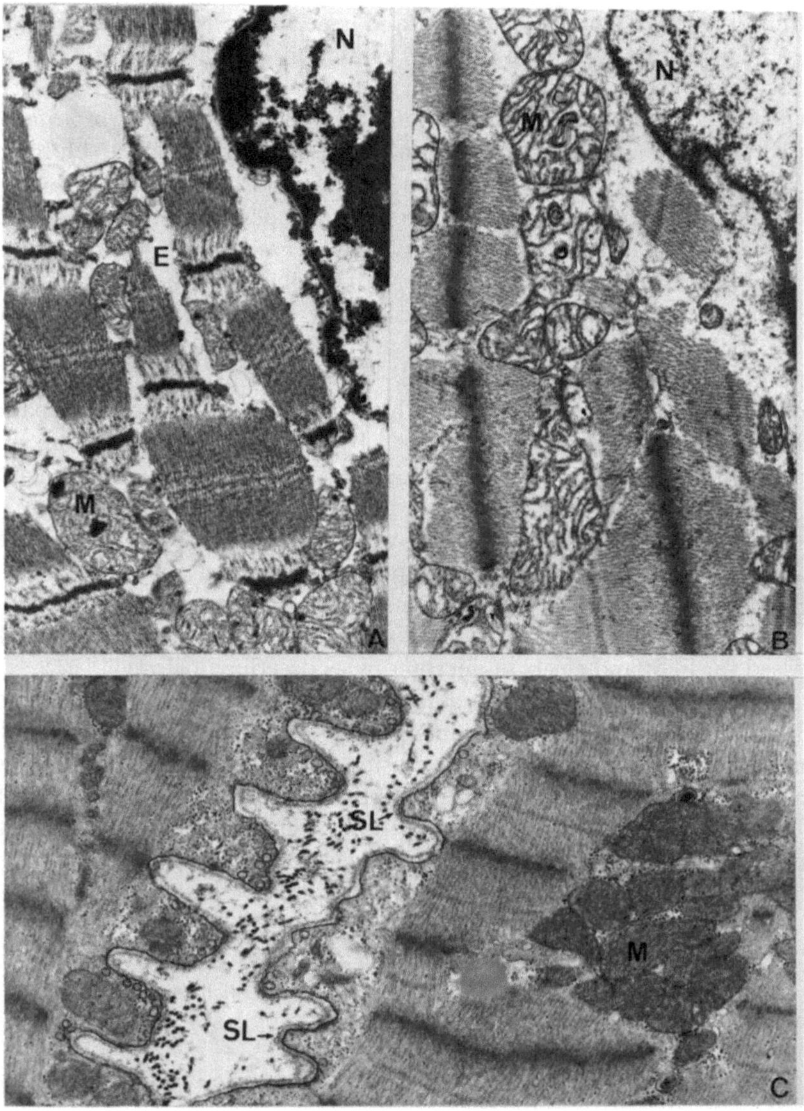

Figure 1. *Panel A*: Electron micrograph from a subendocardial biopsy specimen taken from the center of a 2-hour-old anterior wall infarction, before reperfusion. N=Nucleus, E=Edema; M=Mitochondrion. Note the signs of irreversible cell damage: clumping of the nuclear chromatin and amorphous dense bodies in the mitochondrial matrix. Magnification × 12,870.
Panel B: Electron micrograph from a subepicardial biopsy specimen taken from the same patient as presented in A. Note the slight ischemic damage to the myocytes: clearing of the mitochondrial matrix (M) without nuclear damage (N). Magnification × 12,870.
Panel C: Electron micrograph from a subepicardial biopsy specimen taken from the same area in the same patient as described in B, but after 1 hour of reperfusion . The subcellular structure is completely normal. M=Mitochondrion; SL=Sarcolemma composed of a phospholipid bilayer coated with the glycocalyx. (From Flameng et al. [4])

13 were still necrotic, three were ischemic, and two were normal.

In these 18 patients mean duration of occlusion of the infarction-related vessel was 161 minutes (range 80 to 360 minutes). In the three patients with the longest occlusion duration (210 to 360 minutes) all subendocardial samples were necrotic before and after reperfusion. Patients with subepicardial necrosis also had subendocardial necrosis.

All patients had a complete akinesia in the area of the blocked artery, also during the whole intra-operative reperfusion phase as could be observed devisu and by transesophagal echo-cardiography. This demonstrates that in spite of a completely normal structure of at least the subepicardium (see Figure 1c) myocardial stunning is observed upon reperfusion.

At 2–24 months postoperatively myocardial scintigraphy (Tl–201 at rest in 3 views) and an equilibrium gated radionuclide blood pool study in the resting state (human albumin labelled with Tc–99m) was performed in surgical patients. For comparison a prospective matched control group (n=45) of patients admitted with a first acute myocardial infarction and receiving conventional treatment was studied in the same way. The reasons why not all patients entered radionuclide follow-up were: the EMI had to be the first infarction (otherwise postoperative radionuclide abnormalities could not be related to EMI only, main stem lesions had to be excluded – valid controls

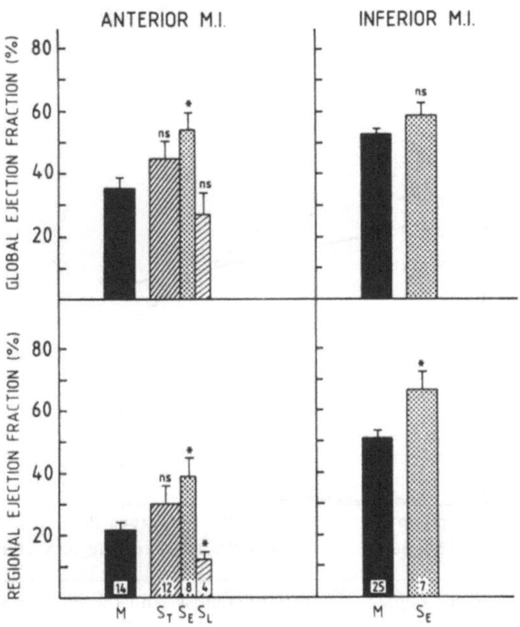

Figure 2. Left ventricular function 2 months after acute infarction in medically (M) and surgically (S) treated patients. Global and regional ejection fraction was measured by technetium 99m scintigrapghy.

are lacking) and the patients must have survived. This reduces the number of patients to 19 in the surgical group and to 39 in the control group.

The patients are divided into 2 groups according to the localisation of the infarction (anterior, inferior): the T1–201 defects after revascularization were smaller than in controls ($p \leqslant 0{,}001$). After early revascularization, i.e., within 4 hours, T1–201 defects are extremely small: 573±146. When revascularization was performed after more than 4 hours, the T1–201 defect was similar to controls: 2083±453 and larger than after early revascularization ($p \leqslant 0{,}05$). In the group with inferoposterior infarction all the surgically treated patients had early revascularization, i.e., within 4 hours. The size of the T1–201 defect was significantly smaller than in controls ($p \leqslant 0{,}05$).

Regional ejection fraction of the involved segment (anterior or inferoposterior) was higher after early revascularization than in controls ($p \leqslant 0{,}05$). Global ejection fraction in surgically treated patients was significantly higher in early revascularized anterior infarctions than in the controls ($p \leqslant 0{,}001$) (see Figure 2). These results show clearly that in the early port-reperfusion phase after acute ischemia the entire area at risk is completely stunned, even akinetic as could be seen on transesophagal echo. Late after reperfusion segmental wall motion recovered significantly, although infarction was present in all patients to a certain degree. Compared with a matched medically treated group of patients early revascularisation after acute ischemia was beneficial in terms of reduction of infarct size and recovery of contractile function.

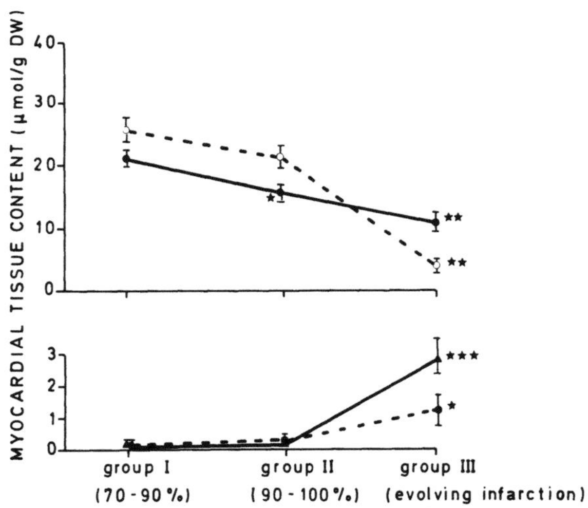

Figure 3. Relation between the degree of coronary stenosis and the high energy phosphate pool (*upper panel*) and purine catabolites (*lower panel*) in the myocardium.
Values are means ± SEM; *$p \leqslant 0.05$ versus group I; **$p \leqslant 0.01$ versus group I; ***$p \leqslant 0.001$ versus group I. Σ adenylates = sum of adenylates (adenosine tri-, di- and monophosphate); DW = dry weight. *Upper panel:* Σ adenylates (●); creatine phosphate (O); *Lower panel*: adenosine + inosine (▲); hypoxanthine + xanthine (●). (From Flameng et al. [18])

C. CHRONIC ISCHEMIA: THE HIBERNATING MYOCARDIUM

Severe, long lasting coronary artery stenosis is associated with a 30% reduction in myocardial nucleotide content and regional wall motion (see Figure 3 and Table 2) [18]. The observation that reduction in the adenylate pool parallels the reduction in local contractility does not necessarily imply that the depression of local function is caused by this reduction in adenylate pool. Indeed, the ADP/ATP ratio, the energy charge and the creatine phosphate levels are in the normal range (see Figure 4) and this is very suggestive for an intact mitochondrial function, that is, a normal energy production. Such a situation resembles well that of the 'stunned myocardium', but now induced by chronic intermittent ischemia. However, recurrent episodes of ischemia not only may induce stunning and purine loss but also may activate proteolytic systems responsible for *myofibrillar lysis*.

Myofibrillar lysis is a typical finding in myocardial cells from chronically hypo or akinetic areas. Most interesting is the finding that myocardial degeneration without fibrosis is related to chronic ischemia [19,20]. In segments with severely reduced contractile function but without significant fibrosis, that is in segments without remote infarction, cell degeneration is massive, mainly in the subendocardium (see Table 2). The most striking subcellular alteration is the *loss of contractile material* which is replaced by large amounts of glycogen, sarcoplasmic reticulum and mitochondria. In many cells only a small rim of sarcomeres arranged marginally is preserved (see Figure 5). It is clear that contractile function of these myocardial cells must be severely reduced. On the other hand, other vital cell components (nucleus, mitochondria cell membranes, etc.) although altered, remained *viable*. Therefore this phenomenon is referred to as *hibernating myocardium*.

In late postrevascularisation studies we showed that contractile function is partially restored in these segments [20] indicating that reversal of early myocytolytic changes may occur when chronic ischemia is reversed in time. A prerequisite for postrevascularization recovery of contractile function in segments showing hibernating myocardium however, is the absense of myocardial fibrosis, i.e., postinfarction scar (see Figure 6). Furthermore, posto-

Table 2. Relationship between degree of coronary artery stenosis Anterior wall motion and histology.

Stenosis	AWM (%)	% normal myocites Epi	Endo	Total	Fibrosis
70–90% (n=17)	49±9	84±14	79±18	82±14	0 of 16 (0%)
90–100% (n=27)	35±10*	59±33*	51±30*	55±30*	3 of 27 (11%)

* $p \leqslant 0.05$ or less versus 70±90% stenosis-group. None of the patients had EGG-signs of previous infarction.

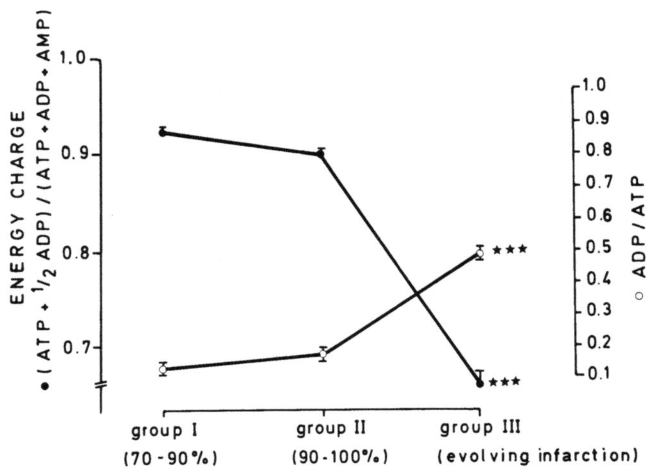

Figure 4. Relation between the degree of coronary stenosis and myocardial mitochondrial function as assessed by the ADP/ATP ratio (○) and the energy charge (●).
Values are means ± SEM. ***$p \leqslant 0.001$ versus Group I. Abbreviations as in Figure 3. (From Flameng et al. [18])

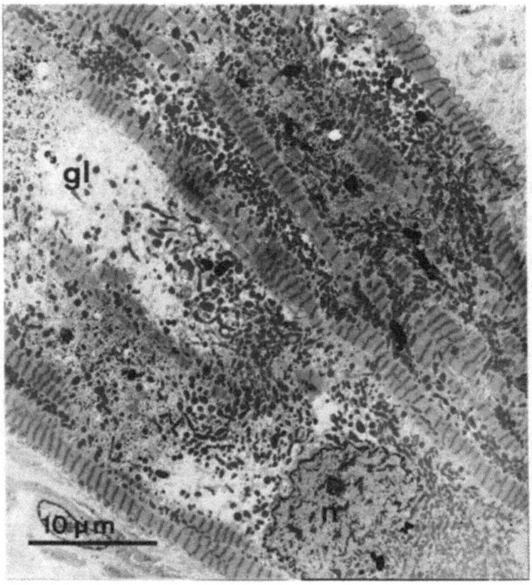

Figure 5. Electron micrograph from a subendocardial biopsy sample of a hypokinetic anterior wall in a patient from group II. This section shows a severely altered myocyte. There is considerable reduction of the myofibrillar volume fraction in the center of the myocardial cell. The sarcolemma appears intact whereas the nucleus (n) is tortuous; most mitochondria are small in size and large areas of glycogen (gl) fill up the cytosol. Magnification × 1688. (From Flameng et al. [18])

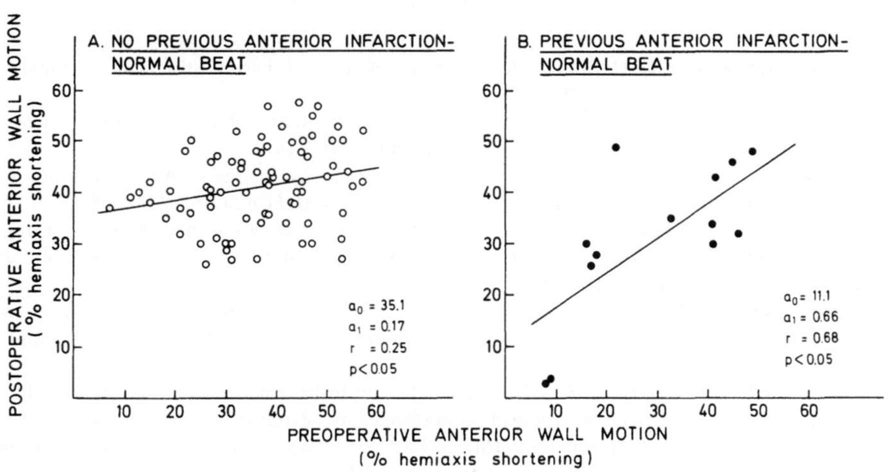

Figure 6. Relationship between pre- and post-operative anterior wall motion in patients with patent LAD-grafts several months after surgery. *Panel A*: Patients without previous anterior wall infarction. Note that preoperative anterior wall motion recovered after surgery. *Panel B*: Patients with previous anterior wall infarction. Note that preoperative anterior wall motion did not recover after succesful revascularization.

perative improvement of wall motion in the hibernating myocardium needs time because recovery of function means regeneration of contractile material within the myocytes.

It is clear that pharmacological treatment of this type of hibernating myocardium with positive inotropic agents must be disappointing, simply because the volume fraction of contractile elements is severely reduced. When heart failure occurs due to large portions of hibernating myocardium, unloading procedures may be more succesful than positive inotropic support. However, when global myocardial function is severely depressed like in end stage coronary artery disease (so called 'bad ventricles' with low ejection fraction), survival after succesful coronary bypass surgery is limited [19]. This poor outcome is related to a high incidence of myocardial cell degeneration associated with myocardial fibrosis [19].

In diffusely hypokinetic, partially fibrotic and chronically ischemic hearts, cardiac transplantation may be the best solution.

Acknowledgements
This work was supported in part by the Nationaal Fonds voor Wetenschappelijk Onderzoek, Belgium.

REFERENCES

1. Braunwald E, Kloner RA (1982) The stunned myocardium: Prolonged postischemic ventricular dysfunction. *Circulation* 60: 1146–1149
2. Braunwald E, Rutherford JD (1986) Reversible ischemic left ventricular dysfunction: Evidence for the 'hibernating myocardium'. *J Am Coll Cardiol* 8: 1467–1470
3. Kammermeier H, Schmidt P, Jungling E (1982) Free energy change of ATP-hydrolysis: A causal factor of early hypoxic failure of the myocardium? *J Mol Coll Cardiol* 14: 267–277
4. Flameng W, Sergeant P, Vanhaecke J, Suy R (1987) Emergency coronary bypass grafting for evolving myocardial infarction. Effects on infarct size and left ventricular function. *J Thorac Cardiovasc Surg* 94: 124–131
5. Hoffmeister HM, Mauser M, Schaper W (1983) Purine nucleotide 'de novo synthesis in postischemic and normal perfused canine myocardium in vivo. *J Mol Cell Cardiol* 15 (Suppl. 7): 13
6. Greenfield RA, Swain JL (1987) Disruption of myofibrillar energy use: Mechanisms that may contribute to postischemic dysfunction in stunned myocardium. *Circ Res* 60: 283–289
7. Schaper W, Buchwald A, Hoffmeister HM, Ito BR (1985) 'Stunned myocardium' is a problem of energy utilization and not of energy supply. *Circulation* 72 (Suppl. 3): 119
8. Ito BR, Tate H, Schaper W (1985) Calcium induced increases in regional contractile function before and after transient coronary occlusion in dog. *Circulation* 72 (Suppl. 3): 68
9. Favaloro RG, Effler DB, Cheanvechai C, Quint RR, SONES FM (1971) Acute coronary insufficiency (impending myocardial infarction and myocardial infarction). Surgical treatment by the saphenous vein graft technique. *Am J Cardiol* 28:598–607
10. Cohn LH, Gorlin R, Herman MV, Collins JJ (1972) Aortocoronary bypass for acute coronary occlusion. *J Thorac Cardiovasc Surg* 64:503–513
11. Dawson IT, Hell RJ, Hallman GL, Cooley DA (1974) Mortality in patients undergoing coronary artery bypass surgery after myocardial infarction. *Am J Cardiol* 33:483–486
12. De Wood AA, Spores J, Berg RJ, Kendall RW Grunwald RP, Sehringer SL, Hensley GR, Sutherland KI, Shiuelds JP (1983) Acute myocardial infarction: A decade of experience with surgical reperfusion in 701 patients. *Circulation* 68 (Suppl. 2): 118–6
13. Spencer FC (1983) Emergency coronary bypass for acute infarction: An improved clinical experiment. *Circulation* 68 (Suppl. 2): 1117–19
14. Mcintosh HD, Buccino RA (1979) Emergency coronary artery revascularization of patients with acute myocardial infarction: You can ...but should you? *Circulation* 60: 247–250
15. Spann JF, Sherry S, Carabello BA, Denenberg BS, Mann RH, Mccann WD, Ganet JH, Gentzler RD, Belber AD, Maurer AH (1984) Coronary thrombolysis by intravenous streptokinase in acute myocardial infarction: Accute and follow-up studies. *Am J Cardiol* 53:655–661
16. Cribier A, Letac B (1983) Intracoronary thrombolysis in evolving myocardial infarction. Sequential angiographic analysis of ventricular performance. *Br Heart J* 50:401–410
17. Flameng W, Van der Vusse GJ, Borgers M (1982) Methods for assessing preservation techniques: invasive methods, pp. 63–80, in: *A Textbook of Clinical Cardioplegia*, ed. by R Engelman and S. Levitsky. New York: Futura
18. Flameng W, Vanhaecke J, Van Belle H, Borgers M, De Beer L, Minten J (1987) Relation between coronary artery stenosis and myocardial purine metabolism, histology and regional function in humans. *JAC* 9: 1235–1242
19. Flameng W, Wouters L, Sergeant P, Levi P, Borgers M, Thone F, Suy R (1984) Multivariate analysis of angiographic, histologic and electrocardiographic data in patients with coronary artery disease. *Circulation* 70: 7–17
20. Flameng W, Suy R, Schwarz F, Borgers M (1981) Ultrastructural correlates of left ventricular contraction abnormalities in patients with chronic ischemic heart disease: Determinants of reversible segmentes asynergy postrevascularization surgery. *Am Heart J* 102: 846–857

8. Heart failure

Newer concepts and origin of symptoms

PHILIP A. POOLE-WILSON

INTRODUCTION

In the last 20 years there have been major advances in the diagnosis, investigation and treatment of chronic heart failure. This has resulted from a greater understanding of the pathophysiology, new techniques for clinical investigation, novel drugs, and cardiac transplantation.

The traditional treatment for heart failure has been digoxin and diuretics. With modern diuretics the elimination of oedema and the prevention of fluid overload is relatively simple. Other considerations are now of greater importance such as the role of newer drugs (vasodilators, angiotensin converting enzyme (ACE) inhibitors, β-blockers, positive inotropes), the origin of symptoms, delay in the progression of myocardial damage, repair of the myocardium after infarction and reduction of mortality.

DEFINITIONS

Heart failure can be defined as a clinical syndrome caused by an abnormality of the heart and recognised by a characteristic pattern of hemodynamic, renal, neural and hormonal responses [1]. This definition is pragmatic and practical having some application at the bedside. The diagnosis is made by doctors with ease, accuracy and consistency. The definition requires an abnormality of the heart to be present and thus excludes some of the high output states regarded by some as heart failure. The definition also emphasises that much of the clinical syndrome is the result of the body's response to heart failure and in particular the retention of sodium and water by the kidney. A shorter definition is ventricular dysfunction with symptoms. The presence of symptoms is important because otherwise left ventricular dysfunction alone could by considered as heart failure and the phrase, heart failure, would include all patients with the most trivial myocardial damage or ventricular incoordination.

The definition of heart failure has been a source of much dispute [2–4]

E. Andries & R. Stroobandt (eds.), Hemodynamics in Daily Practice, 113–127.

Table 1.

Some definitions of heart failure:

A condition in which the heart fails to discharge its contents adequately.
Thomas Lewis, *Diseases of the Heart* (1933)

A state in which the heart fails to maintain an adequate circulation for the needs of the body despite a satisfactory venous filling pressure.
Paul Wood, *Diseases of the Heart and Circulation* (1950)

A pathophysiological state in which an abnormality of cardiac function is responsible for the failure of the heart to pump blood at a rate commensurate with the requirements of the metabolising tissues.
Eugene Braunwald, *Heart Disease* (1980)

Practical definitions:

A clinical syndrome caused by an abnormality of the heart and recognised by an characteristic pattern hemodynamic, renal, neural and hormonal responses.

Ventricular dysfunction with symptoms.

Some past definitions are shown in Table 1. Most are unsatisfactory because they emphasise one or other physiological or biochemical feature of heart failure. The symptoms of heart failure occur on exercise so that definitions based on observations at rest are unsatisfactory. With modern treatment the classical physical signs of overt heart failure may be absent. The symptoms and clinical signs of treated heart failure are subtle. Emphasis should not be placed on the ventricular filling pressure since this may be normal at rest, can be altered by diuretics, varies from moment to moment and in chronic heart failure is not closely related to symptoms [5]. The phrases 'discharge its contents adequately', 'adequate circulation for the needs of the body' or 'requirements of the metabolising tissues' [4] do not have a precise meaning that can easily be tested. The limiting metabolic substrate of most tissues is oxygen and the oxygen content of blood in the femoral vein at peak exercise in heart failure is almost zero while arterial oxygen saturation is unchanged. The whole body oxygen consumption of patients with heart failure at rest or at low work loads is identical to that of normal persons and is only reduced towards the end of of exercise when anaerobic metabolism is activated. Even then the reduction is small because the ability of anaerobic metabolism to generate high energy phosphates within skeletal muscle cell is small in comparison to aerobic metabolism. Thus a definition based on 'the requirements of the metabolising tissues' needs qualification.

Many adjectives have been added to the generic term heart failure. These are high and low output cardiac failure, forward and backward failure, right and left heart failure, congestive heart failure, and acute and chronic heart failure. For practical purposes two entities only need be considered *acute heart failure*, which is a medical emergency closely allied to pulmonary oedema, and *chronic heart failure*. Chronic heart failure should be regarded as a dynamic condition since the function of the heart and the interaction of the heart and circulation vary with time. Many patients with chronic heart failure develop acute exacerbations which are not always due to extraneous causes such as lung infection; they are often precipitated by changes of rhythm. The clinical entity whereby patients spontaneously recover and relapse with chronic heart failure can be called undulating heart failure.

PROGNOSIS AND PREDICTION OF PROGNOSIS

Heart failure is a common in the community but the true prevalence and incidence are dependent on the definition of heart failure. American sources indicate a prevalence of 1% and an incidence of 0.4% [6]. A lower prevalence of 0.4% is found in London using a rather more rigid definition of heart failure based on the treatment of the patient with diuretics for heart failure. If all patients are considered then the mortality at two years is approximately 25% [7]. In patients with moderate or severe heart failure the mortality at two years is approximately 50% and 80% respectively [8, 9]. The prognosis is poor particularly for those with moderate or severe heart failure and is comparable with that in the more malignant forms of cancer. The objectives of treatment are to ameliorate intolerable symptoms, to improve the quality of life, to delay the progression of damage to the ventricular myocardium, and to reduce mortality.

The prognosis of heart failure has been claimed to be dependent upon aetiology. Several studies have demonstrated that patients with ischaemic heart disease appear to fare worse than those with dilated cardiomyopathy [10]. But this conclusion is misleading. Patients with dilated cardiomyopathy often present to the physician later in the course of their disease when there is cardiomegaly. The large heart may be the consequence of past damage and the patient can have an excellent prognosis. Others will have continuing disease due to myocarditis, hypertension, or a continuing intake of excessive alcohol. It is by no means certain that these patients are similar or comparable at the moment when they get entered into studies of the natural history to those who have ischaemic heart disease. Differences usually exist in the ejection fraction at rest and the dimensions of the left ventricle, both important determinants of prognosis.

PREDICTORS OF PROGNOSIS

Many clinical features of patients with heart failure (symptoms, heart size, hemodynamics, plasma hormones, arrhythmias) have prognostic significance. But such predictors show only that those who already have the features of heart failure have a worse prognosis than an asymptomatic person. The diagnosis of heart failure predicts death from heart failure, not a profound statement. Such predictors do not always discriminate in terms of prognosis amongst a group of patients already classified as being in severe heart failure.

Information is becoming available on comparisons between the predictive power of many variables [11–14]. The two most powerful predictors are the ejection fraction at rest and the peak oxygen consumption on exercise [11–14]. Other variables such as heart size, plasma sodium, plasma catecholamines or arrhythmias are of less significance. The resting ejection fraction reflects the extent of myocardial damage and the magnitude of the end-diastolic volume rather than ventricular function. The peak oxygen consumption is a measure of cardiac reserve. This information has important consequences for the investigation of patients, the classification of patients (particularly in clinical trials) and methods for assessment of progression of disease and treatment.

AETIOLOGY OF HEART FAILURE

Abnormalities of cardiac rhythm, valves or pericardium may cause heart failure but the commonest cause is an abnormality of the ventricular myocardium. The myocardium may be abnormal as a consequence of atheromatous coronary artery disease or cardiomyopathy. Cardiomyopathy is divided by clinical descriptors into dilated, hypertrophic and restrictive cardiomyopathies. Since hypertrophic and restrictive cardiomyopathy are relatively rare, the major division is between those patients with coronary artery disease and those with a dilated cardiomyopathy. The patient either has or has not atheroma in the coronary arteries.

This classification of heart failure is oversimplistic. Further subsetting of patients may lead to specific groups of patients who will benefit from particular treatments. An alternative approach to the description of patients is based partly on the work of Linzbach [15]. The commonest cause of heart failure is a reduction of muscle mass available to bring about contraction. This usually results from myocardial infarction. A second common cause is incoordinate contraction of the ventricle. The remaining causes of heart failure are either extracellular of cellular. In the past the presumption has been that patients with heart failure have a cellular abnormality of systolic contraction. It is possible that in many patients heart failure is due to alterations in the architecture of the heart, the shape of the ventricle, slippage of adjacent cells and embedding of cells in a network of fibrosis. There would not need to be any abnormality of the myocyte itself and several groups have failed to show a reduced response to calcium of muscle from patients undergoing cardiac transplantation. Numerous cellular abnormalities have been described including down regulation of beta-receptors [16–18], increased Gi proteins [19], modified contractile proteins, altered function of the sarcoplasmic reticulum and calcium overload. Although a reduction in contractile strength would be expected, experiments on isolated muscle have not bee able to demonstrate a reduced response to a high concentration of extracellular calcium [20,21]. The nature of any systolic abnormality of the myocardium in heart failure must be more complex. Diastolic abnormalities have been identified, notably a delay in relaxation of the myocardium [22].

RESPONSES IN BODY TO HEART FAILURE

The responses of the body to heart failure are shown in Table 2. The most important and least understood is cardiac hypertrophy. Hypertrophy can vary substantially between patients with apparently equal stimuli to hypertrophy such as high blood pressure or volume overload. Many enzymes in the heart and the contractile proteins exist in several isoforms. In general hypertrophy seems to be associated with regression to isoforms common in the neonate. The clinical consequence of these changes is as yet unresolved.

The second response is the increase of cardiac output resulting from an elevated ventricular filling pressure (Starling's Law) associated with the retention sodium and water.

The third response is stimulation of the neurohumoral system [23]. This has received much emphasis in recent years. The sympathetic system is stimulated in mild heart failure and the renin angiotensin system to a lesser degree. Plasma aldosterone, antidiuretic hormone (vasopressin), prostaglandins and atrial natriuretic peptide (ANP) are all increased in severe heart failure. Numerous new peptides (ANP, EDRF, endothelin, NPY, CGRP etc) have been identified and many of these have powerful effects on sodium and water metabolism and on the systemic vascular resistance but their role in heart failure is not yet established. The best known is atrial natriuretic peptide (ANP)

Table 2. Response to heart failure.

1. Hypertrophy of the myocardium
2. Sodium retention and increase of the ventricular filling pressure (Starling's Law)
3. Activation of the neurohumoral system
    - Sympathetic system
    - Renin-angiotensin system
    - Anti-diuretic hormone (vasopressin)
    - Atrial natiuretic peptide
    - Prostaglandins
    - Other hormones
4. Increased arteriolar resistance
    - Sodium retention in smooth muscle
    - Extramural pressure on blood vessels from tissue oedema
    - Endothelial cell swelling or dysfunction
5. Down regulation of beta receptors in the myocardium.

which is released from the atria in response to stretch and causes both natriuresis and vasodilatation. Atrial natriuretic peptide is increased in patients with heart failure and the increase is related to the magnitude of the left and right atrial pressures. Whether the increase of ANP in heart failure is merely a marker of a raised atrial pressure or an important pathological mechanism in heart failure is as yet unknown but the limited effects of ANP infusion suggest a minor role.

The sensor to activate this pattern of neurohumoral response remains unclear. In the absence of a response the blood pressure would fall. Possible sensors are the baroreceptors in the heart and aorta, and low pressure sensors in the ventricles and atria.

The hormonal changes which are described in the literature as being characteristic of heart failure have been measured in patients with treated heart failure. Since diuretics are known to stimulate the renin-angiotensin at least part of the response to heart failure is in reality a response to treatment [24]. Measurements in untreated patients [24, 25] show that in mild heart failure the renin-angiotensin system is hardly activated, if at all, whereas the sympathetic system is stimulated. This may be partly due to suppression of initial activation of the renin-angiotensin system in heart failure by expansion of the circulating volume and sodium retention. Treatment with diuretics increases the plasma renin activity but reduces the plasma noradrenaline concentration. Activation of the sympathetic system is the earliest neuroendocrine perturbation in heart failure.

The fourth response to heart failure is controversial. Even in the presence of inhibitors of many of the neuroendocrine systems the systemic vascular resistance is still elevated at rest and blood flow to skeletal muscle on exercise is markedly reduced [26]. This suggests that in these vascular beds there are additional abnormalities limiting blood flow. The nature of such abnormalities is not clear. A popular and old hypothesis is that sodium is retained within smooth muscle causing vasoconstriction [27]. An alternative cause is endothelial cell swelling or an abnormality of endothelial cell function. Until the putative abnormality is corrected the resistance to blood flow during exercise in the skeletal muscle bed remains high and exercise performance is diminished because maximal blood flow to exercising skeletal muscle is reduced. This mechanism may be the reason why most inotropic drugs, vasodilators and the angiotensin converting enzyme inhibitors do not bring about an increase in exercise capacity when given acutely, but can, particularly the angiotensin converting enzyme inhibitors, after treatment has been continued for several weeks. A principle which may be emerging is that no improvement in symptoms will occur unless the blood flow to the exercising skeletal muscle is increased [28, 29]. Since peak blood pressure is little altered by treatment, this means that the resistance in the vascular bed must be lowered.

The fifth response to heart failure is at a molecular level and affects the likely response to some therapeutic agents. Plasma catecholamines are elevated in patients with heart failure. The increase relates to the severity of heart failure. The catecholamines are reduced in the heart and there is a defect in the synthesis of noradrenaline. No simple relationship exists between the plasma catecholamines and the myocardial catecholamines [30] and the abnormality is more common in the endocardium rather than the epicardium. However the response of the heart to β-1 adrenoceptor stimulation is reduced (desensitisation). This loss of sensitivity can be because of internalisation of receptors (a rapid and reversible mechanism) or, more usually, down-regulation (a loss of the proteins making up the receptor). The abnormality may be homologous affecting only the adrenoceptors or heterologous when many different types of receptor are affected. The simple idea that down regulation is a response to elevated plasma catecholamines and is a cause of the progression of heart failure is being challenged. In some patients abnormalities of receptors may be a consequence of heart failure rather than a cause.

The responses of the body to heart failure are similar to the response to exercise, stress and haemorrhage. Harris has argued that the evolutionary origins of the response and the major factor initiating the response is the requirement to maintain a blood pressure sufficient to allow an immediate reaction to stress [32, 33].

ISCHEMIC SYNDROMES

Atheromatous disease in the coronary arteries is the commonest cause of heart failure. This is usually explained by a reduction in the mass of myocardium available for contraction or incoordinate contractility. Recently, several other syndromes have been described or at least given catchy names, 'stunned myocardium' [34], 'hibernating myocardium' [35], 'stuttering ischaemia' [36], 'mummified myocardium'. Many of these entities are rather similar to what used to be called 'chronic ischemia'. The implication is that improved perfusion of the myocardium would lead to clinical benefits. The biochemical basis for stunned, hibernating or mummified myocardium is not understood. Stunned myocardium has been attributed to damage from free radicals. Part of the reduced contractile activity may reflect myocytolysis in selected cells. The extent to which such cells can recover is unknown. The diagnosis in patients is difficult, if not impossible, to make.

SYSTOLIC AND DIASTOLIC HEART FAILURE

Diastolic heart failure is an old idea described rather elegantly over 65 years ago:

> ...the rate of relaxation of the heart... is quite as important... as the systolic contraction...
>
> If an old man's heart relaxes slowly, his capacity for physical exertion is thus limited.
>
> (Yendell Handerson, 1923)

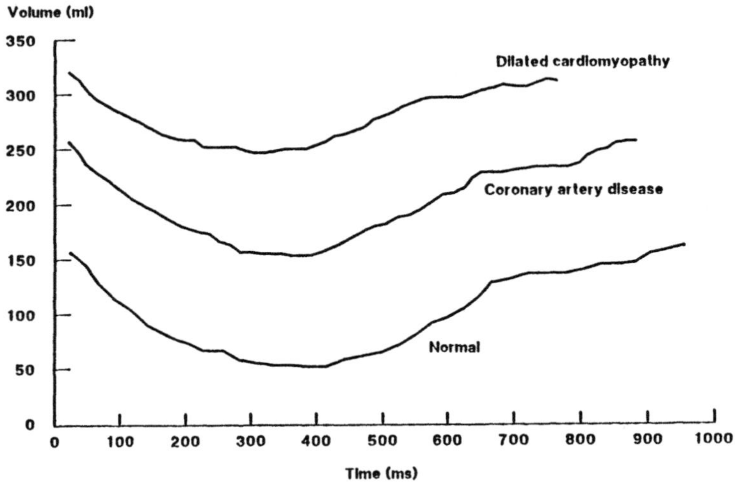

Figure 1. Ventricular volumes, based on Lavine et al. *Int. J. Cardiol.* (1985) 8: 423

Diastolic heart failure occurs particularly in the context of hypertrophied muscle in the presence of a small heart and a fast heart rate. This situation commonly exists in hypertrophic cardiomyopathy, hypertensive heart disease, following aortic valve surgery and in many patients with coronary artery disease. The abnormality is due to slow relaxation of the heart, so that at the end of diastole the left ventricular end diastolic pressure is raised and filling of the ventricle is not complete.

The events during diastole (Figure 1) are complex and diastole is comprised of periods of isovolumic relaxation, rapid filling, passive filling, and atrial contraction. Many papers have been published [38] in which diastolic heart failure is regarded as existing in those patients who have a normal ejection fraction at rest (indicating broadly that the heart size was normal) and in whom there is a reduced rapid filling of the ventricle. The latter, of course, can easily be measured using radionuclide techniques. This does not, however, identify patients with diastolic heart failure as defined above. For the clinician, the problem remains as to which patients, whether with small or enlarged hearts, truly have inadequate ventricular filling at the end of diastole. That is instant prolongation of the diastolic interval would lead to considerably greater filling of the heart. Such a situation may well exist in patients with ischemic heart disease and incoordinate contraction. But this author considers such a mechanism unlikely in patients with grossly dilated hearts. More precise techniques are needed.

The mechanism by which the cardiac output increases on exercise in heart failure varies according to the cause of the failure [39]. In dilated cardiomyopathy the end-diastolic volume changes hardly at all and the stroke volume increases because of a smaller end-systolic volume, i.e., an increase of ejection fraction. By contrast in patients with coronary artery disease the end-diastolic volume tends to increase and end-systolic volume is almost unaltered, i.e. a negligible change of ejection fraction. These volume changes are compatible with the idea that in dilated cardiomyopathy the end-diastolic volume is maximal whereas in some patients with heart failure due to ischemic heart disease the volume at end-diastole may be submaximal.

CAUSE OF SYMPTOMS

The major symptoms of patients with heart failure are shortness of breath and fatigue. With the proper use of modern diuretics shortness of breath can be minimised and the major symptom is fatigue. The origin of these symptoms remains controversial (Table 3) [5, 40, 41]. In acute heart failure shortness of breath is directly related to the left atrial pressure or the left ventricular end-diastolic pressure. Reduction of this pressure by therapeutic intervention brings immediate relief to the patient. In patients with chronic heart failure treated with diuretics the origins of breathlessness are less clear and more complex. The use of diuretics guided by clinical assessment of the patient normalises the plasma, extracellular volumes and the total body sodium [42]. Symptoms are not related to fluid overload. There is no simple correlation in this group of patients between peak oxygen consumption (a measure of exercise capacity) and estimates of left atrial pressure at peak exercise. Drugs which acutely reduce the left atrial pressure or alter hemodynamics do not increase exercise capacity in such patients. Different types of exercise test give rise to different symptoms terminating exercise despite the left atrial pressure at peak exercise being identical. Changes of blood pH, plasma potassium and other metabolic signals almost certainly are contributory factors to shortness of breath in patients with chronic heart failure in addition to changes in the lungs such as increased stiffness and particularly an increased physiological dead space.

The cause of fatigue is even more bewildering. Patients with chronic heart failure have an increased resistance to blood flow in skeletal muscle at rest

Table 3. Origin of symptoms on exercise in chronic heart failure.

1. Lungs	– increased physiological deadspace
	– raised left atrial pressure
	– increased lung stifness
	– respiratory rate
2. Circulation	– reduced blood flow to skeletal muscle
	– increase production of metabolites
3. Skeletal muscle	– rest atrophy
	– specific biochemical abnormality

and on exercise [26]. Metabolic signals may arise from the leg muscles due to stimulation of anaerobic metabolism. In addition skeletal muscle atrophies and the maximal strength of contraction is reduced. A metabolic defect in skeletal muscle has been postulated and demonstrated by magnetic resonance [43, 44]. Such abnormalities would result in the earlier onset of anaerobic metabolism in a particular muscle group for a given workload. The interpretation of the data is complicated by the fact that muscle atrophy is present so that any particular muscle may be functioning under different loading conditions compared to the same muscle in a normal person. But the metabolic abnormality is evident even when the total circulation is occluded [43]. The function and histology of skeletal muscle in patients with heart failure is also abnormal [45–47].

Some important principles are emerging. In most patients with heart failure it is not the cardiovascular system which ultimately limits exercise capacity. This has been a hotly debated topic in normals and athletes for many years [48]. In most normals and in all patients with heart failure a maximum oxygen consumption is never reached. The limiting factor is an abnormality of the muscle itself either of the energy generating system in the muscle or of the excitation-contraction sequence. In patients with chronic heart failure optimally treated with diuretics the blood pressure at peak exercise is marginally reduced. However blood flow is greatly reduced. Thus the resistance is increased. This abnormality is a consequence of the original defect of the function of the heart but is not directly related to central hemodynamics. The blood flow through a muscle on exercise is determined by the resistance in the vascular bed and not by the cardiac output because there is no great change in the blood pressure. A consequence is that an improvement of exercise capacity in patients with heart failure will not occur unless there is a reduction in the resistance (oxygen extraction is maximal) and improvement in symptoms will only result if blood flow to skeletal muscle on exercise is increased [28, 29]. Some minor improvement could result from alteration of the fibre type in the muscle but this will have only a very limited effect since the anaerobic capacity of skeletal muscle in the leg is small.

SPIRAL OF HEART FAILURE

In the 1970s treatment with vasodilators was advocated for patients with heart failure [49]. The rationale was two-fold. First, hemodynamics were altered in a manner which was considered to be beneficial (this was an unjustified assumption, see below) and second, the unloading of the left ventricle might alter the progression of heart disease within the myocardium.

The latter hypothesis has been tested in animal models where it has been demonstrated that the progression of ventricular dysfunction after myocardial infarction [50] or in response to hypertension can be altered by vasodilators. Some similar data has been obtained in man [51, 52]. The hypothesis is that in heart failure the increase in the systemic vascular resistance increase wall stress on the already damaged myocardium. This causes further damage to the heart muscle, worsening heart failure, activation of neuroendocrine systems and increase of the systemic vascular resistance. The sequence is a vicious spiral of heart failure. The clinical hope was and is that vasodilators in patients might delay the progression of heart disease. The extent to which the theory can be applied to man is uncertain. The progression of heart disease in patients with coronary artery disease is probably dominated by the natural history of atheroma in the coronary arteries and subsequent ischaemic events. In some patients with cardiomyopathy the prognosis is related to the continuing presence of the causal factor, for example alcohol.

The spiral of heart failure could be explained not by an effect on wall stress in the heart but by the continuing retention of salt and water due to acivation of the neurohumoral response. If this were so, an explanation emerges for the apparent greater longterm benefit of ACE inhibitors compared to vasodilators. ACE inhibitors are known to affect sodium balance in the kidney and provided the blood pressure does not fall cause a transient loss of salt and water.

The anticipated benefit to patients from altered hemodynamics as a consequence of vasodilator drugs has not been confirmed in controlled trials [53]. The reason is twofold. First the assumption that left ventricular filling pressure was a major determinant of the symptom of shortness of breath has been shown to be erroneous. Second the increase of cardiac output observed at rest results in more blood being directed to previously constricted tissue beds such as the skin and splanchnic circulations but does not result in any substantial increase of skeletal muscle perfusion on exercise.

EXERCISE TESTING

In recent years the exercise test has been widely used as a means of assessing the patient with heart failure. Exercise capacity confirms the severity of disability suspected from the clinical history, categorises the severity of heart failure, predicts the prognosis and is useful in the subsequent assessment of therapy. The purpose of the exercise test in patients with heart failure is different to that when exercising patients with overt or suspected coronary artery disease in order to ascertain the presence or severity of coronary artery disease.

Many uncertainties still exist with regard to exercise testing in heart failure including the most appropriate type of test (treadmill, erect or supine bicycle), the nature of the exercise protocol (fast or slow test, ramp or step increases in workload, fixed workload or patient selected workload), reproducibility and sensitivity. A placebo effect of repeat exercise testing has been described but of more significance is the increased confidence of both patient and doctor as familiarity with the test increases. Exercise time is not, contrary to often stated opinion, an objective measurement and is influenced strongly by the doctor/patient relationship and by other factors such as anxiety and, in tests of long duration, boredom.

Sophisticated techniques exist for recording gas exchange during exercise. The measurement of peak oxygen consumption was introduced as an objective test for heart failure [54]. That it is not. If patients can be persuaded to exercise further after they believe that they have achieved their maximum exercise capacity, oxygen consumption is increased. Patients with heart failure never achieve a plateau in their oxygen consumption and even athletes rarely do so [48]. Nevertheless the measurement of oxygen consumption is useful in that if changes of exercise time and peak oxygen consumption between two tests performed on different occasions are not similar then it is probable that one or both of the exercise tests has been influenced by factors other than heart failure and possibly by anxiety and the use of additional muscle groups during exercise to hold onto the frame of the exercise machine. Peak oxygen consumption is influenced by the muscle mass being used during exercise. Furthermore if a patient fails to reach a respiratory quotient of one during an exercise test for heart failure it is unlikely that the cardiovascular system is the limiting factor for that patient.

In an attempt to circumvent these problems the concept of 'anaerobic threshold' [55] has been applied to measurements of oxygen consumption and carbon dioxide production as an objective indicator of exercise performance in patients with heart failure. This concept is flawed since skeletal muscle contains mixed fibres with different metabolic pathways and anaerobic metabolism is not initiated in all muscle types at the same moment or to the same extent during exercise. The relationship between oxygen consumption and carbon dioxide production is curvilinear and not comprised of two straight lines. The relationship is affected by hyperventilation.

Newer techniques are being developed which may allow a more objective assessment of patients during heart failure from measurements of gas exchange during exercise [56].

The measurement of maximal exercise capacity is assumed to be an accurate indicator of the capacity of patients to lead a normal life; that may be an erroneous assumption. Other tests such as the six-minute walking test [57] and adaptations of that test [58] have been suggested as having a greater sensitivity for the effect of treatment in certain patients with heart failure. These tests measure the distance walked in a given time, the patient being allowed to choose the speed of walking. The tests may more accurately reflect the symptoms and limitations of patients with heart failure in everyday life.

REFERENCES

1. Poole-Wilson PA (1985) Heart failure. *Medicine International* 2: 866–871
2. Lewis T (1933) *Diseases of the Heart*. London/New York: MacMillan
3. Wood P (1950) *Diseases of the Heart and Circulation*. London: Eyre and Spoltiswoode

4. Braunwald E (1980) *Heart Disease. A Textbook of Cardiovascular Medicine*. Philadelphia/London/Toronto: WB Saunders
5. Lipkin DP, Poole-Wilson PA (1986) Symptoms limiting exercise in chronic heart failure. *Br Med J* 292: 1030–1031
6. McFate Smith W (1985) Epidemiology of congestive heart failure. *Am J Cardiol* 55: A3–8
7. Kannel WB, Plehn JF, Cupples LA (1988) Cardiac failure and sudden death in the Framingham study. *Am Heart J* 115: 869–875
8. Franciosa JA (1986) Epidemiologic patterns, clinical evaluation, and long-term prognosis in chronic congestive heart failure. *Am J Med* 80 (Suppl 2B): 14–21
9. The CONSENSUS Trial Study Group (1987) Effects of enalapril on mortality in severe congestive heart failure. Results of the Cooperative North Scandinavian Enalapril Survival Study (CONSENSUS). *N Engl J Med* 316: 1429–1435
10. Franciosa JA, Willen M, Ziesche S, Cohn JN (1983) Survival in men with severe chronic left ventricular failure due to either coronary heart disease or idiopathic dilated cardiomyopathy. *Am J Cardiol* 51: 831–836
11. Cohn JN, Archibald DG, Francis GS, Ziesche S, Franciosa JA, Harston WE, Tristani FE, Dunkman WB, Jacobs W, Flohr KH, Goldman S, Cobb FR, Shah PM, Saunders R, Fletcher RD, Loeb HS, Hughes VC. BakerB (1987) Veterans Administration Cooperative study on vasodilator therapy of heart failure: Influence of prerandomisation variables on the reduction of mortality by treatment with hydralazine and isosorbide dinitrate. *Circulation* 75 (Suppl 4): 49–54
12. Likoff MJ, Chandler SL, Kay HR (1987) Clinical determinants of mortality in chronic congestive heart failure secondary to idiopathic dilated or to ischaemic cardiomyopathy. *Am J Cardiol* 59: 634–638
13. Szlachic J, Massie BM, Kramer BL, Topic N, Tubau J (1985) Correlates and prognostic implication of exercise capacity in chronic congestive heart failure. *Am J Cardiol* 55: 1037–1042
14. Franciosa JA (1987) Why patients with heart failure die: Hemodynamic and functional determinants of survival. *Circulation* 75 (Suppl 4): 20–27
15. Linzbach AJ Heart failure from the point of view of quantitative anatomy. *Am J Cardiol* 5: 370–380
16. Bristow MR, Ginsburg R, Minobe W, Cubicciotti RS, Sageman S, Lurie K, Billingham ME, Harrison DC, Stinson EB (1982) Decreased catecholamine sensitivity and B-adrenergic-receptor density in failing human hearts. *N Engl J Med* 307: 205–211
17. Brown L, Lorenz B, Erdmann E (1986) Reduced positive inotropic effects in diseased human ventricular myocardium. *Cardiov Res* 20: 516–520
18. Brodde O-E, Schuler S, Kretsch R, Brinkman M, Borst HG, Hetzer R, Reidemeister JC, Warnecke H, Zerkowski H-R (1986) Regional distribution of B-adrenoceptors in the human heart: Coexistence of functional B1- and B2- adrenoceptors in both atria and ventricles in severe congestive cardiomyopathy. *J Cardiov Pharmacol* 8: 1235–1242
19. Neumann J, Scholz H, Doring V, et al. (1988) Increase in myocardial G(i)-proteins in heart failure. *Lancet* 1988/2: 936–937
20. Gwathmey JK, Copelas L, MacKinnon R, Schoen FJ, Feldman MD, Grossman W, Morgan JP (1987) Abnormal intracellular calcium handling in myocardium from patients with end-stage heart failure. *Circ Res* 61: 70–76
21. Ginsburg R, Bristow MR, Billingham ME, Stinson EB, Schroeder JS, Harrison DC (1983) Study of the normal and failing isolated human heart: Decreased response of failing heart to isoproterenol. *Am Heart J* 106: 535–540
22. Feldman MD, Copelas L, Gwathmey JK, Phillips P, Warren SE, Schoen FJ, Grossman W, Morgan JP (1987) Deficient production of cyclic AMP: Pharmacologic evidence of an important cause of contractile dysfunction in patients with end-stage heart failure. *Circulation* 75: 331–339
23. Francis GS (1985) Neurohumoral mechanisms involved in congestive heart failure. *Am J Cardiol* 55: A15–21

24. Bayliss J, Norell M, Canepa-Anson R, Sutton G, Poole-Wilson P (1987) Untreated heart failure: Clinical and neuroendocrine effects of introducing diuretic. *Br Heart J* 57: 17–22
25. Anand IS, Ferrari R, Kalra GS, Wahi PL, Poole-Wilson PA, Harris P (1988) Edema of cardiac origin: Studies of body water and sodium, renal function, hemodynamics and plasma hormones in untreated congestive heart failure. *Circulation*, in press
26. LeJemtel TH, Maskin CS, Lucido D, Chadwick BJ (1986) Failure to augment limb blood flow in response to one-leg versus two-leg exercise in patients with severe heart failure. *Circulation* 74: 245–251
27. Zelis R, Delea CS, Coleman H, Mason DT (1970) Arterial sodium content in experimental congestive heart failure. *Circulation* 41: 213–216
28. Mancini DM, Davis L, Wexler JP, Chadwick B, LeJemtel TH (1987) Dependence of enhanced maximal exercise performance on increased peak skeletal muscle perfusion during long-term captopril therapy. *JACC* 10: 845–850
29. Drexler H, Banhardt U, Meinertz T, Wollschlager H, Lehmann M, Just H (1989) Contrasting peripheral short-term and long-term effects of converting enzyme inhibition in patients with congestive heart failure. *Circulation* 79: 491–502
30. Pierpont GL, Francis GS, DeMaster EG, Olivari MT, Ring WT, Goldenberg IF, Reynolds S, Cohn JN (1987) Heterogeneous myocardial catechiolamine concentrations in patients with congestive heart failure. *Am J Cardiol* 60: 316–321
31. Murphree SS, Saffitz JE (1989) Distribution of B-adrenergic receptorsin failing human myocardium. *Circulation* 79: 1214–1225
32. Harris P (1987) Congestive cardiac failure: Central role of the arterial blood pressure. *Br Heart J* 58: 190–203
33. Harris P (1988) Role of arterial pressure in the oedema of heart failure. *Lancet* 1988/1: 1036–1038
34. Braunwald E, Kloner RA (1982) The stunned myocardium: prolonged, postischemic ventricular dysfunction. *Circulation* 66: 1146–1149
35. Rahimtoola SH (1985) A perspective on the three large multicenter randomised clinical trials of coronary bypass surgery for chronic stable angina. *Circulation* 72 (Suppl 5): 123–135
36. Pole-Wilson PA (1983) Angina - pathological mechanisms, clinical expression and treatment. *Postgrad Med J* 59 (Suppl 3): 11–21
37. Henderson Y (1923) Volume changes of the heart. *Phys Rev* 3: 165–208
38. Soufer R, Wohlgelernter D, Vita NA, Amuchestegui M, Sostman D, Berger HJ, Zaret BL (1985) Intact systolic left ventricular function in clinical congestive heart failure. *Am J Cardiol* 55: 1032–1036
39. Shen WF, Roubin GS, Hirasaw K, Choong C Y–P, Hutton BF, Harris PJ, Fletcher PJ, Kelly DT (1985) Left ventricular volume and ejection fraction response to exercise in chronic congestive heart failure: Difference between dilated cardiomyopathy and previous myocardial infarction. *Am J Cardiol* 55: 1027–1031
40. Poole-Wilson PA (1988) The origin of symptoms in patients with chronic heart failure. *Eur Heart J* 9 (Suppl H): 49–53
41. Poole-Wilson PA, Buller NP (1988) Cause of symptoms in chronic congestive heart failure and implications for treatment. *Am J Cardiol* 62: A31–34
42. Anand IS, Veall N, Kalra GS, Ferrari R, Sutton G, Harris P, Poole-Wilson PA (1989) Treatment of heart failure with diuretics: body compartments, renal function and plasma hormones. *Eur Heart J* 10: 445–450
43. Massie BM, Conway M, Rajagopalan B, Yonge R, Frostick S, Ledingham J, Sleight P, Radda G (1988) Skeletal muscle metabolism during exercise under ischaemic conditions in congestive heart failure. Evidence for abnormalities unrelated to blood flow. *Circulation* 78: 320–326
44. Wiener DH, Fink LI, Maris J, Jones RA, Chance B, Wilson JR (1986) Abnormal skeletal muscle bioenergetics during exercise in patients with heart failure: Role of reduced muscle blood flow. *Circulation* 73: 1127–1136
45. Buller NP, Jones D, Poole-Wilson PA (1987) Evidence for an intrinsic defect of skeletal metabolism in patients with chronic heart failure. *Clin Sci* 72 (Suppl 16): 60P

46. Lipkin DP, Jones DA, Round JM, Poole-Wilson PA (1988) Abnormalities of skeletal muscle in patients with chronic heart failure. *Int J Cardiol* 18: 187–195
47. Poole-Wilson PA, Buller NP, Lipkin DP (1988) Regional blood flow, muscle strength and skeletal muscle histology in severe congestive heart failure. *Am J Cardiol* 62: E49–52
48. Noakes T (1988) Implications of exercise testing for prediction of athletic performance: a contemporary perspective. *Med Sci Sports Exerc* 20: 319–330
49. Braunwald E, Colucci WS (1984) Vasodilator therapy of heart failure. Has the promissory note been paid? *New Engl J Med* 310 (7): 459–461
50. Pfeffer J, Pfeffer MA, Braunwald E (1985) Influence of chronic captopril therapy on the infarcted left ventricle of the rat. *Circ Res* 57: 84–95
51. Pfeffer MA, Lamas GA, Vaughan DE, Parisi AF, Braunwald E (1988) Effect of captopril on progressive ventricular dilatation after anterior myocardial infarction. *N Engl J Med* 319: 80–86
52. Sharpe N, Murphy J, Smith H, Hannan S (1988) Treatment of patients with symptomless left ventricular dysfunction after myocardial infarction. *Lancet* 1988/1: 255–259
53. Lipkin DP, Poole-Wilson PA (1985) Treatment of chronic heart failure: a review of recent trials. *Br Med J* 291: 993–996
54. Weber KT, Janicke JS (1985) Cardiopulmonary exercise testing for evaluation of chronic heart failure. *Am J Cardiol* 55: 22A–31A
55. Wasserman K, McIlroy MB (1964) Detecting the threshold of anaerobic metabolism in cardiac patients during exercise. *Am J Cardiol* 14: 844–852
56. Buller NB, Poole-Wilson PA (1988) 'Extrapolated maximum oxygen consumption': A new method for the objective analysis of respiratory gas exchange during exercise. *Br Heart J* 59: 212–217
57. Lipkin DP, Scriven AJ, Crake T, Poole-Wilson PA (1968) Six minute walking test for assessing exercise capacity in chronic heart failure. *Br Med J* 292: 653–655
58. Parameshwar J, Dambrink J-HE, Sparrow J. Wright C, Park A, Tweed J, Poole-Wilson PA (1989) A new exercise test for the assessment of heart failure: Use of a self powered treadmill. *Br Heart J* 61: 421–425

9. Guidelines for the evaluation of treatment in congestive heart failure

WOLFGANG KÜBLER*

Treatment of congestive heart failure is based on two aims: (1) *Reduction in mortality.* This can only be proven in rather large randomized trials, such as the CONSENSUS-trial, and (2) *Improvement of symptoms and signs of congestive heart failure.* This effect has be be evaluated in the individual patient.

Up to the seventies treatment of congestive heart failure was mainly based on the restriction of physical activity and of sodium intake, and on the application of diuretics and/or digitalis. The acute efficacy of diuretic treatment was easily evaluated by the increase in urine volume, the loss in body weight, disappearance of lung congestion, and of peripheral edema. Although digitalis glycosides have now been in use for the treatment of heart failure for more than 200 years, their therapeutic efficacy is still not yet established apart from atrial fibrillation.

There might be two reasons for discussing the evaluation of treatment in congestive heart failure:

1. *Methodological problems.* A large number of invasive and non-invasive methods for the evaluation of left and/or right ventricular function are now available. Mention of all these methods and discussion or their relative pros and cons is neither very interesting nor very informative. Left ventricular function before and after treatment can be adequately assessed by using a Swan-Ganz-catheter and by monitoring cardiac index and pulmonary artery pressure (PA-pressure) as an index of left ventricular filling pressure.
2. *Biological problems.* By introducing a new therapeutic approach, i.e., afterload reduction by vasodilators not only new biological and pharmacological problems were encountered, but also new insights into the pathophysiology of heart failure were gained.

* Own investigations were supported by a grant from the Deutsche Forschungsgemeinschaft within the SFB 320 *Herzfunktion und ihre Regulation*, University of Heidelberg, Germany.

E. Andries & R. Stroobandt (eds.), Hemodynamics in Daily Practice, 129–135.

The effect of a vasodilator may be attenuated by several mechanisms:

1. *Unsufficient reabsorption*, e.g., in right heart failure with congestions of the bowels.
2. *Tolerance*, i.e., diminishing efficacy during long term treatment. This has been reported for many vasodilators, such as e.g. nitrates, prazosin, hydralazine, etc...
3. *Non optimal choice of the drug*. A pure arterial vasodilator induces only a minimal increase in cardiac index in the normal or in the patient with heart failure and normal left ventricular enddiastolic pressure (LVEDP). In patients with elevated LVEDP, however, cardiac output is markedly increased. In contrast, a pure venous dilator may improve congestive symptoms by reducing elevated PA-pressure, but has little effect on cardiac output. In patients with normal LVEDP – e.g. following diuretic therapy – a pure venous dilator may even reduce cardiac output. Hence the effects of vasodilator therapy depend likewise on its preferential side of action, i.e. arterial or venous side, as well as on LVEDP.
4. *Counterregulation* to vasodilatation by activating pressure systems, such as the sympathetic system, the renin-angio tensin-system, and the vasopressin-system. Activation of any of these pressure systems may reduce stroke volume due to an increase in afterload.

The contribution of the different pressure systems to counter-regulation in vasodilator therapy may best be evaluated in patients treated with hydralazine, as this substance is a rather pure vasodilator. In the responders group – characterized by an unchanged or even reduced heart rate after treatment – plasma noradrenaline (NA) levels are significantly reduced after hydralazine, whereas in the non-responders – with an increase in heart rate after treatment – the NA levels are augmented. The reduction of plasma NA after hydralazine is related to the NA levels before the treatment, i.e., the higher the pre-treatment NA levels, the greater the reduction after treatment. In contrast to NA plasma renin activity is not significantly changed in responders but increased in non-responders, probably due to the increased sympathetic tone. Vasopressin showed only a marked increase in those patients with a decrease in mean blood pressure of at least 15 mmHg after treatment. In these patients the fall in blood pressure and the reduction in sympathetic tone may lead to an activation of the vasopressin system: the more pronounced the fall in blood pressure, the higher the vasopressin levels.

From these data it follows that it is mainly the activity of the sympathoneuronal system which allows to distinguish responders from non-responders after treatment. The renin-angiotensin system may even exhibit an activation in the responders.

The activity of the sympathoneuronal system can either be evaluated by determination of plasma-NA-levels, or more easily and less expensive by evaluation of the changes in heart rate, which are closely related to plasma-NA-levels, especially in patients with sinus rhythm.

Non-responders to acute hydralazine therapy remain non responders even after chronic treatment for 4 weeks with a marked rise in heart rate and plasma-NA-levels, and only a small increase in stroke index.

Non-responders to acute hydralazine, however, whose treatment was changed to captopril turned to become responders, as indicated by a reduction in heart rate and in plasma-NA-levels and a marked increase in stroke index. Hence, patients who are non-responders to one vasodilator, e.g. hydralazine, cannot be expected to become responders due to chronic treatment. Non-responders to one vasodilator, e.g. hydralazine, however, may well respond to another, e.g. an ACE, inhibitor.

Serious ventricular tachyarrhythmias are not only related to sudden death, but may also further deteriorate LV-function. In patients with coronary artery disease or aortic valve disease, the number of ventricular PB's is significantly increased at an EF $\leqslant$ 40%. In patients with dilative cardiomyopathy a high number of ventricular PB's is present in those with an EF $\geqslant$ 40% or $\leqslant$ 40%.

Also the Lown-classification increases with more severe impairment of LV-function. The incidence of Lown IVb, i.e., short runs of ventricular ectopy, is significantly increased in patients with an EF $\leqslant$ 40%. Hence, mainly in the patients with severely impaired LV-function potentially life-threatening ventricular tachyarrhythmias occur. They should be evaluated on a quantitative basis by Holter monitoring before antiarrhythmic treatment may be considered.

The evaluation of the efficacy of treatment can be based on the clinical assessment, on the results of non-invasive and invasive techniques, and on laboratory tests. The main indicators for a favourable result are:

- Improvement of the NYHA classification,
- Reduction in sympathetic tone, either evaluated by a reduction in heart rate and/or by determination of plasma-NA-levels,
- Reduction in lung congestion, either seen on the chest X-ray or determined with a Swan-Ganz catheter,
- Improvement of LV-function either evaluated non-invasively by 2–D echocardiography or more expensively by radio-isotope cardiography or invasively with a Swan-Ganz catheter.
- Reduction in the number and in the classification of ventricular ectopics as shown by Holter monitoring.

Figure 1 offers a proposal how one might proceed in an individual patient: If clinical assessment and non-invasive techniques clearly indicate a favourable result and Holter monitoring yields no severe ventricular tachyarrhythmias, i.e., no Lown IVb, the patient may be discharged. He should, however, reevaluated after some months, as late tolerance e.g. may occur.

If clinical assessment and non-invasive tests yield questionable or even negative results, one may proceed to invasive techniques, i.e., the Swan-Ganz catheter. In addition evaluation of plasma NA levels may be considered as heart rate may be misleading, e.g. due to sinus node dysfunction. After gaining positive results of these tests and of Holter monitoring, the patient may likewise be discharged.

If the results, however, are still negative, heart failure refractory to medical

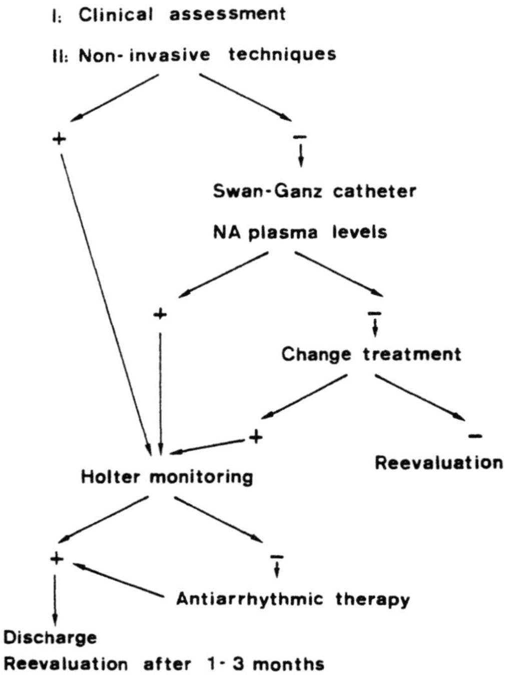

Figure 1. Congestive heart failure: Evaluation of efficacy of treatment.

treatment can only be accepted when all possible errors in diagnosis and/or in appropriate treatment can be excluded.

The possible causes include:

A. *Diagnostic problems*
   1. Unknown cause of heart failure.
   2. Unrecognized concomitant cardiac diseases.
   3. Unrecognized complications of heart failure.
   4. Wrong diagnosis.

B. *Therapeutic problems*
   5. Unsufficient drug treatment.
   6. Side-effects of the drugs.
   7. Unsufficient efficacy of the drugs used.

Ad 1. Unknown cause of heart failure. The diagnosis of heart failure is ultimately based on a combination of certain symptoms and signs. The etiology of the disorder remains often obscure. In heart failure the usual symptoms and signs can be disguised, clinical diagnosis may then become more difficult. In coronary artery disease large ischemic areas may rather induce the symptom of dyspnea instead of angina. This applies mainly to patients with left stem stenosis and/ or severe 3-vessel-disease. In younger patients heart failure may be due to coronary anomalies, such as, e.g., the Bland-White-Garland syndrome. In congestive heart failure signs of valvular diseases may be attenuated due to diminished cardiac output: In aortic stenosis the systolic ejection murmur will become lower and the systolic thrill in the 2nd intercostal space in the jugulum or over the carotid arteries will disappear. In congestive heart failure with mitral stenosis its diastolic murmur may be likewise rather low. Acute severe aortic incompetence may impose special problems, as the diastolic murmur may be rather short, and the typical signs in the ECG and in the chest X-ray may be missing.

Ad 2. Unrecognized concomitant cardiac diseases. If heart failure persists despite adequate treatment, a concomitant cardiac disease has to be considered as listed in Table 1.

Table 1. *Concomitant cardiac diseases causing refractory heart failure.*

Arterial hypertension	
Hyperthyroidism	
Additional	cardiac disease, e.g.
	- carditis
	- pericardial effusion
	- additional congenital or acquired heart disease, cardiomyopathy, or coronary artery disease

Ad 3. Unrecognized complications of heart failure. A further cause of heart failure refractory to conventional therapy is the occurrence of complications, mainly due to pulmonary embolism. Although they are found at post mortem in more than 50% of the deceased patients, the correct diagnosis was made intra vitam in less than 30% of the patients. Hence, anticoagulants may be given to patients with heart failure on a rather large scale. Furthermore, any otherwise unexplained deterioration in a patient with heart failure may be suspect of pulmonary embolism.

Ad 4. Wrong diagnosis. Heart failure refractory to treatment may also be based on a wrong diagnosis – its main causes are listed in Table 2. If heart failure

Table 2. *Refractory heart failure wrong diagnosis.*

'Fluid lung' in renal failure	
Nephrotic syndrome	
Ankle edema, e.g.	
	- deep vein thrombosis
	- peripheral lymphedema
	- hormonal disorders
	- mediastinal tumors

stays refractory to treatment despite all diagnostic efforts the efficacy of the drug regime has to be reevaluated.

Ad 5. Unsufficient drug treatment. The main cause for inefficiency of drug treatment in heart failure may be either unreliable drug intake by the patient, wrong dosage or inappropriate choice of drugs. In our country unreliable drug intake by the patient has been reported in 35% under clinical conditions and in 65% in outpatients.

As may be shown e.g. for digitalis glycosides a too low dosage may be ineffective, whereas a too high dosage may even aggravate the symptoms and signs of heart failure. In clinical practice the determination of the plasma digitalis levels may not be very rewarding. The effects of digitalis are probably related to its binding on specific receptors, probably the Na^+–K^+-ATPase. This binding, however, is modulated by drugs, such as e.g. diphenylhydantoine, or ions, such as e.g. K^+. Furthermore during longterm treatment with digitalis the number of the receptors may increase with the theoretical consequence of reduced efficiency of the treatment.

Failure of treatment can also be due to an inappropriate choice of the drug. The so-called potassium-sparing diuretics induce only a rather weak diuresis, thiazides are not effective in renal failure. Heart failure refractory to treatment can therefore only be accepted if loop diuretics, such as furesomide, are likewise ineffective even in higher dosage.

If the leading symptom is not due to backward failure inform of pulmonary congestion but rather forward failure as e.g. in severe aortic stenosis, diuretics may only be given with great caution, as the reduction in preload may induce further reduction in cardiac output. Immediate prosthetic replacement of the aortic valve may be the treatment of choice under these conditions.

Ad 6. Side-effects of the drugs. Due to unwanted side effects the drugs applied may even aggravate heart failure. Digitalis glycosides even in the therapeutic range may induce ventricular tachyarrhythmias which may further impede LV-function.

Whereas bradyarrhythmias may well be controlled in heart failure by implantation of a pacemaker (if possible of the DDD-type), the treatment of ventricular tachyarrhythmias is still an unsolved problem. Most of the antiarrhythmic drugs are more or less negative inotropic, they may even induce life threatening ventricular tachyarrhythmias due to a proarrhythmic effect, which occurs in about 10–20% of cases. It has in addition to be taken into account that depressed LV-function is an independent risk factor for sudden death. Prognosis in these patients may be improved either by individual 'optimizing' antiarrhythmic treatment by programmed electrical stimulation and/or by Holter monitoring, or by implantation of a defibrillator.

Ad 7. Unsufficient efficacy of the drugs used. Despite adequate dosage the drugs used may be at least partially ineffective. The diuretics act mainly via secretion of Na^+, so that in heart failure with low plasma sodium their effect is greatly attenuated. Plasma sodium may be reduced due to intake of free water, increased secretion of ADH, transmineralisation with increase in the intracellular and decrease of the extracellular sodium concentration, and lastly due to the excessive use of diuretics. In these cases: fluid restriction, application of sodium and/or glucose-insuline-potassium-infusions may be of benefit.

The vasodilators may be ineffective due to malabsorption, tolerance, and counter regulation by pressure systems as already discussed.

The effect of positive inotropic drugs may be attenuated due to the increased sympathoneuronal and sympathoadrenal activity, which by itself exerts a marked increase in contractility.

Conclusions

Heart failure can be considered as the endstage of many cardiac diseases. The main therapeutic goal is therefore its prevention. Whenever possible cardiac surgery should be advised before heart failure has developed, which not only increases perioperative mortality, but also affects longterm prognosis. Furthermore all diseases predisposing to heart failure, such as e.g. arterial hypertension or hyperthyroidism should be adequately controlled in order to avoid the terminal stage of many heart diseases.

REFERENCES

1. Kübler W, Hennig E, Manthey J, Mäurer W, Mehmel HC, Schuler G (1982) Die sogenannte 'therapierefraktäre' Herzinsuffizienz, pp. 39–48, in: Kommerell B, Hahn P, Kübler W, Mörl H, and Weber E. (eds.), *Fortschritte in der Inneren Medizin*. Berlin/Heidelberg/New York: Springer
2. Kübler W, Manthey J, Osterziel KJ (1988) Personal view Congestive Heart Failure: how to evaluate efficacy of treatment. *Eur Heart J* 9: 602–609

10. Management of patients with hypertrophic cardiomyopathy

ROBERT O. BONOW, BARRY J. MARON, MARTIN B. LEON, RICHARD O. CANNON III & STEPHEN E. EPSTEIN

Patients with hypertrophic cardiomyopathy (HCM) commonly manifest a spectrum of abnormalities of left ventricular morphology and function, including a variety of patterns of myocardial hypertrophy, impaired early diastolic relaxation and filling [1–7], reduced end diastolic volume [8, 9], elevated end diastolic pressure [1, 8, 10], reduced coronary vasodilator reserve [11–13], hyperdynamic systolic function [8, 14] and, in some patients, subaortic obstruction [8, 14–18]. The complex interaction of these alterations in left ventricular anatomy and function may result in myocardial ischemia, elevated left ventricular filling pressures, and reduced stroke volume, thereby producing the clinical manifestations of angina, dyspnea, fatigue, and syncope. In addition, both supraventricular and ventricular arrhythmias occur not uncommonly in patients with HCM [19–21]. Succesful medical or surgical treatment of this disease must ameliorate the underlying pathophysiological mechanism or mechanisms operative in each patient [22, 23]. Hence, the management of patients with HCM must be based on an understanding of these disease processes.

1. PATHOPHYSIOLOGY OF HYPERTROPHIC CARDIOMPATHY

1.1 Left ventricular diastolic function

Altered diastolic function of the hypertrophied left ventricle is a common characteristic of patients with HCM and may contribute importantly to its clinical manifestations. Increased ventricular stiffness and reduced ventricular filling during diastole may lead to elevated pulmonary venous pressures, reduced stroke volume, and myocardial ischemia. Diastolic dysfunction results both from altered passive elastic properties leading to reduced compliance [1, 10] and impairment of active ventricular relaxation [4, 6, 7]. Reduced left ventricular compliance in HCM arises from increased left ventricular muscle mass, as well as increased stiffnes of the muscle itself (which may result form fibrosis and cellular disorganization [24–30]).In addition to these disorders

E. Andries & R. Stroobandt (eds.), Hemodynamics in Daily Practice, 137–157.

of ventricular chamber stiffness, prolonged or incomplete left ventricular relaxation has been well demonstrated in HCM [4, 6, 7], leading to a reduced rate of diastolic pressure decline and persistant myocardial tension development during the filling phase of diastole. The mechanism for reduced left ventricular relaxation is two-fold. The inactivation process, by which calcium ions are sequestered in the sarcoplasmic reticulum [31], is impaired in hypertrophic conditions, which may lead to intracellular calcium overload; this might result either from primary abnormalities in transmembrane calcium flux [32–34] or from myocardial ischemia [31, 35]. Relaxation may also be disturbed on the basis of load dependent mechanisms, including left ventricular restoring forces (end systolic pressure and volume), afterload, coronary blood flow, regional asynchrony, and wall stress after mitral valve opening [36–38]. Impaired relaxation leads both to a reduced rate and extent of left ventricular rapid filling and elevated left ventricular pressures at any level of ventricular diastolic volume. Thus, the diastolic pressure-volume relations that determine ventricular stiffness are governed not only by the passive properties of the left ventricle but also by the complex interplay between left ventricular relaxation and filling [39, 40].

1.2 Myocardial ischemia

There is growing awareness that myocardial ischemia, in the absence of coronary artery disease, occurs commonly in patients with HCM. Several lines of evidence support this concept. Angina pectoris is a common symptom: although angina may occur at rest, it characteristically develops with increases in myocardial oxygen demand during exercise or with atrial pacing in the catheterization laboratory [12, 13]. These latter studies demonstrate reduced coronary vasodilator capacity, such that incremental increases in myocardial demand are not balanced by appropriate increases in coronary flow: this imbalance is associated with disproportionate increases in left ventricular filling pressures and reduction in myocardial lactate consumption [11–13]. The

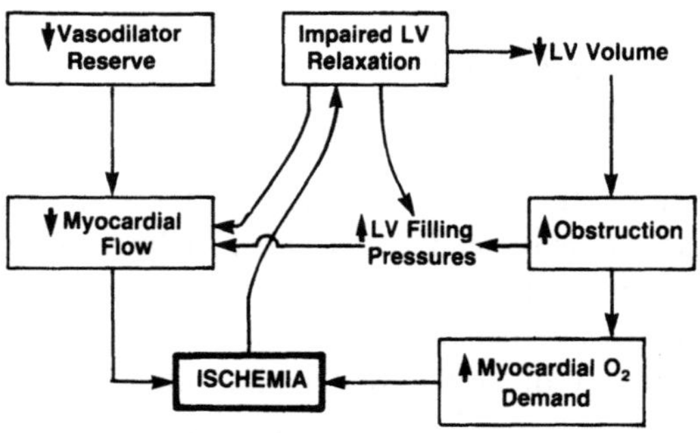

Figure 1. Influence of reduced coronary vasodilator reserve, impaired left ventricular relaxation, and subaortic obstruction on myocardial ischemia in hypertrophic cardiomyopathy.

increased demands of exercise are often associated with reversible, segmental thallium-201 perfusion defects, compatible with transient ischemia [41–43]. Finally, necropsy examinations demonstrate foci of fibrous tissue deposition, ranging from patchy fibrosis to large regions of transmural scar [26, 28, 30], likely the consequence of an ischemic process.

Myocardial ischemia may develop both from inadequate myocardial blood flow and increased myocardial demand (Figure 1). Inappropriately reduced coronary flow may result from left ventricular diastolic dysfunction, as increases in myocardial wall tension arising from prolonged or imcomplete relaxation will restrict early diastolic coronary flow, and elevated left ventricular cavity pressures in late diastole will have a compressive effect upon the intramyocardial coronary arteries that further limits blood supply [13], especially in the subendocardial regions. In addition, patients with HCM manifest diminished coronary vasodilator reserve [11–13]. Although this may represent a nonspecific effect of myocardial hypertrophy [44–46], reduction in vasodilator capacity could also develop in HCM because of abnormalities of the small intramural coronary arteries [47, 48], which are only rarely present in other forms of hypertrophy. The intramyocardial coronary arteries in HCM are characterized by thickening of the intima or media (or both) of the arterial walls, often with apparent luminal compromise [48]. Myocardial oxygen demands may also be a causative factor for ischemia. Demand in increase in HCM is related to excessive oxygen requirements of the hypertrophied ventricular myocardium and, in many patients, the added demands of greatly elevated systolic pressures resulting form outflow tract obstruction. Once ischemia develops, it may be self-perpetuating, as ischemia results in further impairment of left ventricular relaxation [31, 35] and further increase in end-diastolic pressure, resulting in a greater compromise of myocardial blood flow (Figure 1).

1.3 Left ventricular systolic function

In the vast majority of patients with HCM, indexes of left ventricular systolic performance are normal or supranormal [8, 14, 50]. This appears to represent the influence of reduced afterload rather than augmented contractility, as some clinical studies suggest that left ventricular contractility in HCM may actually be depressed, rather than increased [51]. The increased ventricular mass in HCM results in reduced systolic wall stress (and hence, reduced afterload), allowing for enhanced ventricular ejection [51]. In an important subset of patients, this hyperdynamic systolic function in combination with reduced cross-sectional area of the left ventricular outflow tract (probably resulting from a combination of basal ventricular septal hypertrophy and anterior displacement of the mitral valve apparatus within the small ventricular chamber) results in systolic pressure gradients within the outflow tract [8, 14, 17, 18]. Such subaortic gradients are dynamic and may be exacerbated by interventions that reduce ventricular volume or increase ventricular inotropic state [8, 22, 52]. The subvalvular gradient develops as blood is ejected at high velocities through the narrowed outflow tract, establishing Venturi forces that pull the anterior mitral leaflet in contact with the ventricular septum, creating an impediment to further ejection and, in many patients, mitral regurgitation [22, 23, 53–60]. The timing and magnitude of systolic anterior motion (SAM) of the mitral valve, which can be visualized by angiography or echocardiography, correlates with the timing and magnitude of the outflow gradient [22, 23, 60–69]. Although the nature and clinical importance of outflow tract gradients in HCM remain the subjects of ongoing debate [22, 23, 52, 54–61, 67, 68, 70–78] (despite over 20 years of investigation), we believe that the evidence indicates overwhelmingly that the outflow gradient represents an obstruction to left ventricular ejection, and that such obstruction is deleterious. For example, patients with obstructive HCM have evidence of increased myocardial oxygen demands [49], and these increased myocardial demands are reduced when the outflow gradient is obliterated by surgical therapy [79]. It must be emphasized, however, that patients with and without obstruction may experience symptoms of equal severity. In nonobstructive patients, symptoms may develop purely on the basis of abnormalities of diastolic function or myocardial ischemia. Patients with subaortic obstruction may also have similar disturbances, but in addition have the burden of markedly elevated intraventricular pressures superimposed upon these more general abnormalities.

In a small subset of patients with HCM, the disease process is characterized by progressive impairment of left ventricular systolic function [80]. The evidence suggests that the evolution of the natural history of these patients is characterized by progressive myocardial scarring, leading to myocardial wall thinning, left ventricular cavity dilatation, and reduced systolic performance [26, 80–83]. Such patients almost invariably have no outflow tract gradients, as they lack the morphologic and functional conditions required to generate high outflow velocities and elevated systolic pressures [80]. Patients in this subgroup are usually severely symptomatic on the basis of both systolic and diastolic dysfunction. The management options for such patients are distinctly different from those considered for the more typical patients with hyperdynamic systolic function.

1.4 Arrhythmias

Both supraventricular and ventricular arrhythmias are prevalent in HCM. Although all forms of ventricular arrhythmias, supraventricular arrhythmias, and conduction disturbances may develop in this disease [19–21, 84–86], atrial fibrillation and ventricular tachycardia have the most important therapeutic implications, as these are the most hemodynamically devastating and life threatening rhythm complications. Several features of atrial fibrillation in HCM are analogous to its occurrence in mitral stenosis: (1) it develops on the basis of elevated left atrial filling pressures, leading to atrial dilatation, (2) patients usually develop episodes of paroxysmal atrial fibrillation before the development of chronic sustained atrial fibrillation, and (3) patients with atrial fibrillation are at risk of systemic embolization [87, 88]. Patients with HCM may develop hemodynamic decompensation with the onset of atrial fibrillation [75, 87, 89, 90], since atrial systole contributes importantly to left ventricular filling in the setting of impaired relaxation and reduced compliance [91]. Thus, reduced cardiac output during atrial fibrillation results not only from the very rapid and irregular heart rate but also from loss of the important contribution of atrial function to left ventricular stroke volume.

Ventricular tachycardia is the most common factor associated with sudden death in HCM [19–21, 92–95]. The finding that sudden death often occurs either during or shortly after vigorous exercise [93, 94, 96] suggests that inducible myocardial ischemia or hemodynamic abnormalities (such as increased outflow obstruction) may play a causative role in the pathogenesis of ventricular tachycardia. However, the mechanism responsible for this arrhythmia in HCM has not been established.

2. MEDICAL THERAPY

2.1 Beta-blocking drugs

Beta adrenergic blocking agents are effective in alleviating symptoms in many symptomatic patients with HCM [52, 97–104]. The mechanism for this therapeutic effect appears to be mediated by reduction in heart rate, reduction in inotropic state, and inhibition of sympathetic stimulation of the heart during physical or emotional stress [11, 98]. Thus, beta-blocker therapy may be effective in decreasing outflow tract gradients, reducing myocardial oxygen demand and, by virtue of the reduced heart rate, prolonging the diastolic portion of the cardiac cycle during which ventricular filling occurs. Although early observations indicated that propranolol might enhance left ventricular relaxation and diastolic pressure-volume relations in patients with HCM [105, 106], subsequent data demonstrate that beta-blocking agents usually have no clinically important primary effects on left ventricular relaxation and filling [5, 107, 108]. However, in individual patients, such therapy could theoretically lead to beneficial effects on diastolic function, either indirectly via reduction in myocardial ischemia or by decreasing the heart rate. At reduced heart rates, the diastasis period of diastole is prolonged, allowing for a greater extent of passive ventricular filling.

Although symptoms are improved satisfactorily in approximately 50% of patients after the initiation of standard doses of beta-blockers (equivalent to propranolol 160–320 mg/d) many patients develop recurrent symptoms during longer term therapy. In such patients, or in patients who do not respond initially to standard doses, higher doses of beta-blocking drugs (equivalent to propranolol 640 mg/d) may be effective. Such doses are usually well tolerated with relatively few cardiovascular adverse reactions other than bradycardia, but at this dosage range many patients will also experience important beta-blocker side effects. Even higher doses (in the range of propranolol 1 gm/d) have been advocated for patients who fail to respond adequately to the more usual doses [104]. However, such extreme doses are often poorly tolerated because of side effects and usually do not provide additional therapeutic effects beyond those observed with more standard doses.

2.2 Calcium-channel blocking drugs

Calcium-channel blocking agents have been studied intensively in patients with HCM for the past decade. The greatest clinical experience, and the only studies of long-term oral administration, have been obtained using verapamil. Verapamil reduces symptoms and increases exercise tolerance in the majority of patients during short-term therapy [109–113], with sustained clinical improvement in over 50% of patients during long-term treatment (up to 4 years) [109, 111–113]. Some investigators now favor verapamil for use as first line drug therapy rather than beta-blocking agents. The possible mechanisms responsible for beneficial clinical results are related to verapamil's negative chronotropic effects, negative inotropic effects, and effects on left ventricular relaxation and diastolic filling. Hemodynamic studies demonstrate that the acute intravenous administration of verapamil in patients with HCM produces a decrease in left ventricular contractility, manifested by reduction in ejection fraction as well as a downward and rightward shift in the end systolic pressure-volume relation [114]. This negative inotropic effect is sufficient in most patients to substantially reduce (and in many cases, obliterate) the outflow tract gradient [114, 115]. However, it is uncertain whether these negative inotropic properties are an important mechanism for the salutary clinical effects of verapamil, as evidence of reduced systolic function or decreased outflow gradient is usually not evident during oral therapy [5, 91, 113, 116, 117]. In contrast, numerous studies indicate that enhanced left ventricular diastolic function results from both intravenous and oral administration of verapamil [5, 91, 108, 113, 114, 117–120]. Verapamil improves indices of impaired left ventricular relaxation and increases the rate and magnitude of early rapid diastolic filling. In most patients, these effects result in increased left ventricular stroke volume and increased end diastolic volumes without an associated increase in left ventricular end diastolic pressure or pulmonary wedge pressure [114, 117, 119, 120], and in a subset of patients, the increased end diastolic volume after verapamil is associated with a decrease in end diastolic pressure (Figure 2) [114], evidence for a beneficial effect on left ventricular stiffness stemming from enhanced relaxation. These alterations in left ventricular filling characteristics correlate with objective symptomatic improvement; approximately 70% of patients manifesting an improvement in left ventricular filling during verapamil have an associated increase in exercise tolerance by treadmill testing, whereas a similar improvement in exercise tolerance is observed in only 10% of patients in whom left ventricular filling is not increased [113].

Several factors may explain the improvement in left ventricular relaxation and filling by verapamil. These include a reduction in ischemia, increased coronary blood flow, reduced regional left ventricular asychrony [121], and beneficial changes in left ventricular loading conditions. In addition, there

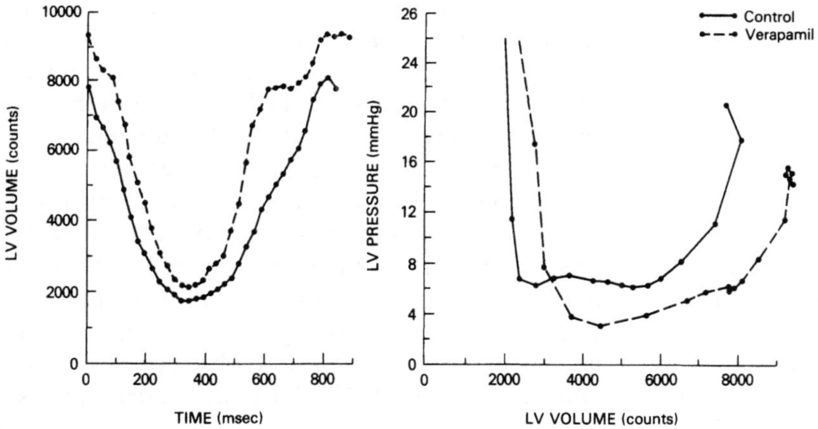

Figure 2. Effect of intravenous verapamil on left ventricular diastolic function in a patient with hypertrophic cardiomyopathy studied at chateterization. The left ventricular volume curves (*left panel*) demonstrate an increase in the rate and extent of rapid diastolic filling after verapamil administration, associated with increased end-diastolic volume and stroke volume. This results in a downward and rightward shift in the diastolic pressure-volume relation (*right panel*), such that increased end-diastolic volume is achieved at reduced end-diastolic pressure. In this study, volume data were obtained using a nonimaging scintillation probe. (Reproduced from Bonow et al. [114] with permission of the American Heart Association)

is experimental evidence for disturbed calcium ion flux in hypertrophied myocardium resulting in intracellular calcium overload [32–34]. If this mechanism is operative in HCM, it could contribute to incomplete myocardial relaxation; verapamil may therefore have a direct effect on improving myocardial relaxation by reducing intracellular calcium ion concentration. Such direct effects at the cell membrane level are difficult to substantiate in clinical studies, but evidence for such direct effects of verapamil on improving cellular relaxation in the setting of calcium ion overload has been demonstrated in cultured myocytes [122].

Verapamil should be initiated in patients with HCM at low doses (240–360 mg/d) and then increased over the course of several days or weeks to higher doses (480 mg/d) as needed if symptoms persist. The majority of patients experience only mild symptomatic improvement at lower doses and achieve more acceptable reduction in symptoms at these higher doses. In some patients, bradycardia or orthostatic hypotension may limit dose titration, such that doses of 320–360 mg/d must be employed. Others may not respond to usual therapeutic doses and may require high doses of verapamil (640 mg/d) for symptomatic relief. It must be emphasized that verapamil, especially at high doses, may be associated with adverse cardiovascular reactions, in the form of sinus bradycardia, atrioventricular block, or hypotension. In a minority of patients, varapamil administration may precipitate pulmonary edema [123]. This particular complication appears to develop primarily in patients with outflow obstruction and elevated pulmonary wedge pressures (⩾ 20 mm Hg). The mechanism for pulmonary edema in these patients may be related to the peripheral vasodilating action of verapamil which exacerbates the outflow gradient, thereby further increasing the already high pulmonary venous pressures. This postulated mechanism is supported by hemodynamic data indicating that the only patients in whom intravenous verapamil results in no change or worsening of outflow obstruction are those patients who manifest the greatest decrease in systemic blood pressure with verapamil [115]. Although pulmonary edema is rare after verapamil administration, it is a severe and life-threatening complication, such that initiating outpatient drug therapy is relatively contraindicated in patients with outflow obstruction at rest and pulmonary wedge pressures ⩾ 20 mm Hg [123]. Since such patients are usually candidates for operation, the risks of surgical therapy appear to be less than the risk of verapamil therapy. In patients in whom the risks of surgery may be higher than usual because of unsuitable septal anatomy, age, or associated medical illnesses, verapamil may be given carefully along with diuretics. If the postulated mechanism for pulmonary edema with verapamil is correct, then patients with no outflow obstruction (either at rest or with provocation) would appear to be at lower risk of this complication, even if left ventricular filling pressures are elevated. Since these particular patients are not candidates for surgery, and since the elevated filling pressures presumably occur because of diastolic dysfunction, treatment with verapamil may be attempted. Such therapy, however, should be given judiciously, beginning at low doses and accompanied by diuretics, and with careful monitoring of the clinical state.

Other calcium channel blocking agents have also been studied in HCM, but the data are much less extensive than for verapamil. Nifedipine has been demonstrated to improve left ventricular relaxation and filling characteristics [124, 125]. The magnitude of enhanced relaxation with nifedipine is greater than would be anticipated on the basis of its potent vasodilating properties alone [125]. Data demonstrating clinically important improvement in left ventricular diastolic function with nifedipine have been inconsistent [126], and there have been no studies demonstrating symptomatic or objective improvement with long-term oral administration. In addition, nifedipine may exacerbate outflow obstruction on the basis of reduced peripheral resistance [126]. Data assessing the efficacy of diltiazem therapy are quite limited, but the available studies suggest that this drug may affect left ventricular hemodynamics favorably [127, 128]. As yet, no clinical trials with diltiazem have been reported.

2.3 Additional drug therapy in symptomatic patients

a. *Disopyramide.* In addition to its antiarrhythmic properties, this drug (in doses of 600–800 mg/d) has been advocated for symptomatic patients with HCM [22, 129]. The mechanism related to the efficacy of disopyramide in improving effort tolerance and reducing symptoms appears to arise purely from a reduction in left ventricular contractility [130]. Thus, this drug may be especially helpful in patients with outflow obstruction, as its negative inotropic effects are associated with reduction in the outflow gradient [129, 130]. However, studies demonstrating long-term relief of symptoms in such patients are lacking. There are also insufficient data with regard to its effects in patients without obstruction.

b. *Amiodarone.* Another antiarrhythmic agent with hemodynamic properties of potential benefit in HCM is amiodarone. Recent studies suggest that amiodarone may result in sustained reduction in symptoms and increased exercise tolerance [131]. After a loading period of high dose amiodarone (800–1200 mg/d), patients may be treated at rather low maintenance dose of 200–400 mg/d. The mechanism underlying the beneficial clinical results has not been established, but could relate to reduced heart rate, peripheral vascular effects, negative inotropic effects, or enhanced left ventricular diastolic performance [131, 132]. Studies demonstrating a salutary clinical effect have been performed in patients whose symptoms were refractory to both beta-blocking drugs and calcium channel blocking drugs, suggesting that amiodarone may play a role in the treatment of patients who do not respond to more conventional forms of medical therapy. However, hemodynamic effects have been inconsistent [133], and in more mildly symptomatic patients, amiodarone has been shown to increase left ventricular filling pressures and reduce exercise capacity [134]. Moreover, several of our patients have died suddenly within 4 months of initiation of amiodarone. This inconsistency in results underscores the complex nature of amiodarone and, along with the numerous significant side effects experienced by patients receiving this drug, suggests that its use should be reserved only for patients who are not candidates for surgery and have not responded to either beta-blocking or calcium channel blocking agents. However, amiodarone may be an attractive form of therapy for symptomatic patients with concomitant supraventricular or ventricular arrhythmias wherein it may have a dual role in treating both cardiac symptoms and disturbing arrhythmias [135, 136].

c. *Diuretics.* The noncompliant left ventricle in HCM may require elevated filling pressures to maintain stroke volume. Beta-blocking drugs or calcium channel-blocking drugs alone may be effective in reducing pulmonary venous pressures, and thereby relieving dyspnea, but many patients continue to experience shortness of breath (especially with exertion) despite such therapy. Although treatment with diuretic agents is associated with the theoretic possibility that reduced filling pressures may result in worsening symptoms because of an increase in outflow gradient or low cardiac output, in clinical practice the combination of diuretics with beta blockers or calcium channel blockers is usually quite effective in reducing the severity of dyspnea. Thus, if dyspnea remains an important component of an individual patient's symptom complex during treatment with beta blockers or verapamil, diuretics should be added before it is concluded that the patient's symptoms are refractory to conventional medical therapy and that more aggressive therapy, in the form of investigational drugs or surgery, is warranted. Intravenous diuretics are also valuable, and may be life saving, in the treatment of pulmonary edema related to HCM, as they would be in the treatment of pulmonary edema stemming from other forms of heart disease.

d. *Anticoagulants.* Patients with HCM and episodes of paroxysmal or sustained atrial fibrillation have a similar risk of systemic embolization as do patients with mitral stenosis [87]. Once atrial fibrillation is demonstrated, even if the episodes are brief and infrequent, anticoagulant therapy should be begun and maintained on a long-term basis.

2.4 Antiarrhythmic therapy

Patients with asymptomatic nonsustained ventricular tachycardia during ambulatory monitoring represent a high risk group for sudden death, with an annual mortality rate of approximately 9% [19, 20, 92]. Neither propranolol nor verapamil is effective at suppressing ventricular tachycardia [20, 135]. Although there have been no well controlled studies to assess the efficacy of propranolol or verapamil in preventing sudden death, it is clear that many patients who have died suddenly were receiving propranolol at the time of death [93]. Recently, amiodarone was reported to reduce the risk of sudden death substantially in patients with ventricular tachycardia [137], but this study was not randomized and used historic rather than concurrent controls. In our experience, amiodarone treatment does not confer immunity from sudden death, perhaps because of drug induced ventricular arrhythmias [138].

At present, there are important uncertainties regarding the appropriate evaluation and management of patients with asymptomatic ventricular tachycardia on 24-hour monitoring, since the morbidity of chronic amiodarone therapy in a large number of asymptomatic young patients may be substantial [139]. Although a strong case can be made for aggressive management of ventricular tachycardia when it is either sustained, frequent or associated with symptoms, the goals are less clear in asymptomatic patients with infrequent brief episodes of nonsustained ventricular tachycardia. The role of invasive electrophysiologic testing in guiding antiarrhythmic therapy has also not been established [140–143]. Finally, there are no controlled data comparing ghe efficacy of standard Type I antiarrhythmic drugs to that of amiodarone in preventing sudden death. Until issues are resolved, it would appear reasonable to treat patients with frequent episodes of nonsustained asymptomatic ventricular tachycardia with standard antiarrhythmic agents and to manage patients with sustained or symptomatic ventricular arrhythmias, or those resuscitated from sudden death, with either amiodarone or electrophysiologic guided antiarrhythmic therapy. Possible deleterious effects of amiodarone must always be kept in mind when considering its use.

Supraventricular arrhythmias in HCM are managed in similar fashion to those arising in patients with other forms of heart disease. Atrial fibrillation may require prompt treatment, such as electrical cardioversion, if this rhythm is associated with hemodynamic compromise. Patients with episodes of paraoxysmal atrial fibrillation, in addition to receiving anticoagulants, should be treated with Type I antiarrhythmic agents in an attempt to prevent future occurrences. Although such patients frequently also receive propranolol or verapamil for purposes of rate control when atrial fibrillation again develops, chronic oral doses of propranolol or verapamil are often unsatisfactory in controlling the ventricular response when atrial fibrillation supervenes, and intravenous administration of either propranolol or verapamil may be necessary. In many patients, digitalis is required either acutely or chronically to obtain adequate ventricular rate control. This is the one circumstance in which a cardiac glycoside may be useful in patients with outflow obstruction; the benefits of slowing of heart rate in this situation clearly outweigh the potential disadvantage of enhanced contractility and worsening obstruction.

2.5. Patients with impaired systolic performance

Patients who manifest progressive myocardial scarring, wall thinning, cavity dilatation, and depressed left ventricular systolic function are often severely symptomatic from both systolic and diastolic left ventricular dysfunction, and often these symptoms are refractory to all forms of medical management. Management options in these patients are distinctly different from patients with the more typical, hyperdynamic left ventricular. Drugs with negative inotropic effects, such as beta-blockers, verapamil or disopyramide, may aggravate symptoms and are relatively contraindicated in patients with severe heart failure symptoms. In most cases, patients at this end of the spectrum of HCM require treatment similar to other forms of congestive heart failure with poor systolic function, including combinations of diuretics, nitrates, and peripheral arterial dilators. Cardiac glycosides (or other inotropic agents) may also be added, but we have not been impressed that substantial improvement results. Patients in this subgroup in whom symptoms remain refractory to all forms of medical therapy may be candidates for cardiac transplantation.

2.6 Asymptomatic patients

In patients with HCM and no symptoms, there are no definitive data with which to recommend chronic medical therapy. The rationale for such therapy would be to alter the natural history or to prevent sudden death. Although definitive information is lacking, we believe that it is reasonable to recommend that young asymptomatic patients with either a strong family history of sudden death [95], marked left ventricular hypertrophy, or marked subaortic obstruction be treated prophylactically with beta-blockers or verapamil. All asymptomatic patients should be monitored for arrhythmias and urged to refrain from heavy physical activities or competitive athletics [144].

3. SURGICAL TREATMENT

In a sizeable percentage of patients with HCM, symptoms persist despite vigorous medical treatment. Patients with subaortic obstruction in whom severe symptoms or unacceptable lifestyle limitations continue with standard medical management may be considered candidates for surgical intervention. In such patients, surgical therapy in the form of septal myotomy and myectomy offers an excellent management alternative [145–153]. Long-term postoperative follow-up studies indicate that the majority of patients (70%) are alive with substantial symptomatic improvement during a mean follow-up period of 5 years (Figure 3) [149]. This reduction in symptoms after operation has been substantiated by treadmill exercise studies which demonstrate a significant increase in exercise capacity after operation [154, 155].

Myotomy and myectomy should not be considered a curative procedure, as it does not reverse many of the underlying morphologic and pathophysiologic features of HCM. Factors such as severe left ventricular hypertrophy, cellular disorganization, thickening of the small coronary arteries, hyperdynamic systolic function, and increased left ventricular stiffness are unaffected by surgery. However, myotomy and myectomy is successful in abolishing or reducing the subaortic pressure gradient [145–153, 156–159], thereby eliminating an important pathophysiologic factor that may be superimposed upon certain of these other features of the disease process. The improvement in symptoms stemming from surgical relief of dynamic obstruction probably accrues via several mechanisms. The reduction in left ventricular systolic pressures results in greatly diminished myocardial oxygen demands associated with reduced left ventricular filling pressures and more normal coronary flow

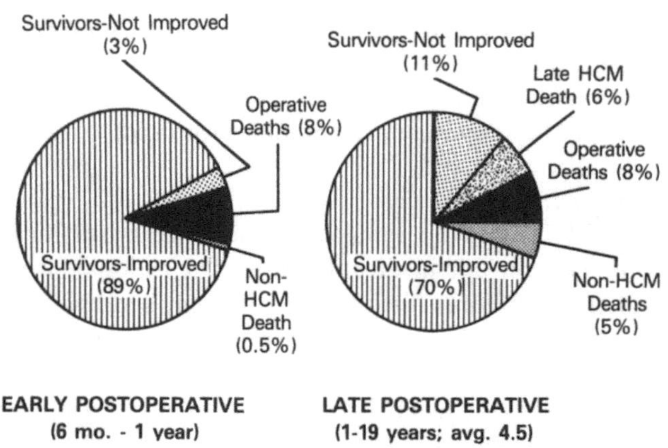

Figure 3. Short-term and long-term clinical results of operation for hypertrophy cardiomyopathy (HCM) in 240 patients. (Reproduced from Maron et al. [149] with permission of the European Heart Journal)

patterns at rest and during pacing tachycardia [79]. Thus, the dynamic interplay between myocardial ischemia and impaired left ventricular diastolic function, which is exacerbated by outflow obstruction (Figure 1), is alleviated by surgical relief of the outflow gradient. The mechanism by which surgery reduces outflow obstruction appears to be an increase in the cross-sectional area of the left ventricular outflow tract [151, 152, 158], and not due to any impairment in left ventricular systolic performance [50]. Echocardiographic studies demonstrate a relation between the enlargement of the outflow tract cross-sectional area and the postoperative reduction in gradient [151]. The increase in outflow area permits stroke volume to be ejected at reduced velocities, such that the Venturi forces that generate SAM do not develop [22, 151, 159–162].

It must be emphasized that myotomy and myectomy has been shown to reduce symptoms, but there are no definitive data to demonstrate an improvement in long-term survival compared to medical therapy. Hence, surgery is rarely indicated in asymptomatic individuals. Moreover, because of the operative risk (4–8%) [145, 146, 148–150, 157, 158] and the fact that symptoms persist or recur in some survivors [148, 149], myotomy and myectomy should be reserved for those patients in whom symptoms impose unacceptable lifestyle limitations despite medical management. Thus, two criteria must be met before recommending surgery: (1) an outflow gradient in excess of 50 mm Hg at rest or with provocation, and (2) moderate to severe symptomatic limitation (New York Heart Association Functional Class III–IV) despite treatment with beta-blockers and then verapamil. Exceptions to these criteria are patients with outflow obstruction and elevated pulmonary venous pressures (wedge pressure $\geqslant$ 20 mmHg or a history of orthopnea and paroxysmal nocturnal dyspnea); in such patients, who are otherwise ideal candidates for surgery, the risk of verapamil therapy may be greater than the risk of surgery [123], and these patients become operative candidates if their symptoms are refractory to beta-blockers.

4. CONCLUSIONS

HCM is a heterogeneous and multifaceted disease process. Because of the multiple pathophysiologic mechanisms that may be operative, a single form of treatment should not be expected to be successful in all patients. In an individual patient, the physician may be required to attempt several different avenues of therapy before symptom relief is attained. When viewed in the context of the complex interaction of the various pathophysiologic features that may produce symptoms, however, these symptoms may be controlled by interventions that enhance diastolic performance, reduce ischemia, or relieve dynamic obstruction. Either beta blockers or calcium channel blockers (alone or in combination with diuretics) are effective in the majority or patients. If these prove to be ineffective, then many patients respond favorably to either operation or investigational drug regimens.

REFERENCES

1. Gaasch WH, Levine HJ, Quinones MA, Alexander JK (1976) Left ventricular compliance: Mechanisms and clinical implications. *Am J Cardiol* 38: 645–653
1. Sanderson JE, Gibson DG, Brown DJ, Goodwin JF (1977) Left ventricular filling in hypertrophic cardiomyopathy: An angiographic study. *Br Heart J* 39: 661–670
2. St. John Sutton MG, Tajik AJ, Gibson DG, Brown DJ, Seward JB, Giuliani ER (1978) Echocardiographic assessment of left ventricular filling and septal and posterior wall dynamics in idiopathic hypertrophic subasortic stenosis. *Circulation* 57:512–560
3. Hanrath P, Mathey DG, Siegert B, Bleifeld W (1980) Left ventricular relaxation and filling pattern in different forms of left ventricular hypertrophy: An echocardiographic study. *Am J Cardiol* 45:15–23
4. Bonow RO, Rosing DR, Bacharach SL, et al. (1981) Effects of verapamil on left ventricular systolic function and diastolic filling in patients with hypertrophic cardiomyopathy. *Circulation* 64:787–796
5. Alvares RF, Shaver JA, Gamble WH, Goodwin JF (1984) Isovolumic relaxation period in hypertrophic cardiomyopathy. *J Am Coll Cardiol* 3:71–81
6. Betocchi S, Bonow RO, Bacharach SL, Rosing DR, Maron BJ, Green MV (1986) Isovolumic relaxation period in hypertrophic cardiomyopathy: Assessment with radionuclide angiography. *J Am Coll Cardiol* 7:74–81
7. Braunwald E, Lambrew CT, Rockoff SD, Ross J Jr, Morrow AG (1964) Idiopathic hypertrophic subaortic stenosis, I: A description of the disease based upon an analysis of 54 patients. *Circulation* 30 (Suppl. IV): IV–3–119
8. Klein MD, Lane FJ, Gorlin R (1965) Effect of left ventricular size and shape upon the hemodynamics of subaortic stenosis. *Am J Cardiol* 15:773–782
10. Grossman W, McLaurin LP (1976) Diastolic properties of the left ventricle. *Ann Int Med* 84:316–326
11. Thompson DS, Nagvi N, Juul SM, et al. (1980) Effects of propranolol on myocardial oxygen consumption: Substrate extraction and hemodynamics in hypertrophic cardiomyopathy. *Br Heart J* 44:488–498
12. Pasternac A, Noble J, Streulens Y, Elie R, Henschke C, Bourassa MG (1982) Pathophysiology of chest pain in patients with cardiomyopathies and normal coronary arteries. *Circulation* 65:778–789
13. Cannon RO, Rosing DR, Maron BJ, et al. (1985) Myocardial ischemia in patients with hypertrophic cardiomyopathy: Contribution of inadequate vasodilator reserve and elevated left ventricular filling pressures. *Circulation* 71:234–243
14. Wigle ED, Heimbecker RO, Gunton RW (1962) Idiopathic ventricular septal hypertrophy causing muscular subaortic stenosis. *Circulation* 26:325–340
15. Brock R (1957) Functional obstruction of the left ventricle (acquired aortic subvalvular stenosis). *Guy's Hosp Rep* 106:221–238
16. Barcu BA, Diettert GA, Danforth WH, Ahlvin RC, Belliveau RR (1958) Pseudoaortic stenosis produced by ventricular hypertrophy. *Am J Med* 25:814–818
17. Goodwin JF, Hollman A, Cleland WP, Teare D (1960) Obstructive cardiomyopathy simulating aortic stenosis. *Br Heart J* 22:403–414
18. Morrow AG, Braunwald E (1959) Functional aortic stenosis: A malformation characterized by resistance to left ventricular outflow without anatomic obstruction. *Circulation* 20:181–189
19. McKenna WJ, England D, Doi YL, Deanfield DE, Oakley CM, Goodwin JF (1981) Arrhythmia in hypertrophic cardiomyopathy, I: Influence on prognosis. *Br Heart J* 46:168–172
20. McKenna WJ, Chetty S, Oakley CM, Goodwin JF (1980) Arrhythmia in hypertrophic cardiomyopathy: Exercise and 48-hour ambulatory electrocardiographic assessment with and without beta adrenergic blocking therapy. *Am J Cardiol* 45:1–5
21. Canedo MI, Frank MJ, Abdulla AM (1980) Rhythm disturbances in hypertrophic cardi-

omyopathy: Prevalence, relation to symptoms and management. *Am J Cardiol* 45:848–855
22. Wigle ED, Sasson Z, Henderson MA, et al. (1985) Hypertrophic cardiomyopathy: The importance of the site and the extent of hypertrophy. A review. *Prog Cardiovasc Dis* 28:1–83
23. Maron BJ, Bonow RO, Cannon RO, Leon MB, Epstein SE (1987) Hypertrophic cardiomyopathy: Interrelations of clinical manifestations, pathophysiology, and therapy (two parts). *N Engl J Med* 316:780–789, 844–852
24. Teare D (1958) Asymmetrical hypertrophy of the heart in young patients. *Br Heart J* 20:1–8
25. Van der BelKahn J (1977) Muscle fiber disarray in common heart diseases. *Am J Cardiol* 40:355–364
26. Maron BJ, Epstein SE, Roberts WC (1979) Hypertrophic cardiomyopathy and transmural myocardial infarction without significant atherosclerosis of the extramural coronary arteries. *Am J Cardiol* 43:1086–1102
27. Maron BJ, Roberts WC (1979) Quantitative analysis of cardiac muscle cell disorganization in the ventricular septum of patients with hypertrophic cardiomyopathy. *Circulation* 59:689–706
28. St John Sutton MG, Lie JT, Anderson KR, O'Brien PC, Frye RL (1980) Histopathological specificity of hypertrophic obstructive cardiomyopathy. Myocardial fibre disarray and myocardial fibrosis. *Br Heart J* 44:433–443
29. Maron BJ, Anan TJ, Roberts WC (1981) Quantitative analysis of the distribution of cardiac muscle cell disorganization in the left ventricular wall of patients with hypertrophic cardiomyopathy. *Circulation* 63:882–894
30. Tanaka M, Fujiwara H, Onodera T, Wu DJ, Hamashima Y, Kawai C (1986) Quantitative analysis of myocardial fibrosis in normals, hypertensive hearts, and hypertrophic cardiomyopathy. *Br Heart J* 55:575–581
31. Nayler WC, Willams A (1978) Relaxation in heart muscle: Some morphological and biochemical considerations. *Eur J Cardiol* 7 (Supp I): 35–50
32. Sordahl LA, McCollum WB, Wood WG, Schwartz A (1973) Mitochondria and sarcoplasmic reticulum function in cardiac hypertrophy and failure. *Am J Physiol* 224:497–502
33. Ito Y, Suko J, Chidsey CA (1974) Intracellular calcium and myocardial contractility, V: Calcium uptake of sarcoplasmic reticulum fractions in hypertrophied and failing rabbit hearts. *J Mol Cell Cardiol* 6:237–247
34. Lecarpentier Y, Martin JL, Gastineau P, Hatt PY (1982) Load dependence of mammalian heart relaxation during cardiac hypertrophy and heart failure. *Am J Physiol* 242:H855–861
35. Mann T, Goldberg S, Mudge GH, Grossman W (1979) Factors contributing to the altered left ventricular diastolic properties during angina pectoris. *Circulation* 59:14–20
36. Gaasch WH,Blaustein AS, Andrias CW, Donahue RP, Avitall B (1980) Myocardial relaxation, II: Hemodynamic determinants of the left ventricular isovolumic pressure decline. *Am J Physiol* 239:H1–6
37. Brutsaert DL, Housmans PR, Goethals MA (1980) Dual control of relaxation: its role in the ventricular function in the mammalian heart. *Circ Res* 47:637–652
38. Brutsaert DL, Rademakers FE, Sys SU (1984) Triple control of relaxation: implications in cardiac disease. *Circulation* 69:190–196
39. Gaasch WH, Cole JS, Quinones MA, Alexander JK (1975) Dynamic determinants of left ventricular diastolic pressure-volume relations in man. *Circulation* 51:317–323
40. Grossman W, Barry WH (1980) Diastolic pressure-volume relations in the diseased heart. *Federation Proc* 39:148–155
41. Rubin KA, Morrison J, Padnick MB et al. (1979) Idiopathic hypertrophic subaortic stenosis: Evaluation of anginal symptoms with thallium-201 myocardial imaging. *Am J Cardiol* 44:1040–1045
42. Pitcher D, Wainwright R, Maisey M, Curry P, Sowton E (1980) Assessment of chest pain in hypertrophic cardiomyopathy using exercise thallium-201 myocardial scintigraphy. *Br Heart J* 44:650–656
43. Hanrath P, Mathey D, Montz R, et al. (1981) Myocardial thallium-201 imaging in hypertrophic

obstructive cardiomyopathy. *Eur Heart J* 2:177–185

44. Marcus ML, Doty DB, Hiratzka LF, Wright CB, Eastham CL (1982) Decreased coronary reserve: A mechanism for angina pectoris in patients with aortic stenosis and normal coronary arteries. *N Engl J Med* 307:1362–1366
45. Bailey IK, Come PC, Kelly DT, et al. (1977) Thallium-201 myocardial perfusion imaging in aortic valve stenosis. *Am J Cardiol* 40:889–899
46. Opherk D, Mall G, Zebe H, et al. (1984) Reduction of coronary reserve: A mechanism for angina pectoris in patients with arterial hypertension and normal coronary arteries. *Circulation* 69:1–7
47. James TH, Marshall TK (1975) De subitaneis mortibus, XII: Asymmetrical hypertrophy of the heart. *Circulation* 51:1149–1166
48. Maron BJ, Wolfson JK, Epstein SE, Roberts WC (1986) Intramural ('small vessel') coronary artery disease in hypertrophic cardiomyopathy. *J Am Coll Cardiol* 8:545–557
49. Cannon RO, Schenke WH, Maron BJ, et al. (1987) Differences in coronary flow and myocardial metabolism at rest and during pacing between patient with obstructive and patients with nonobstructive hypertrophic cardiomyopathy. *J Am Coll Cardiol* 10:53–62
50. Borer JS, Bacharach SL, Green MV, et al (1979) Effect of septal myotomy and myectomy on left ventricular systolic function at rest and during exercise in patients with IHSS. *Circulation* 60 (Suppl I):I 82–87
51. Pouleur H, Rousseau MF, van Eyll C, Brasseur LA, Charlier AA (1983) Force-velocity-length in hypertrophic cardiomyopathy: Evidence of normal or depressed myocardial contractility. *Am J Cardiol* 52:813–817
52. Epstein SE, Henry WL, Clark CE, et al. (1974) Asymmetric septal hypertrophy. *Ann Intern Med* 81:650–680
53. Grose R, Strain J, SpindolaFranco H (1986) Angiographic and hemodynamic correlations in patients with hypertrophic cardiomyopathy and intracavity pressure gradients. *Am J Cardiol* 58:1085–1092
54. Maron BJ, Gottdiener JS, Arce J, Rosing DR, Wesley YE, Epstein SE (1985) Dynamic subaortic obstruction in hypertrophic cardiomyopathy: Analysis by pulsed Doppler echocardiography. *J Am Coll Cardiol* 6:1–8
55. Gardin JM Dabestani A, Glasgow GA (1985) Echocardiographic and Doppler flow observations in obstructed and nonobstructed hypertrophic cardiomyopathy. *Am J Cardiol*
56. Jenni R, Ruffman A, Vieli M, Anliker M, Krayenbuehl HP (1985) Dynamics of aortic flow in hypertrophic cardiomyopathy. *Eur Heart J* 6:391–398
57. Yock PG, Hatle L, Popp RL (1986) Patterns and timing of Doppler-detected intracavitary and aortic flow in hypertrophic cardiomyopathy. *J Am Coll Cardiol* 8:1047–1058
58. Maron BJ, Epstein SE (1986) Clinical significance and therapeutic implications of the left ventricular outflow tract pressure gradient in hypertrophic cardiomyopathy. *Am J Cardiol* 58:1093–1096
59. Pierce GE, Morrow AG, Braunwald E (1964) Idiopathic hypertrophic subaortic stenosis, III: Intraoperative studies of the mechanism of obstruction and its hemodynamic consequences. *Circulation* 30 (Suppl IV): IV 152–213
60. Wigle ED (1987) Hypertrophic cardiomyopathy: A 1987 viewpoint. *Circulation* 73:311–322
61. Wigle ED, Auger P, Marquis Y (1967) Muscular subaortic stenosis: The direct relation between the intraventricular pressure difference and the left ventricular ejection time. *Circulation* 36:36–44
62. Shah PM, Gramiak R, Kramer DH (1969) Ultrasound localization of left ventricular outflow obstruction in hypertrophic obstructive cardiomyopathy. *Circulation* 40:3–11
63. Popp R, Harrison D (1969) Ultrasound in the diagnosis and evaluation of therapy of idiopathic hypertrophic subaortic stenosis. *Circulation* 40:905–914
64. Henry WL, Clark CE, Glancy DL, Epstein SE (1973) Echocardiomyopathic measurement of the left ventricular outflow gradient in idiopathic hypertrophic subaortic stenosis. *N Engl J Med* 288:989–993
65. Ibrahim M, Silie M, Delahaye JP, Froment R (1973) Systolic time intervals in valvular aortic

stenosis and idiopathic hypertrophic subaortic stenosis. *Br Heart J* 35:276–283
66. Boughner DR, Schuld RL, Persaud DA (1975) Hypertrophic obstructive cardiomyopathy: Assessment by echocardiographic and Doppler ultrasound techniques. *Br Heart J* 37:917–923
67. Pollick C, Morgan CD, Gilbert BW, Rakowski H, Wigle ED (1982) Muscular subaortic stenosis: The temporal relationship between systolic anterior motion of the anterior mitral leaflet and the pressure gradient. *Circulation* 66:1087–1094
68. Pollick C, Rakowski H, Wigle ED (1984) Muscular subaortic stenosis: The quantitative relationship between systolic anterior motion and the pressure gradient. *Circulation* 69:43–49
69. Spirito P, Maron BJ (1984) Patterns of systolic anterior motion of the mitral valve in hypertrophic cardiomyopathy: Assessment by twodimensional echocardiography. *Am J Cardiol* 54:1039–1046
70. Hernandez RR, Greenfield JC, McCall BW (1964) Pressure-flow studies in hypertrophic subaortic stenosis. *J Clin Invest* 43:401–407
71. Criley JM, Lewis KB, White RI, Ross RS (1965) Pressure gradients without obstruction: A new concept of 'Hypertrophic Subaortic Stenosis'. *Circulation* 32:881–887
72. Ross J, Braunwald E, Gault JH, Mason DT, Morrow AG (1966) The mechanism of the intraventricular pressure gradient in idiopathic hypertrophic subaortic stenosis. *Circulation* 34:558–578
73. Wigle ED, Marquis Y, Auger P (1967) Muscular subaortic stenosis: Initial left ventricular inflow tract pressure in the assessment of intraventricular pressure differences in man. *Circulation* 35:1100–1147
74. Murgo JP, Alter BR, Dorethy JF, Altobelli SA, McGranaham Sm (1980) Dynamics of left ventricular ejection in obstructive and nonobstructive hypertrophic cardiomyopathy. *J Clin Invest* 66:1369–1382
75. Goodwin JF (1982) The frontiers of cardiomyopathy. *Br Heart J* 48:1–18
76. Sugrue DD, McKenna WJ, Dickie S, et al. (1984) Relation between left ventricular gradient and relative stroke volume ejected in early and late systole in hypertrophic cardiomyopathy: Assessment with radionuclide cineangiography. *Br Heart J* 52:602–609
77. Siegel RJ, Criley JM (1985) Comparison of ventricular emptying with and without a pressure gradient in patients with hypertrophic cardiomyopathy. *Br Heart J* 53:283–291
78. Criley JM, Siegel RJ (1985) Has 'obstruction' hindered our understanding of hypertrophic cardiomyopathy? (editorial). *Circulation* 72:1148–1154
79. Cannon RO, McIntosh CL, Schenke WH, Maron BJ, Bonow RO, Epstein SE (1989) Effect of surgical reduction of left ventricular outflow obstruction on hemodynamics, coronary flow, and myocardial metabolism in hypertrophic cardiomyopathy. *Circulation* 79:766–775
80. Ciro E. Maron BJ, Bonow RO, Cannon RO, Epstein SE (1984) Relation between marked changes in outflow tract gradient and disease progression in patients with hypertrophic cardiomyopathy. *Am J Cardiol* 53:1103–1109
81. Ten Cate FJ, Roelandt J (1979) Progression to left ventricular dilatation in patients with hypertrophic obstructive cardiomyopathy. *Am Heart J* 97:762–765
82. Spirito P, Maron BJ, Bonow RO, Epstein SE (1986) Severe functional limitation in patients with hypertrophic cardiomyopathy and only mild localized left ventricular hypertrophy. *J Am Coll Cardiol* 8:537–544
83. Spirito P, Maron BJ, Bonow RO, et al. (1987) Occurrence and significance of progressive left ventricular wall thinning and relative cavity dilatation in patients with hypertrophic cardiomyopathy. *Am J Cardiol* 60:123–129
84. Krikler DM, Davies MJ, Rowland E, Goodwin JF, Evans RC, Shaw DB (1980) Sudden death in hypertrophic cardiomyopathy: Associated accessory atrioventricular pathways. *Br Heart J* 43:245–245
85. Frank MJ, Watkins LO, Prisant LM, Stefadouras MA, Abdulla AM (1984) Potentially lethal arrhythmias and their management in hypertrophic cardiomyopathy. *Am J Cardiol* 53:1608–1613

86. Louie EK, Maron BJ (1986) Familial spontaneous complete heart block in hypertrophic cardiomyopathy. *Br Heart J* 55:469–474
87. Henry WL, Morganroth J, Pearlman AS, et al. (1975) Relation between echocardiographically determined left atrial size and atrial fibrillation. *Circulation* 53:273–279
88. Furlan AJ, Craciun AR, Raju NR, Hart N (1984) Cerebrovascular complications associated with idiopathic hypertrophic subaortic stenosis. *Circulation* 15:282–284
89. Glancy DL, O'Brien KP, Gold HK, Epstein SE (1970) Atrial fibrillation in patients with idiopathic hypertrophic subaortic stenosis. *Br Heart J* 32:652–659
90. Goodwin JF (1970) Congestive and hypertrophic cardiomyopathy: A decade of study. *Lancet* 1970/1: 731–739
91. Bonow RO, Frederick TM, Bacharach SL, et al. (1983) Atrial systole and left ventricular filling in patients with hypertrophic cardiomyopathy: effect of verapamil. *Am J Cardiol* 51:1386–1391
92. Maron BJ, Savage DD, Wolfson JK, Epstein SE (1981) Prognostic significance of 24-hour ambulatory electrocardiographic monitoring in patients with hypertrophic cardiomyopathy: A prospective study. *Am J Cardiol* 48:252–257
93. Maron BJ, Roberts WC, Epstein SE (1982) Sudden death in hypertrophic cardiomyopathy: Profile of 78 patients. *Circulation* 65:1388–1394
94. Maron BJ, Roberts WC, Edwards JE, McAllister HA, Foley DD, Epstein SE (1978) Sudden death in patients with hypertrophic cardiomyopathy: Characterization of 26 patients without functional limitation. *Am J Cardiol* 41:803–810
95. Maron BJ, Lipson LC, Roberts WC, Savage DD, Epstein SE (1978) 'Malignant' hypertrophic cardiomyopathy: Identification of a subgroup of families with unusually frequent premature death. *Am J Cardiol* 41:1133–1140
96. Maron BJ, Roberts WC, McAllister HA, Rosing DR, Epstein SE (1980) Sudden death in young athletes. *Circulation* 62:218–229
97. Harrison DC, Braunwald E, Glick G, Mason DT, Chidsey CA, Ross J (1964) Effects of beta adrenergic blockade on the circulation, with particular reference to observations in patients with hypertrophic subaortic stenosis. *Circulation* 26:84–98
98. Cohen LS, Braunwald E (1967) Amelioration of angina pectoris in idiopathic hypertrophic subaortic stenosis with beta-adrenergic blockade. *Circulation* 35:847–851
99. Flamm MD, Harrison DC, Hancock EW (1968) Muscular subaortic stenosis. Prevention of outflow obstruction with propranolol. *Circulation* 38:846–858
100. Adelman AG, Shah PM, Gramiak R, Wigle ED (1970) Long-term propranolol therapy in muscular subaortic stenosis. *Br Heart J* 32:804–811
101. Adelman AG, Wigle ED, Ranganathan N, et al. (1972) The clinical course in muscular subaortic stenosis: A retrospective and prospective study of 60 hemodynamically proved cases. *Ann Intern Med* 77:515–525
102. Shah PM, Adelman AG, Wigle ED, et al. (1973) The natural (and unnatural) course of hypertrophic obstructive cardiomyopathy: A multicenter study. *Circ Res* 34 and 35 (Suppl. II): II 179–195
103. Stenson RE, Flamm MD, Harrison DC, Hancock EW (1973) Hypertrophic subaortic stenosis: Clinical and hemodynamic effects of long-term propranolol therapy. *Am J Cardiol* 31:763–773
104. Frank JM, Abdulla AM, Canedo MI, Saylors RE (1978) Long-term medical management of hypertrophic obstructive cardiomyopathy. *Am J Cardiol* 42:993–1001
105. de la Calzada CS, Ziady GM, Hardarson TM, Curiel R, Goodwin JF (1976) Effect of acute administration of propranolol on ventricular function in hypertrophic obstructive cardiomyopathy measured by noninvasive techniques. *Br Heart J* 38:798–803
106. Swanton RH, Brooksby IAB, Jenkins BS, Webb-Peploe MM (1977) Hemodynamic studies of beta blockade in hypertrophic obstructive cardiomyopathy. *Eur J Cardiol* 5:327–341
107. Speiser KW, Krayenbuehl HP (1981) Reappraisal of the effect of acute betablockade on left ventricular filling dynamics in hypertrophic obstructive cardiomyopathy. *Eur Heart J* 2:21–29

108. Hess OM, Grimm J, Krayenbuehl HP (1983) Diastolic function in hypertrophic cardiomyopathy: Effects of propranolol and verapamil on diastolic stiffness. *Eur Heart J* 4 (Suppl F): 47–56
109. Kaltenbach M, Hopf R, Kober G, Bussmann WD, Keller M, Person Y (1979) Treatment of hypertrophic obstructive cardiomyopathy with verapamil. *Br Heart J* 42:35–42
110. Rosing DR, Kent KM, Maron BJ, Epstein SE (1979) Verapamil therapy: A new approach to the pharmacologic treatment of hypertrophic cardiomyopathy, II: Effects on exercise capacity and symptomatic status. *Circulation* 60:1208–1213
111. Rosing DR, Condit JR, Maron BJ, et al. (1981) Verapamil therapy: a new approach to the pharmacologic treatment of hypertrophic cardiomyopathy, III: Effects of longterm administration. *Am J Cardiol* 48:545–553
112. Rosing DR, IdanpaanHeikkla U, Maron BJ, Bonow RO, Epstein SE (1985) Use of calcium channel blocking drugs in hypertrophic cardiomyopathy. *Am J Cardiol* 55:185B–195B
113. Bonow RO, Dilsizian V, Rosing DR, Maron BJ, Bacharach SL, Green MV (1985) Verapamil-induced improvement in left ventricular diastolic filling and increased exercise tolerance in patients with hypertrophic cardiomyopathy: Short- and long-term effects. *Circulation* 72:853–864
114. Bonow RO, Ostrow HG, Rosing DR, et al. (1983) Verapamil effects on left ventricular systolic and diastolic function in patients with hypertrophic cardiomyopathy: Pressure-volume analysis with a nonimaging scintillation probe. *Circulation* 68:1062–1073
115. Rosing DR, Kent KM, Borer JS, Seides SF, Maron BJ, Epstein SE (1979) Verapamil therapy: a new approach to the pharmacologic treatment of hypertrophic cardiomyopathy, I: Hemodynamic effects. *Circulation* 60:1201–1207
116. Bonow RO, Rosing DR, Epstein SE (1983) The acute and chronic effects of verapamil on left ventricular function in patients with hypertrophic cardiomyopathy. *Eur Heart J* 4 (Suppl F): 57–65
117. Anderson DM, Raff GL, Ports TA, Brundage BH, Parmley WW (1984) Hypertrophic obstructive cardiomyopathy: Effects of acute and chronic verapamil treatment on left ventricular systolic and diastolic function. *Br Heart J* 51:523–529
118. Hanrath P, Mathey DG, Kremer P, Sonntag F, Bleifeld W (1980) Effect of verapamil on left ventricular isovolumic relaxation time and regional left ventricular filling in hypertrophic cardiomyopathy. *Am J Cardiol* 45:1258–1264
119. Hanrath P, Schluter M, Sonntag F, Diemert J, Bleifeld W (1983) Influence of verapamil therapy on left ventricular performance at rest and during exercise in hypertrophic cardiomyopathy. *Am J Cardiol* 51:544–548
120. Hess OM, Murakami T, Krayenbuehl HP (1986) Does verapamil improve left ventricular relaxation in patients with myocardial hypertrophy? *Circulation* 74:530–543
121. Bonow RO, Vitale DF, Maron BJ, Bacharach SL, Frederick TM, Green MV (1987) Regional left ventricular asynchrony and impaired global filling in hypertrophic cardiomyopathy: Effect of verapamil. *J Am Coll Cardiol* 9:1108–1116
122. Lorell BH, Barry WH (1984) Effects of verapamil on contraction and relaxation of cultured chick embryo ventricular cells during calcium overload. *J Am Coll Cardiol* 3:341–348
123. Epstein SE, Rosing DR: Verapamil (1981) Its potential for causing serious complications in patients with hypertrophic cardiomyopathy. *Circulation* 64:437–441
124. Lorell BH, Paulus WJ, Grossman W, Wynne J, Cohn PF (1982) Modification of abnormal left ventricular diastolic properties by nifedipine in patients with hypertrophic cardiomyopathy. *Circulation* 65:499–507
125. Paulus WJ, Lorell BH, Craig WE, Wynne J, Murgo JP, Gorssman W (1983) Comparison of the effects of nitroprusside and nifedipine on diastolic properties in patients with hypertrophic cardiomyopathy: Altered left ventricular loading or impaired muscle inactivation? *J Am Col Cardiol* 2:879–886
126. Betocchi S, Cannon RO, Watson RM, et al. (1985) Effects of sublingual nifedipine on hemodynamics and systolic and diastolic function in patients with hypertrophic cardiomyopathy. *Circulation* 72:1001–1007

127. Nagao M, Yasue H, Omote S, et al. (1980) Diltiazem-induced decrease of exercise-elevated pulmonary artery pressure on hypertrophic cardiomyopathy patients. *Am Heart J* 102:789–790
128. Suwa M, Hirota Y, Kawamura K (1984) Improvement in left ventricular diastolic function during intravenous and oral diltiazem therapy inpatients with hypertrophic cardiomyopathy: an echocardiographic study. *Am J Cardiol* 54:1047–1053
129. Pollick C (1982) Muscular subaortic stenosis hemodynamic and clinical improvement after disopyramide. *N Engl J Med* 307:997–999
130. Pollick C, Detsky A, Ogilvie R, Wilansky S (1985) Disopyramide and propranolol in hypertrophic cardiomyopathy: Double-blind randomized trial. *Circulation* 72(Suppl III): III-155 (abstract)
131. Leon MB, Rosing DR, Maron BJ, Bonow RO, Lesko LJ, Epstein SE (1984) Amiodarone in patients with hypertrophic cardiomyopathy and refractory cardiac symptoms: An alternative to current medical therapy . *Circulation* 70 (Suppl II): II–18 (abstract)
132. Leon MB, Bonow RO, Tracy CM, Green MV, Bacharach SL, Rosing DR (1985) Amiodarone improves rapid diastolic filling in patients with hypertrophic cardiomyopathy. *Circulation* 72 (Suppl III): III–445 (abstract)
133. Sugrue DD, Dickie S, Myers MJ, Lavender JP, McKenna WJ (1984) Effect of amiodarone on left ventricular ejection and filling in hypertrophic cardiomyopathy as assessed by radionuclide angiography. *Am J Cardiol* 54:1054–1058
134. Paulus WJ, Nellens P, Heyndrickx GR, Andries E (1986) Effects of long-term treatment with amiodarone on excercise hemodynamics and left ventricular relaxation in patients with hypertrophic cardiomyopathy. *Circulation* 74:544–554
135. McKenna WJ, Harris L, Perez G, et al. (1981) Arrhythmia in hypertrophic cardiomyopathy, II: Comparison of amiodarone and verapamil in treatment. *Br Heart J* 46:173–178
136. McKenna WJ, Harris L, Rowland E, et al. (1984) Amiodarone for long-term management of patients with hypertrophic cardiomyopathy. *Am J Cardiol* 54:802–810
137. McKenna WJ, Oakley CM, Krikler DM, Goodwin JF (1981) Improved survival with amiodarone in patients with hypertrophic cardiomyopathy and ventricular tachycardia. *Br Heart J* 53:412–416
138. Sclarovsky S, Lewin RF, Kracoff O, Strasberg B, Arditti A, Agmon J (1983) Amiodarone-induced polymorphous ventricular tachycardia. *Am Heart J* 105:6–12
139. Harris L, McKenna WJ, Rowland E, Holt DW, Storey GCA, Krikler DM (1983) Side effects of long-term amiodarone therapy. *Circulation* 67:45–51
140. Coltart DJ, Meldrum SJ (1970) Hypertrophic cardiomyopathy: An electrophysiologic study. *Br Med J* 4:217–218
141. Ingham RE, Mason JW, Rossen RM, Goodwin DJ, Harrison DC (1978) Electrophysiologic findings in patients with idiopathic hypertrophic subaortic stenosis. *Am J Cardiol* 41:811–816
142. Kowley PR, Eisenberg R, Engel TR (1984) Sustained arrhythmias in hypertrophic obstructive cardiomyopathy. *N Engl J Med* 310:1566–1569
143. Anderson KP, Stinson EB, Derby GC, Oyer PE, Mason JW (1983) Vulnerability of patients with obstructive hypertrophic cardiomyopathy to ventricular arrhythmia induction in the operation room. *Am J Cardiol* 51:811–816
144. Maron BJ, Gaffney FA, Jeresaty RM, McKenna WJ, Miller WW (1985) Hypertrophic cardiomyopathy, other myopericardial diseases and mitral valve prolapse. [Bethesda Conference, No. 16: Cardiovascular abnormalities in the athlete: Recommendations regarding elgibility for competition.] *J Am Coll Cardiol* 6:1215–1217
145. Morrow AG, Reitz BA, Epstein SE, et al. (1975) Operative treatment in hypertrophic subaortic stenosis: Techniques, and the results of pre and postoperative assessment in 83 patients. *Circulation* 52:88–102
146. Agnew TM, BarrattBoyes BC, Brandt PWT, Roche AHG, Lowe JB, O'Brien KP (1977) Surgical resection in idiopathic hypertrophic subaortic stenosis with a combined approach through aorta and left ventricle. *J Thorac Cardiovasc Surg* 74: 307–316

147. Reis RL, Hannah H. Carley JE, Pugh DM (1977) Surgical treatment of idiopathic hypertrophic subaortic stenosis (IHSS): Postoperative results in 30 patients following ventricular septal myotomy and myectomy (Morrow procedure). *Circulation* 56 (Suppl II): II–128–132
148. Maron BJ, Merrill WH, Freier PA, Kent KM, Epstein SE, Morrow AG (1978) Long-term clinical course and symptomatic status of patients after operation for hypertrophic stenosis. *Circulation* 57: 1205–1213
149. Maron BJ, Epstein SE, Morrow AG (1983) Symptomatic status and prognosis of patients after operation for hypertrophic obstructive cardiomyopathy: Efficacy of ventricular septal myotomy and myectomy. *Eur Heart J* 4 (Suppl F): 175–185
150. Beahrs MM, Tajik AJ, Seward JB, Giuliani ER, McGoon DC (1983) Hypertrophic obstructive cardiomyopathy: 10–21 year follow-up after partial septal myectomy. *Am J Cardiol* 51: 1160–1166
151. Spirito P, Maron BJ, Rosing DR (1984) Morphologic determinants of hemodynamic state following ventricular septal myotomy-myectomy in patients with hypertrophic cardiomyopathy: M-mode and two-dimensional echocardiographic assesment. *Circulation* 70: 984–995
152. Schapira JN, Stemple DR, Martin RP, Rakowski H, Stinson EB, Popp RL (1978) Single and two-dimensional echocardiographic visualization of the effects of septalmyectomy in idiopathic hypertrophic subaortic stenosis. *Circulation* 58: 850–860
153. Bolton MR, King JF, Polumbo RA, et al. (1974) The effects of operation on the echocardiographic features of idiopathic hypertrophic subaortic stenosis. *Circulation* 50: 897–900
154. Redwood DR, Goldstein RE, Hirshfeld J. et al. (1979) Exercise performance after septal myotomy and myectomy in patients with obstructive hypertrophic cardiomyopathy. *Am J. Cardiol* 44: 215–220
155. Losse B, Kuhn H, Loogen F, Schulte HD (1983) Exercise performance in hypertrophic cardiomyopathy. *Eur Heart J* 4 (Suppl F): 197–208
156. Fighali S, Krajcer Z, Leachman RD (1984) Septal myomectomy and mitral valve replacement for idiopathic hypertropic subaortic stenosis: Short and long-term follow-up. *J Am Coll Cardiol* 3: 1127–1134
157. Bircks W, Schulte HD (1983) Surgical treatment of hypertrophic obstructive cardiomyopathy with special reference to complications and to atypical hypertrophic obstructive cardiomyopathy. *Eur Heart J* 4 (Suppl F): 187–190
158. Turina J, Jenni R, Krayenbuehl HP, Turina M, Rothlin M (1986) Echocardiographic findings late after myectomy in hypertrophic obstructive cardiomyopathy. *Eur Heart J* 7: 685–692
159. Wigle ED, Trimble AS, Adelman AG, Bigelow WG (1967) Surgery in muscular subaortic stenosis. *Prog Cardiovasc Dis* 11: 83–112
160. Shah PM, Gramiak R, Adelman AG, et al. (1972) Echocardiographic assesment of the effects of surgery and propranolol on the dynamics of outflow obstruction in hypertrophic subaortic stenosis. *Circulation* 45: 516–521
161. Henry WL, Clark CE, Griffith JM, et al (1975) Mechanism of left ventricular outflow obstruction in patients with obstructive asymmetric septal hypertrophy (idiopathic hypertrophic subaortic stenosis). *Am J Cardiol* 35: 337–345
162. Spirito P, Maron BJ (1983) Significance of left ventricular outflow tract cross-sectional area hypertrophic cardiomyopathy: A two-dimensional echocardiographic assesment. *Circulation* 67: 1100–1108

11. Antiarrhythmic therapy in heart failure*

J. BRACHMANN, C. SCHMITT, T. BEYER, B. WALDECKER, T. HILBEL, M. SCHWEIZER & W. KÜBLER

It has been well established that death due to progressive heart failure constitutes a major risk in cardiac patients. However, the exact mechanism of death remains subject to controversy. While the contribution of arrhythmias alone is questioned, the widely accepted fact is that most patients finally die due to malignant arrhythmias [1, 2, 3]. Even more doubts arise around the problem of drug therapy directed to suppress arrhythmias in patients with impaired ventricular function. The results of the CAST trial that are presented in this book elsewhere have contributed to doubts regarding the value of non-discriminative prophylactic therapy againstspontaneous ectopy guided by Holter monitoring [4]. In contrast, results of the consensus trial have supported the assumption that improvement of LV function by means of afterload reduction can improve the clinical outcome either by hemodynamic improvement alone or by direct antiarrhythmic action [5].

The experimental set-up to analyse the latter controversy more precisely consists of a conscious dog model which investigates the late postmyocardial infarction period 3 to 8 days after proximal ligation of the left anterior descending coronary artery. Details are described elsewhere [6]. The dogs were anesthetized by 30 mg/kg pentobarbital and a left thoracotomy was performed. The left anterior descending coronary artery was exposed and just distal of the septal artery a two-stage ligation was accomplished. Epicardial composite electrodes were fixed to record potentials from the infarct zone and adjacent normal myocardium to identify abnormal electrical activity potentially involved in reentrant arrhythmias. The thoracotomy was closed and the animals subsequently permitted to recover.

After 3 to 8 days, the animals were studied using recordings of the surface electrogram and the composite electrograms by means of programmed electrical stimulation. Induction of sustained ventricular tachycardia was repeated to demonstrate reproducibility unless external cardioversion had been employed

*This study was supported by the SFB 320 'Herzfunktion und ihre Regulation' with the Deutsche Forschungsgemeinschaft.

E. Andries & R. Stroobandt (eds.), Hemodynamics in Daily Practice, 159–166.

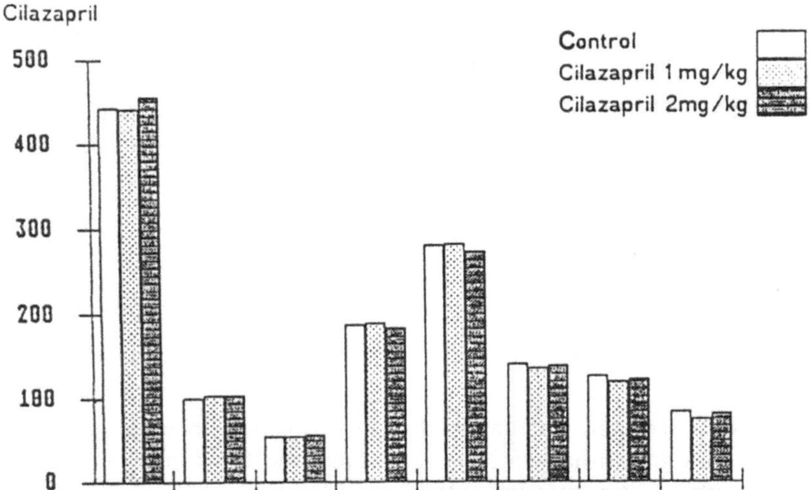

	CI-SR	PQ	QRS	QT	QTc	CI-SVT	BS•	BD•
Kon	442•15	99•8	53•3	186•5	280•7	141•17	126•8	83•9
Cil 1mg	440•14	102•9	53•2	188•5	282•6	134•8	119•14	74•12
Cil 2mg	455•17	103•9	54•2	183•10	272•11	139•15	122•8	81•13

values are in msec (mean ± SD), • = mmHg

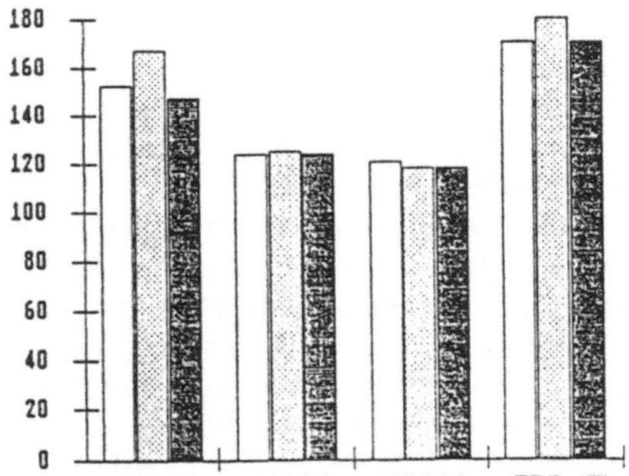

	AS300	VS330	VS250	ERP-IZ
Kon	152•26	124•8	121•8	170
Cil 1mg	167•20	125•7	118•7	180
Cil 2mg	147•27	124•8	118•7	170

values are in msec (mean ± SD)

Figure 1. Effect of the ACE inhibitor metabolite cilazaprilat 1 and 2 mg/kg in 10 conscious dogs in the late postmyocardial infarction period. All values are presented as mean ± SD, differences between the increasing doses of cilazaprilate were analyzed by analysis of variance. None of the electrophysiological parameters was significantly changed, while systolic and diastolic blood pressure significantly fell after application of cilazaprilat. Cl-SR, cycle length of sinus rhythm; PQ, PQ-interval; QRS, QRS interval; QT, QT interval; QT_c, QT_c interval corrected for sinus rate; CL-SVT, cycle length of the sustained ventricular tachycardia; BS, systolic blood pressure; BP, diastolic blood pressure; AS 300, atrial stimulation at 300 ms; VS 330, ventricular stimulation at 330 ms; VS 250, ventricular stimulation at 250 ms cycle length; ERP_{IZ}, effective refractory period of the infarct zone.

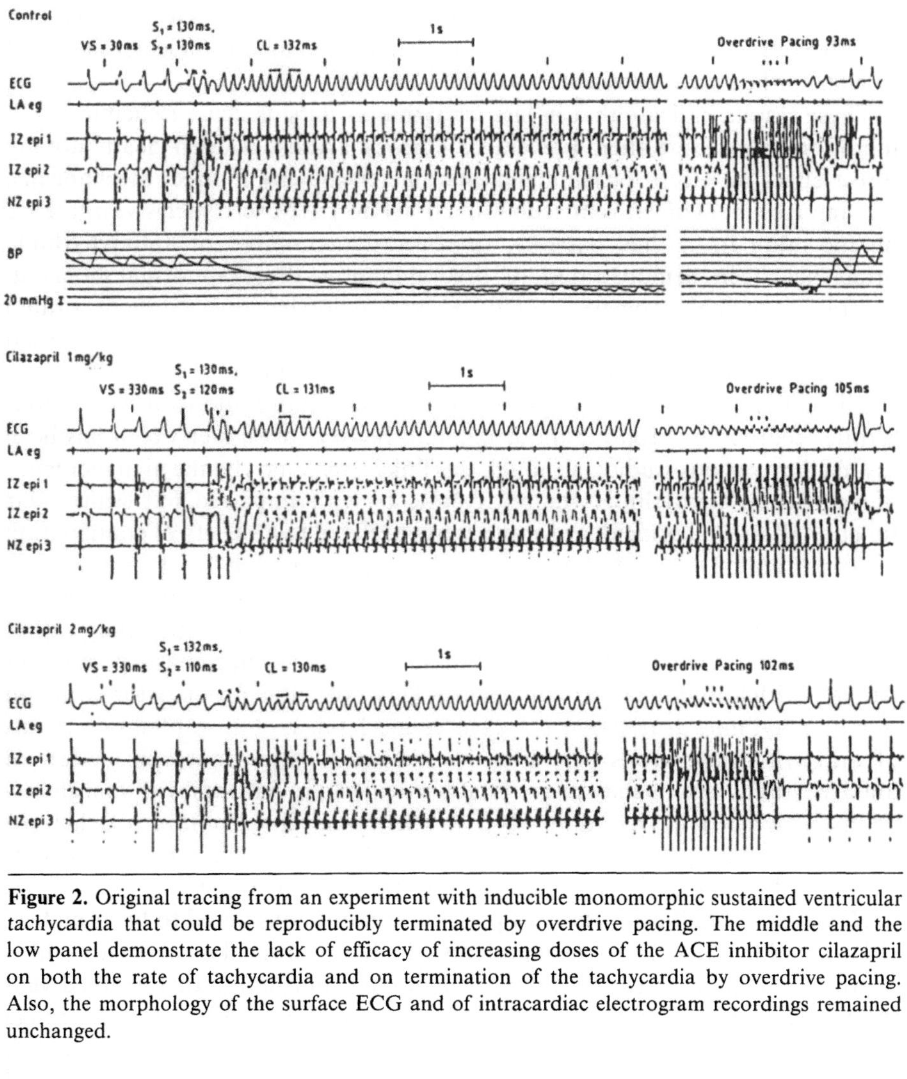

Figure 2. Original tracing from an experiment with inducible monomorphic sustained ventricular tachycardia that could be reproducibly terminated by overdrive pacing. The middle and the low panel demonstrate the lack of efficacy of increasing doses of the ACE inhibitor cilazapril on both the rate of tachycardia and on termination of the tachycardia by overdrive pacing. Also, the morphology of the surface ECG and of intracardiac electrogram recordings remained unchanged.

for termination of the arrhythmia. Thereafter, the new inhibitor of the angiotensin converting enzyme (ACE-inhibitor) cilazapril and its active metabolite cilazaprilat were administered intravenously at 1 and 2 mg/kg at different days. This dosis was found to be hemodynamically effective in earlier experiments. The results are summarized in Figure 1, and representative tracings are presented in Figure 2. In these experiments, no significant alteration of either electrophysiological parameters or inducibility of ventricular tachyarrhythmias was observed both by cilazapril and its active metabolite. Similar results were obtained in a dose-response curve recorded in action potentials from isolated preparations by means of standard microelectrode techniques.

All parameters including resting potential, action potential amplitude and duration at 50% and 90% repolarization, maximum upstroke velocity and effective refractory period did not exhibit a significant alteration when cilazapril or cilazaprilate were administered at 10^{-8}–10^{-4} M.

These results indicate that in late arrhythmias outside acute ischemia, ACE inhibitors may exert their preventive efficacy against sudden death not by direct effect on electrophysiological parameters but by indirect mechanisms, e.g., improvement of left ventricular function known to exert a decisive influence on mortality in cardiac patients. In contrast, a number of antiarrhythmic drugs has been demonstrated to predominantly affect abnormal fibers in contrast to normal myocytes [7]. This selective action has yet to be incorporated into clinical practice and may provide guidelines toward a more individual approach to antiarrhythmic drug therapy in cardiac failure.

Clinically, an association between the prevalence of spontaneous ventricular ectopy recorded by Holter monitoring and the risk for sudden death has been assumed by various studies, although this link is weakened by the high incidence of ventricular arrhythmias in most patients with impaired left ventricular function [8–10]. This incidence appears to be related to a variety of contributing factors (Table 1). No firm data have been presented so far to establish a correlation between reduction of ectopy by antiarrhythmic drugs and improvement of prognosis. The results of the above-mentioned CAST study rather suggest an extremely cautious use of these drugs in asymptomatic postinfarct patients with low grade ventricular ectopy [11]. Although proarrhythmic action of antiarrhythmic drugs is the most feared mechanism of unwanted side effects of antiarrhythmic drugs [12, 13], the known negative inotropic action of antiarrhythmic agents may prove fatal particularly in patients with marginally compensated left heart failure [14]. A schematic representation of this potentially vicious cycle is presented in Figure 3, while a comparison of hemodynamic effects of antiarrhythmic drugs is presented in Table 2.

However, a significant group of patients remains considered to be at highest risk for sudden death, e.g., such patients who have survived an aborted sudden death or emergency treatment due to ventricular fibrillation or sustained ventricular tachycardia. In this high risk group, annual mortality rates may range between 20 and 70% resulting overwhelmingly from sudden cardiac death [15]. This poor prognosis has prompted the aggressive use of programmed electrical stimulation to provoke the clinically documented arrhythmia by induction

Table 1. Some factors involved in the pathogenesis of arrhythmias in dilative cardiomyopathy.

1.	Mechanical factors (regional wall motion stress)
2.	Scarring
3.	High catecholamines (increased sympathetic outflow/high levels of circulating catecholamines)
4.	Electrolyte depletion: K^+ & Mg^{++}
5.	Drugs: Diuretics, Digitalis, Phosphodiesterase inhibitors, and Antiarrhythmic drugs

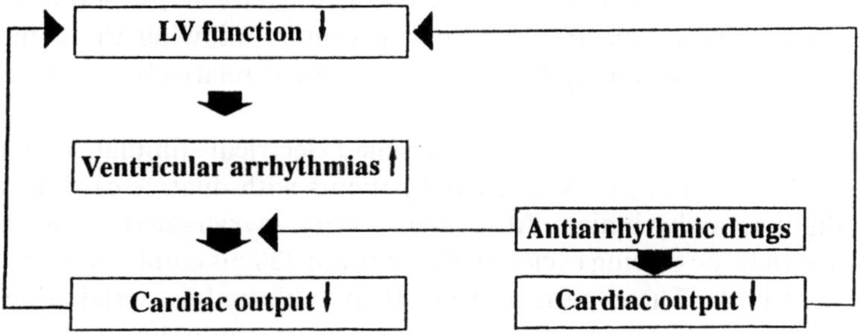

Figure 3. Schematic diagram representing the impossible benefici al and detrimental effects of antiarrhythmic drugs in patients with ventricular arrhythmias and heart failure.

Table 2. Schematic representation of the *hemodynamic effects* of antiarrhythmic drugs on inotropy, peripheral resistance and cardiac output.

Classification*			Intropy	Peripheral resistance	Cardiac output
I	A	Quinidine	↓	↓↓	ø–(↓)
		Disopyramide	↓↓	↑	↓↓
		Procainamide	↓	↓	(↓)
	B	Lidocaine	(↓)	ø	ø
		Mexiletine	(↓)	ø	ø–(↓)
	C	Propafenone	↓	ø	(↓)
		Flecanide	↓	ø–(↑)	(↓)
II		β-receptor antagonists	↓↓	ø–(↑)	↓↓
III		Amiodarone	(↓)	↓	ø
		Sotalol	↓	ø	↓
		d-Sotalol	ø–(↓)	ø	ø
IV		Ca antagonists	↓	↓	ø–(↓)

*Antiarrhythmic drugs are listed according to the classification by Vaughan Williams. Note that most antiarrhythmic drugs present a more or less negative inotropic action while effects on peripheral resistance and cardiac output may differ quite considerably.

of ventricular extrastimuli following a basic pacing train via temporary pacing catheters [16, 17].

The underlying concept is not only to investigate spontaneous ectopy occurring more frequently but most likely only triggering the malignant event but to analyze electrical properties of the arrhythmia substrate which is considered to provide in most patients conditions suitable for a sustained reentrant mechanism. The concept is to suppress susceptibility to malignant arrhythmias by altering the electrical parameters of the assumed reentrant circuit by directly investigating the influence of antiarrhythmic drugs. Because no drug has been shown to be effective in all patients, a serial approach is preferred by many electrophysiological centers allowing the comparative testing of various antiarrhythmic drugs within a relatively short period of time.

In order to test the efficacy of programmed electrical stimulation in patients with poor LV function, we studied 103 patients with dilative cardiomyopathy and malignant arrhythmias. All patients were investigated using a pacing protocol with basic driving cycles of 550, 400 and 330 ms employing a maximum of 3 extrastimuli. These patients were then subjected to serial drug testing consisting of the following antiarrhythmic drugs: quinidine (10 mg/kg iv), propafenone (3 mg/kg iv), mexiletine (5 mg/kg iv), d-Sotalol (1,5 mg/kg iv), flecainide (2 mg/kg iv), amiodarone (1 g/day for 10 days orally). After either intravenous or oral treatment, the exact protocol of programmed stimulation at control was repeated. Only if no sustained arrhythmia defined as lasting for at least 30 s or requiring termination because of hemodynamic side effects was induced, the drug was coined effective. Patients which remained inducible served as control group. The overall success rate according to the electrophysiological criteria was 58% of the patients in whom longterm antiarrhythmic therapy was initiated. The remaining patients received the antiarrhythmic agent that was causing the most prominent slowing of induced tachycardias, mostly amiodarone which was supplied at individual doses of 200 – 600 mg/d.

The clinical outcome between both groups which did not differ significantly with respect to age (53 ± 12 vs 55 ± 17, responders vs non-responders), ejection fraction (31 ± 13% vs 27 ± 16%) and clinical history is demonstrated in Table 3. The responders did significantly better with a lower recurrence rate while the nonresponder group was suffering from a high recurrence rate. Similarly, sudden death was lower in the nonresponder group (4%/year) than in the nonresponder group (18%/year). This result which is similar to other studies in patients with coronary artery disease can be interpreted in two ways. Firstly, the drugs may truely exert a beneficial action in preventing sudden death, with their individual efficacy established by programmed stimulation, while

Table 3. Prognosis of patients with delative cardiomyopathy using serial drug testing. Patients without suppression of inducibility had a significantly worse prognosis as compared to a patient who responded to at least one antiarrhythmic drug.

Group of patients	Prognosis	Rate %/year
Suppression of inducibility of VT/VF	Low rate of recurrence	6
	Low incidence of sudden death	4
No suppression of inducibility of VT/VF	High rate of recurrence	32
	High incidence of sudden death	18

the same group of drugs may simply fail or even exaggerate arrhythmias in the non-responder group. Secondly, this response to arrhythmias may just provide the selection criterium for patients with good and poor prognosis. This would imply that these patients could also do well when left without any antidysrhythmic therapy. However, no study has been presented as of now to corroborate this assumption but may be a fascinating project. One has to keep in mind, however, that all patients in this group already experienced one or more clinical episodes of malignant arrhythmias that were frequently aborted only by rather fortunate circumstances. Also, as mentioned before, most historical studies without antiarrhythmic drugs reported an extremely high mortality rate. However, not only antiarrhythmic regimens have changed but also medical therapy in general has been markedly improved most notably by indroduction of ACE inhibitors which already have been unequivocally shown to reduce mortality. Thus, the present use of antiarrhythmic drugs in patients with impaired cardiac function should be constrained to patients with documented high degree arrhythmias and may only serve to identify ineffective medication but may identify those who will benefit most either from cardiac transplant or implantable defibrillators with advanced antitachycardia function which may prevent sudden death in the highest risk group currently at the expense of major surgery and costs [18]. More research is required to finalize the role of drugs in this field for years to come.

REFERENCES

1. Packer M (1985) Sudden unexpected death in patients with congestive heart failure: A second frontier. *Circulation* 72: 681–685
2. Anderson KP, Freedman RA, Mason JW (1987) Sudden death in idiopathic cardiomyopathy. *Ann Intern Med* 107: 104–106
3. Von Ohlshausen K, Schafer A, Mehmel HC,Schwarz F, Senges J, Kübler W (1984) Ventricular arrhythmias in idiopathic dilated cardiomyopathy. *Br Heart J* 51: 195
4. The Cardiac Arrhythmia Suppression Trial (CAST) Investigators (1989) Preliminary report: effect of encainide and flecainide on mortality in a randomized trial of arrhythmia suppression after myocardial infarction. *N Engl L Med* 321: 406–412
5. The CONSENSUS Trial Study Group (1987) Effects of enalapril on mortality in severe congestive heart failure. Results of the Cooperative North Scandinavian Enalapril Survival Study (CONSENSUS). *N Engl Med* 316: 1429–1435
6. Brachmann J, Kabell G, Scherlag BJ, Harrison L, Lazzara R (1983) Analysis of inerectopic activation patterns during sustained ventricular tachycardia. *Circulation* 67: 449–456
7. Lazzara R, El-Sherif N, Hope RR, Scherlag BJ (1978) Ventricular arrhythmias and electrophysiological consequences of myocardial ischemia and infarction. *Circ Res* 42: 740–749
8. Dargie HJ, Cleland GF, Leckie BJ, Inglis CG, East BW, Ford I (1987) Relation of arrhythmias and electrolyte abnormalities to survival in patients with severe chronic heart failure. *Circulation* 75: IV–98
9. Meinertz T, Hofman T, Kasper W, Treese N, Bechtold H, Stienen U, Pop T, Leitner E-RV, Anderson D, Myer J (1984) Significance of ventricular arrhythmias in dilated cardiomyopathy: Observations in 35 patients. *Am J Cardiol* 51: 507
10. Wilson JR, Schwartz S, Sutton MS, Ferraro N, Horowitz LN, Reichek N, Josephson ME (1983) Prognosis in severe heart failure: Relation to hemodynamic measurements and

ventricular ectopic activity. *J Am Coll Cardiol* 2: 403

11. Francis GS (1988) Should asymptomatic ventricular arrhythmias in patients with congestive heart failure be treated with antiarrhythmic drugs? *J Am Coll Cardiol* 12: 274
12. Brachmann J, Aidonidis I, Schöls W, Senges J, Kübler W (1986) Paradoxical arrhythmogenic properties of antiarrhythmic drugs: Experimental and clinical finding. In: *Cardiac Arrhythmias*. Amsterdam: Elsevier
13. Minardo JD, Heger JJ, Miles WM, Zipes DP, Prystowsky EN (1988) Clinical characteristics of patients with ventricular fibrillation during antiarrhythmic therapy. *N Engl J Med* 319: 257
14. Woosley RL (1987) Pharmacokinetics and pharmacodynamics of antiarrhythmic agents in patients with congestive heart failure. *Am Heart J* 114: 1280
15. Wilbur DJ, Garan HS, Finkelstein D, Kelly E, Newell J, McGovern B, Ruskin JN (1988) Out-of-Hospital cardiac arrest, Use of electrophysiologic testing in the prediction of long term outcome. *N Engl J Med* 318: 19
16. Fisher JD, Cohen HL, Mehra R, et al (1977) Cardiac pacing and pacemakers, II: Serial electrophysiologic-pharmacologic testing for control of recurrent tachyarrhythmias. *Am Heart J* 93: 658–668
17. Josephson ME, Horowitz LN (1979) Electrophysiologic approach to therapy of recurrent sustained ventricular tachycardia. *Am J Cardiol* 43: 631–642
18. Tchou PJ, Kadri N, Anderson J, Caceres JA, Jazayeri M, Akhtar M (1988) Automatic implantable cardioverter defibrillators and survival of patients with left ventricular dysfunction and malignant ventricular arrhythmias. *Ann Intern Med* 109: 529

12 Non-invasive evaluation of cardiomyopathies

JOS R.T.C. ROELANDT, FOLKERT J. ten CATE &
GEORGE R. SUTHERLAND

No other diagnostic techniques than M-mode, two-dimensional, and Doppler echocardiography have had a more profound effect on the pathophysiologic understanding and clinical assessement of the cardiomyopathies. Cardiomyopathies are heart muscles diseases of unknown cause and are divided into dilated (congestive), hypertrophic, and restrictive types [1]. Despite progress in our understanding of the pathophysiology of these disorders has been striking, due in part to the use of Doppler echocardiography, the etiologies of these myocardial diseases remain elusive and our therapeutic approaches unsatisfactory. Nevertheless, the cardiomyopathies continue to be a subject of fascination and frustration. Since both the etiologic and pathophysiologic classification of cardiomyopathies based on clinical findings and haemodynamic evaluation are limited (Table 1), echo/Doppler by providing detailed information on altered structure and function plays a major role in both the diagnosis and follow-up of patients with cardiomyopathy.

Table 1. Classification of cardiomyopathies.

Classification	LV volume	LV EF	Heart failure
Dilated	↑↑	< 40%	Systolic function ↓
Restrictive	Nl or ↓	> 30–70%	Restriction to filling
Hypertrophic	Nl or ↓	45 – 95%	Resistance to filling

EF: ejection fraction; LV: left ventricle.

A. DILATED CARDIOMYOPATHY

1. Pathology of dilated cardiomyopathy

The most common of the idiopathic or primary cardiomyopathies is the dilated type. The heart in these patients shows dilatation of all cardiac chambers. Heart rate is increased while myocardial thickness is variable, increased in

E. Andries & R. Stroobandt (eds.), Hemodynamics in Daily Practice, 167–183.

some, and decreased or normal in others. The myocardium is pale and flabby. Scarring is grosly visable in about 20% at necropsy, despite absence of significant atherosclerotic coronary artery stenosis [2] and a mural thrombus is found in 60% of patients. The valve leaflets are intrinsically normal, while pure atrioventricular valve regurgitation is common (Table 2).

Table 2. Structural differences between cardiomyopathies.

	DCM	HCM	RCM
Dilated ventricular cavities	+	–	–
Dilated atrial cavities	+	+	+/–
Asymmetric septal hypertrophy	–	+	–
Increased heart weight	+	+	+/–
Ventricular scarring	–/+	–/+	–
Thickened MV	–	+	–/+
Plaque in LVOT	–	+	–

DCM: dilated cardiomyopathy; HCM: hypertrophic cardiomyopathy; LVOT: left ventricular outflow tract; MV: mitral valcve; RCM: restrictive cardiomyopathy.

Histologic examination shows non-specific findings of end-stage myocardial disease: interstitial and perivascular fibrosis, myocyte hypertrophy, and vacuolated cytoplasm. These non-specific degenerative findings have been accompanied by non-specific and negative immunohistochemical, ultrastructural and microbiologic studies [3]. It appears that the results of endomyocardial biopsy in patients with or suspected of having dilated cardiomyopathy are disappointing.

2. Echocardiography of dilated cardiomyopathy

M-mode and cross-sectional echocardiography allow to detect the presence and assess the severity of the dilation of all four cardiac chambers and provide quantitative assessment of left ventricular (LV) function [4]. An increased LV cavity dimension (greater than 5.6 cm at end-diastole) and a low fractional shortening (smaller than 25%) are found. Cross-sectional echocardiography is used to measure end-dialostic volume which is in excess of 80 ml/m^2. The left ventricular volumes correlate well with those obtained by LV contrast angiography. Left ventricular ejection fraction is readily determined from end-diastolic and end-systolic volumes. Thickening and amplitude of motion of the LV walls are reduced. Mean and peak velocities of dimensional shortening and lengthening are low and the duration of the rapid filling period is shorter than in normnals. The dilatation of the right ventricle which is present in all patients is more difficult to quantify because of its unusual geometry.

In the dilated left ventricle the mitral valve apparatus tends to remain close to the posterior wall and is stretched to an extent that valve mechanics are altered resulting in mitral regurgitation. In addition to the abnormal chordal tension due to lateral displacement of the papillary muscles as a result of

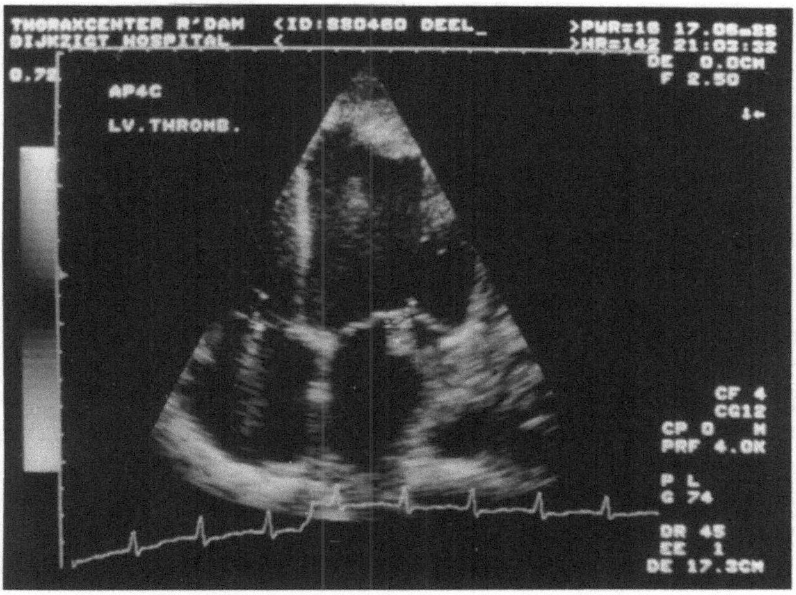

Figure 1. A systolic apical four chamber view of a patient with dilated cardiomyopathy. The left ventricular cavity is dilated and a 'swirling' intracavitary bloodflow pattern is visualised. This indicates slow blood flow as a result of a low output state. Note the apical thrombus. The jets recorded during systole posterior to the atrial ventricular valves indicate mitral and tricuspid regurgitation

progressive ventricular dilatation, the low cardiac output is another factor causing decreased amplitude of opening (less than 20 mm) of the mitral valve. An increased end-diastolic pressure is usually present and is reflected on the mitral valve echogram as a shortened PR-AC interval (less than 50 msec) interrupted by a 'B-notch'. The elevated end-diastolic pressure and mitral regurgitation when present lead to left atrial enlargement. Mural left ventricular thrombi often complicate dilated cardiomyopathy and are generally seen in the left ventricular apex (Figure 1) and occasionally in the right ventricular apex. Sensitivity and specificity of cross-sectional echocardiography for detecting intracavitary left ventricular thrombi is in excess of 90%. Thrombi may also be present in the left atrial appendage in patients with atrial fibrillation. These are best detected by transoesophageal cross-sectional echocardiography.

3. Doppler assessment of dilated cardiomyopathy

The flow velocity profile of the left ventricular outflow and aortic root has been used to assess LV systolic function in dilated cardiomyopathy [5]. The time to peak acceleration of the aortic flow velocity shows a progressive prolongation with decreasing systolic LV function. The duration of systolic flow and its magnitude are decreased reflecting a reduced stroke volume.

Doppler measurements of stroke volume has been estimated from flow velocity integral × the cross-sectional area of the aorta. The velocity profile across the aortic valve and planimetered aortic valve area or flow velocity across the left ventricular outflow tract and the measurement of its cross-sectional area just below the aortic valve are other approaches. Although the yield reliable estimates of stroke volume and cardiac output (Stroke volume × Heart rate), they have limited usefullnes for the diagnosis of dilated cardiomyopathy. They may be useful, however, to assess the short term effects of therapeutic interventions.

Transmitral diastolic inflow velocity provides an indirect measurement of the rate of left ventricular filling and hence its diastolic function. There is little usefull diagnostic information in the Doppler measurements, however, because they reflect an interplay of ventricular diastolic compliance and compensatory haemodynamic variables.

Doppler echocardiography provides objective evidence of the presence and severity of atrio-ventricular regurgitation. Colour flow imaging shows both mitral and tricuspid regurgitation as a mosaic-coloured jet entering into the left or right atrium (Figure 2). The severity of regurgitation can be determined semi-quantitatively by measuring the length, width, and area of the regurgitant

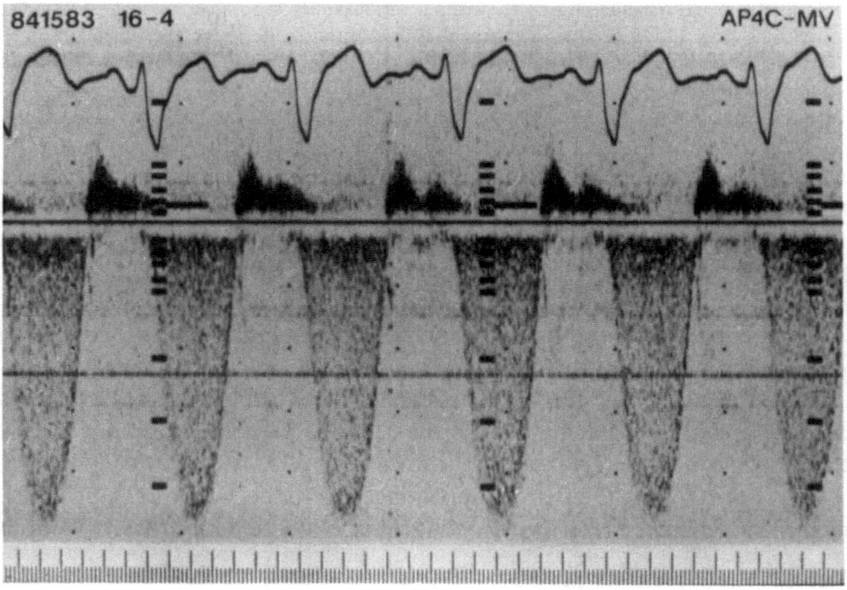

Figure 2. Doppler flow velocity recording of a patient with dilated cardiomyopathy, poor left ventricular function and moderate to severe mitral regurgitation recorded from the apical transducer position with continuous wave Doppler. The maximal velocity is approximately 4.5 m/s indicating a LV-LA pressure difference of about 80 mmHg. The slow rate of rise of the blood velocity curve indicates poor left ventricular function and is the equivalent of a low LV dP/dt. The rapid fall of velocity is consistent with a moderate to large volume regurgitation.

jet in orthogonal planes [6]. Poor left ventricular function is reflected in the low rate of rise of the velocity curve which is the equivalent of a low LV dP/dt. Colour flow imaging helps in determining the right heart pressures and allows the calculation of systolic pulmonary artery pressure from the peak tricuspid regurgitant velocity obtained by colour flow guided continuous wave Doppler interrogation. The transtricuspid systolic Doppler velocity measurement allows calculation of the maximal systolic right ventricular – right atrial pressure drop from the simplified Bernouilli equation: $4 \times (\text{max. velocity})^2$. This right heart pressure is estimated by adding the calculated transtricuspid systolic pressure drop to the estimated right atrial pressure [7, 8]. Similarly, the peak end-dialostic pulmonary regurgitant velocity can be used to determine the pulmonary artery diastolic pressure [9].

4. Clinical implications and problems

The echocardiographic syndrome of 'dilated cardiomyopathy' does not always correspond with the diagnosis of primary or idiopathic dilated cardiomyopathy. It is also found in patients with severe left ventricular dysfunction due to end-stage valvular heart disease or with coronary artery disease. Valvular heart disease is readily diagnosed or excluded by studying the valves. Diffuse wall motion abnormalities are in favour of a primary dilated cardiomyopathy, whereas segmental wall motion abnormalities are more often seen with coronary artery disease. The clinical context may be further helpful but in practice the diagnosis remains one of exclusion. Two important clinical problems remain: (1) Should all patients with a presumptive echo diagnosis of dilated cardiomyopathy undergo endomyocardial biopsy, and (2) Can dilated cardiomyopathy be reliably differentiated from heart failure due to ischemic heart disease by non-invasive investigation without resource to coronary arteriography? It appears that outside the academic institutions with a major research interest in cardiomyopathy or where cardiac transplantation is being carried out, routine endomyocardial biopsy in patients presenting with a clinical picture of dilated cardiomyopathy can hardly be justified.

Attempts to differentiate dilated cardiomyopathy from heart failure due to ischemic heart disease by non-invasive diagnostic methods have not been uniformly successful. It has been argued that this differentiation is academic because the degree of impairment of left ventricular function, irrespective of cause, is the major determinant of prognosis. However, their differentiation is critical for a research point of view. Considering the constraints of costs containment, the role of coronary arteriography must be, in routine practice, at the discretion of the individual clinician.

B. RESTRICTIVE CARDIOMYOPATHY

1. Pathology of restrictive cardiomyopathy

Infiltration or deposition of pathologic substances between myocardial cells and storage of deposits within cells are called infiltrative cardiomyopathies. The most commonly encountered infiltrative disease is amyloidosis (less common are sarcoidosis, neoplasm or mucopolysaccharidosis); whereas hemochromatosis is the most common storgae disease. Others are glycogen, and lipids. In both situations the disease process in its advanced stages results in restrictive hemodynamics. Thus, the terms infiltrative cardiomyopathy and restrictive cardiomyopathy are both used. The prototype and most common infiltrative disorder is cardiac amyloidosis. It is a multi-organ disease in which there is also deposition of the amyloid in the kidney, liver, nerves, skin and tongue [10]. In advanced cases the heart has a firm rubbery consistency and is mildly enlarged with thickened ventricular myocardium, valves, and enlarged atria (Table 2).

2. Echocardiography of restrictive cardiomyopathy

Cross-sectional echocardiography is the procedure of choice for non-invasive detection of cardiac amyloidosis [12]. There is a small or normal LV cavity size, markedly increased thickness of the LV walls with a highly abnormal and typical 'granular' texture appearance (Figure 3). The right ventricular free wall, interatrial septum, papillary muscles and cardiac valves show increased thickness. Left ventricular cavity size may increase while systolic

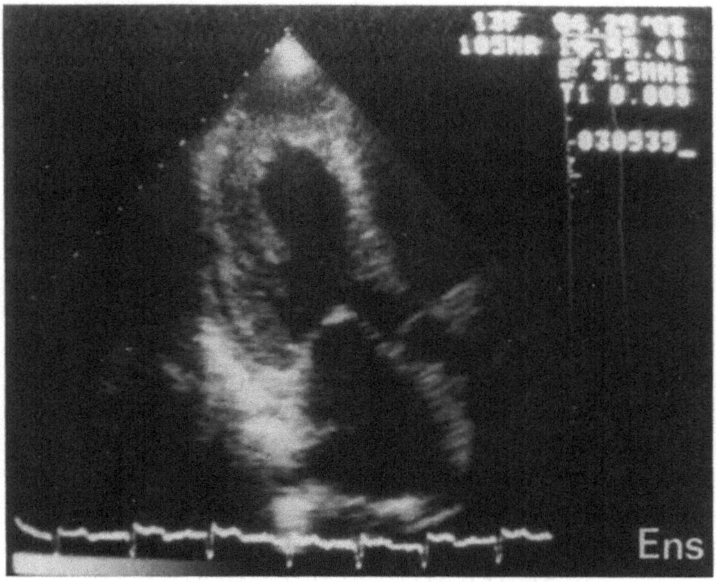

Figure 3. Apical long axis view of a patient with infiltrative cardiomyopathy due to amyloidosis. There is hypertrophy of the LV walls with a 'granular' texture aspect which during real-time has a 'sparkling' appearance.

function decreases in the more advanced stages. The atria are usually moderately enlarged and small to moderate pericardial effusion is common. In a series of 132 patients with biopsy proven systemic amyloidosis, LV mean wall thickness was inversely related with the degree of heart involvement and prognosis [13]. With progression of myocardial involvement, wall thickness increases, thickening decreases as well as the filling rate of the left ventricle.

3. Doppler assessment of restrictive cardiomyopathy

Atrio-ventricular (and semilunar) valve thickening is a frequent finding both at autopsy and echocardiographic examination and is readily detected by Doppler examination. Mild atrio-ventricular regurgitation is common. The major hemodynamic problem of cardiac amyloidosis, however, is impairment of diastolic function leading or restrictive hemodynamics. Restriction to filling is defined as rapid completion of filling as a result of a poorly compliant ventricle early in diastole, with little or no further filling in late diastole. Typically, there is normal or variably depressed systolic function, and a normal LV cavity size. restrictive hemodynamics occurs to a variable degree in many conditions other than restrictive cardiomyopathy and is present in advanced cardiac disease with fibrosis, coronary artery disease, hypertensive heart disease,

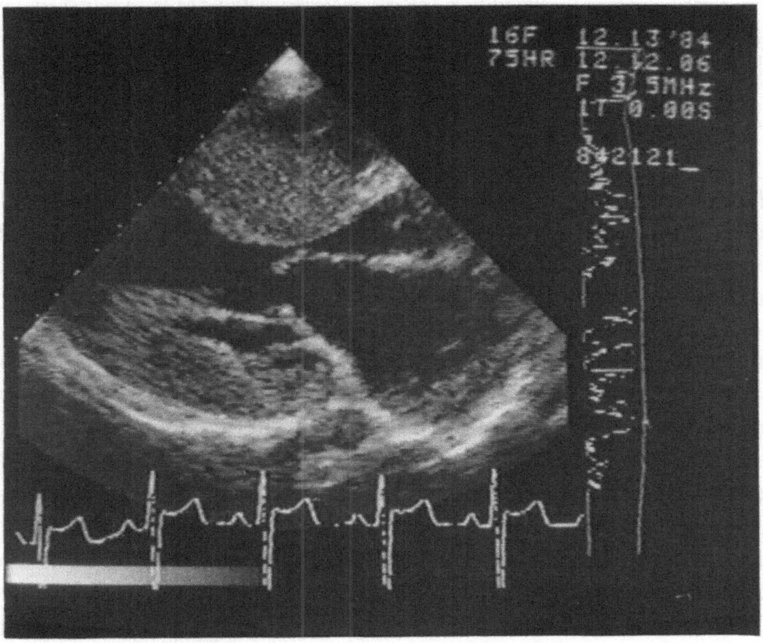

Figure 4. Long axis view of the heart recorded at end-diastole of a patient with hypertrophic obstructive cardiomyopathy and the classical basal septal localisation of the asymmetrical hypertrophy. Note the discrepancy between the thickness of the basal part of the interventricular septum and the left ventricular posterior wall.

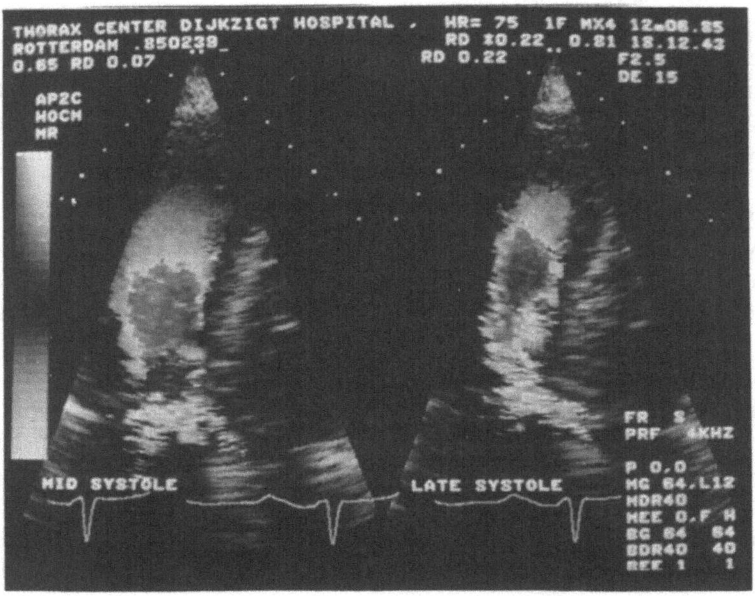

Figure 5. Colour flow maps (represented in black and white) of a patient with hypertrophic obstructive cardiomyopathy. Blood flow velocity increases within the left ventricular cavity and aliasing is seen at mid ventricular level. In mid systole (*left panel*) there is turbulence in the left ventricular outflow tract and mitral regurgitation. In late systole (*right panel*) there are still high velocities with aliasing at mid ventricular level and turbulence in the outflow tract and aorta. Mitral regurgitation has ceased.

etc. Doppler echocardiography has greatly enhanced our understanding of diastolic hemodynamics and function of the left ventricle [14]. Primary restrictive cardiomyopathies, most commonly manifest with their restrictive diastolic filling pattern (Figure 4). This is in contradistinction to the secondary restrictive disorders which initially present with abnormal relaxation hemodynamics (Figure 5). When these secondary disorders progress to a compensatory stage of dilatation, hypertrophy, etc. the diastolic filling patterns normalize (pseudo-normalization), and ultimately change to a restrictive pattern. Thus, it appears that advanced stages of coronary artery disease, hypertensive heart disease, hypertrophic cardiomyopathy demonstrate similar restrictive hemodynamics as is found in restrictive cardiomyopathy. Constrictive hemodynamics have been studied by Doppler echocardiography and have features distinctly different from those of restriction [15]. Restriction and constriction may coexist in the same patient, and clinical and cardiac catherization differentiation have been less than ideal. Restriction (intrinsic) hemodynamics are characterized by rapid early completion of diastolic filling. Constriction (extrinsic) hemodynamics are characterized by a phasic alteration of diastolic filling best appreciated in relationship to the respiratory cycle.

Characteristically, in the presence of constrictive physiology, left ventricular filling and ejection volume are diminished with inspiration while right ventricular filling and ejection are increased. Thus it appears that Doppler echocardiography offers a non-invasive means of accurately recognising and differentiating from constrictive hemodynamics. Colour Doppler flow imaging has limited value for the differentiation between restrictive hemodynamics and abnormal relaxation. The method is superior, however, for the detection of atrioventricular and semilunar valve regurgitation, which are common.

4. Clinical implications and problems

Restrictive cardiomyopathy is still a poorly understood disease. There is a spectrum of abnormalities in these disorders, which reflect both the stage and the duration of heart involvement. Common diseases such as coronary artery disease, hypertensive heart disease may develop restrictive hemodynamics and ressemble restrictive cardiomyopathy. Doppler echocardiography offers the potential to study the specific diastolic pathophysiologic aspects of disorders with restrictive hemodynamics. Elderly patients presenting with atrial fibrillation may have restrictive hemodynamics which has been termed 'senile restrictive disease'. They have normal to mildly depressed systolic function with very slow progression and a good prognosis [16].

C. HYPERTROPHIC CARDIOMYOPATHY

1. Pathology of hypertrophic cardiomyopathy

Hypertrophic cardiomyopathy presents diagnostic challenges to the pathologist. The single most striking and consistent characteristic finding is a hypertrophic non-dilated ventricle in the absence of a heart or systemic disease than can produce LV hypertrophy. Both the site and extent of hypertrophy are important in determining disease manifestations in hypertrophic cardiomyopathy. Asymmetrical hypertrophy of the left ventricle is present in 95% of patients, with septal hypertrophy by far the most common form (95%). In the obstructive form an uncommon variant of hypertrophic cardiomyopathy has been described in which the hypertrophy is confined to the distal portion of the left ventricle, known as apical hypertrophic cardiomyopathy. A fibrotic endocardial lesion just below the aortic valve on the interventricular septum may be present, representing the morphologic equivalent of systolic anterior motion of the mitral valve. Many patients have pure mitral regurgitation. This results form anterior displacement of the antero-lateral and postero-medial papillary muscles, preventing normal mitral leaflet coaptation. Thickened mitral valve leaflets are present in the large majority of patients and may lead to mitral valve prolapse. Quantitative histologic studies have demonstrated distinctive abnormalities in both the obstructive and non-obstructive types of hypertrophic cardiomyopathy and marked ventricular septum fibre disarray is a highly sensitive (86%) and specific (92%) marker (Table 2) [17].

Abnormally thickened intramural coronary arteries were demonstrated in 40 of 48 necropsy patients with hypertrophic cardiomyopathy [18].

2. Echocardiography of hypertrophic cardiomyopathy

Echocardiography is a reliable and certainly the best clinical method to detect the structural abnormalities of hypertrophic cardiomyopathy. A ratio of basal septal thickness to that of the LV posterior wall in the posterobasal region of 1.3 or greater has been reported to be diagnostic for the condition (Figure 4). It should be emphasized that identification of the right side of the interventricular septum (IVS) may be difficult demonstration of asymmetric septal hypertrophy is a sensitive but not a specific marker for the diagnosis of primary hypertrophic cardiomyopathy as it may be found in other conditions.

Table 3. Clinical conditions simulating HCM.

Hypertensive heart disease
Coronary artery disease
Severe aortic stenosis
Coarctation of the aorta
Subaortic stenosis
Chronic hemodyalisis
Endocrine disorders (hyper-, hypothyreoidism, acromegaly, diabetes)

The prevalence of a ratio of IVS/free wall thickness of 1.3 or greater in a general hospital population with heart disease, but without proven cardiomyopathy, is 8% [19]. Fractional and peak reates of thickening of the IVS are decreased while the same parameters of the LV free wall are increased, resulting in a normal or increase overall systolic LV function. The variability of the spectrum of LV dysfunction is better appreciated when diastolic function parameters are considered. Because of the hypertrophy and structural myocardial changes relaxation is prolonged and the resistance to filling increased. Peak left ventricular filling rate is reduced (reflected in a decreased early diastolic closure rate of the aML) and the duration of the early diastolic filling period is prolonged in some patients. Angina pectoris is common in patients with prolonged early diastolic relaxation, as a result of a functional obstruction to inflow in otherwise normal epicardial coronary arteries in addition to the thickened intramural coronary arteries [18]. Angina pectoris might therefore be used as a clinical indicator of severe diastolic LV dysfunction.

Other echocardiographic features of hypertrophic cardiomyopathy are narrowing of the LVOT and the small LV size. To determine the actual shape of the LV and the pattern and extent of myocardial hypertrophy in HCM, two-dimensional echocardiography is the best method. Asymmetrical left ventricular hypertrophy is present in 95% of HCM patients. Four patterns of distribution of hypertrophy can be identified when the parasternal short axis view at mitral valve level is used [20].

Type I: About 10% of patients have myocardial hypertrophy of the IVS confined to its anterior portion. This pattern of local hypertrophy is also seen in about 10% of patients where septal hypertrophy is equal in basal and apical regions.

Type II: In 20% myocardial hypertrophy involves both the anterior and posterior segments of the IVS whereas the LV free wall is essentially normal.

Type III: Most HCM patients (50%) have hypertrophy involving substantial portions of both the IVS and LVPW. Predominant regions of hypertrophy are the anterior or posterior parts of the IVS. These patients have a higher prevalence of obstruction of LV outflow.

Type IV: In this type different of the IVS are involved such as the posterior segment or the apical region of the LV wall. Some patients have hypertrophy only confined to portions of the antero-lateral LV free wall.

It is obvious that in patients in whom there is clinical suspicion of HCM but failure of the M-mode echocardiogram to demonstrate signs of HCM a thorough two-dimensional echocardiographic analysis is mandatory. Among patients with HCM, the thickness of the IVS is not dependent on the presence of LVOT obstruction at rest, and, indeed, IVS thickness is similar in patients with LVOT obstruction at rest and those without. Examination of the basal portion of the LV free wall may permit delineation of these two groups of patients since in the non-obstructive group, the posterolateral basal portion of the LV wall behind the mitral valve is not only thinner than the IVS but also thinner than the LV wall below the tips of the mitral valve. This is contrary to the normal LV and the LV of patients with hypertrophic obstructive cardiomyopathy, where this posterobasal portion fo the LV wall represents the thickest part of the free wall and decreases in thickness form base to apex.

Hypertrophic cardiomyopathy is hemodynamically classified in obstructive and nonobstructive types (Table 4). The subaortic pressure difference in the obstructive type results from LVOT obstruction caused by mitral leaflet septal contact. Colour Doppler flow imaging has revealed an 'ejection-obstruction-regurgitation sequence' during systole [22, 23]. During early systole, there is a rapid, unobstructed ejection of blood from LV into aorta. This rapid ejection through a narrow LVOT results in Venturi forces acting on the mitral valve leaflets to cause systolic anterior motion (SAM). The resulting mitral leaflet – septal contact results in LVOT obstruction and mitral regurgitation (Figure 6) changes in LV contractility and afterload result in changes in magnitude of the LVOT pressure difference and the degree of mitral regurgitation by affecting early systolic ejection velocity, thus altering Venturi forces and hence the degree and duration of SAM. The earlier in systole SAM occurs, the larger the LVOT pressure difference (and mitral regurgitation) and vice-versa [24].

As hypertrophic obstructive cardiomyopathy is a functional disease, SAM may be labile and observed intermittently (e.g. in post-extrasystolic complexes)

Table 4. Hypertrophic cardiomyopathy (HCM) – Hemodynamic classification.

Obstructive (HOCM):	
Systolic pressure gradient across LVOT due to septal-mitral leaflet contact	
Persistent:	Gradient at rest
Labile:	Spontaneously variable
Latent:	Can be provoked
Non-obstructive:	
No pressure gradient at rest or on provocation across LVOT	

H(O)CM: hypertrophic (obstructive) cardiomyopathy; LV: left ventricle; LVOT: left ventricular outflow tract.

or may be latent and evoked by amylnitrate or Valsalva maneuver. On two-dimensional images, SAM is best visualized in the apical long axis view. It is important to differentiate true from pseudo SAM patterns. True SAM demonstrates independent motion which cannot be related to any motion of a structure posterior to it. The anterior mitral leaflet (aML) returns to a closed position at the end of systole before the aortic valve closes. It might therefore be helpful to have the carotid artery tracing or phonocardiogram recorded simultaneously. It should be mentioned that SAM does not always involve the middle part of the aML but may be more pronounced at the level of the chordae or even at its upper part.

SAM may be observed in other conditions than obstructive hypertrophic cardiomyopathy such as aortic stenosis and incompetence, fixed subaortic stenosis, coarctation of the aorta, and in hypercontractile states especially when associated with hypovolemia. Confusing patterns may be seen in the mitral valve prolapse syndrome and in conditions with hyperactivity of the LVPW (e.g., RV volume overload). False SAM is sometimes seen with the swinging heart syndrome in large pericardial effusion. The combination of ASH, a narrow LVOT and SAM are also not a 100% specific for hypertrophic obstructive cardiomyopathy and may exceptionally be seen in restrictive cardiomyopathy.

Echocardiographically, one may seen an increased reflectivity of the mural septal endocardium at the level of the LVOT representing a fibrous plaque. This plaque originates at the areas where the aML touches the IVS and is the anatomic equivalent of SAM. The abnormal LV cavity shape is best recognized by two-dimensional echocardiography. Other echocardiographic findings may be found: (1) increased left atrial size as a response to the impaired LV filling and mitral regurgitation, (2) partial systolic closure of the aortic valve cusps, resulting from decreased forward aortic flow in mid-late systole. A similar pattern can be seen on the pulmonary valve and is related to muscular obliteration of the right ventricular infundibulum during systole. Echocardiography is the method of choice to follow patients with HCM longitudinally in the natural course of their disease and can also be used to determine the effect of therapeutic interventions, considering that a combination of echocardiographic signs rather than a single feature is diagnostic for HCM [25]. Salient echocardiographic features of hypertrophic (obstructive) cardiomyopathy are given in Table 5.

Table 5. Echocardiographic diagnosis of H(O)CM.

Asymmetric LV hypertrophy	Thickened mitral valve
Mural septal plaque	Systolic anterior motion of mitral valve
Abnormal cavity shape	LA dilatation
LV outflow tract dimension	Mid-systolic aorta valve closure

LA: left atrium; LV: left ventricle.

After a myotomy-myectomy an enlarged LVOT van be demonstrated echocardiographically, and the actual excision of septal muscle can be visualized in both the parasternal and apical long axis views. SAM does not always disappear, however.

3. Doppler assessment of hypertrophic cardiomyopathy

Many of the systolic and diastolic function abnormalities of hypertrophic cardiomyopathy are present in other conditions causing hypertrophy of the left ventricle. Doppler echocardiography has substantially added to our understanding of the pathophysiology of these hypertrophic conditions (Table 6).

Table 6. Doppler findings in H(O)CM.

LVOT pressure difference (dynamic)
Mitral regurgitation
Decrease aorta flow velocity in mid-late systole
Transmitral flow velocity
Impaired LV relaxation pattern: prolonged IRP
increased resistance to filling (low E velocity, increased DT, increased A velocity)
Restrictive filling pattern (end-stage): shortened IRP
increased E velocity, decreased DT, decreased A velocity

DT: deceleration time; IRP: isovolumic relaxation time; LVOT: left ventricular outflow tract.

We learned from cross-sectional cardiomyopathy that the systolic function is hyperdynamic frequently obliterating the left ventricular cavity in end-systole. Ejection is rapid, but ejection time is prolonged and an outflow tract gradient may be present. We have already discussed the information obtained for 'ejection-obstruction-regurgitation sequence' during systole [22, 23]. Systolic intracavitary flow dynamics are well demonstrated with colour Doppler flow imaging (Figure 5). During early systole, velocities accelerate in the mid ventricular region and result in aliasing with resultant colour reversal in this region. This is followed by LVOT obstruction as a result of systolic anterior

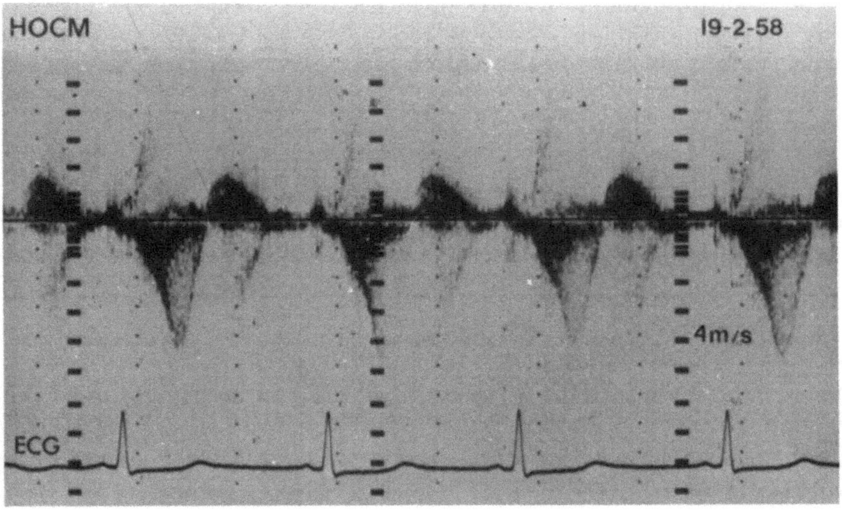

Figure 6. Continuous wave Doppler recording of blood flow velocity in the left ventricular outflow tract representing dynamic obstruction with a late systolic peak velocity of approximately 4.5 m/s representing a calculated maximal pressure difference of 80 mmHg within the outflow tract.

motion on the anterior mitral valve leaflet and a mosaic colour is seen in the area of the outflow tract obstruction. Once the area of increased flow velocities and turbulence have been identified by colour Doppler flow imaging, continuous wave Doppler interrogation allows measurement of the LVOT pressure difference (Figure 6). The velocity profile is characteristic of dynamic outflow tract obstruction. By using continuous wave Doppler intraoperatively, Stewart et al. [24] have provided further support for the notion that the LVOT pressure difference measured by Doppler represents true obstruction by demonstrating the direct relationship between a pressure drop invasively determined simultaneously with Doppler measured flow velocity at the site of obstruction. Mitral regurgitation is seen as a mosaic colour jet in the left atrium during systole (Figure 5). The severity of the mitral regurgitation is also variable and correlates directly with the severity of LVOT obstruction. Because both the LVOT obstruction and mitral regurgitation are dynamic, the dynamics can be altered by manoeuvres which accutely change the preload and afterload or when premature ectopic beats are present (Figure 7). Of course, medical therapy also will change these dynamics. These dynamic changes are best evaluated by Doppler techniques.

Left ventricular hypertrophic results in increased chamber stiffness and impaired relaxation of the left ventricle. The factors affecting diastolic filling are complex and are extensively described in a recent review [22]. Diastolic filling abnormalities include prolongation of the isovolumic relaxation period, delayed and reduced early diastolic filling and velocity, increased deceleration

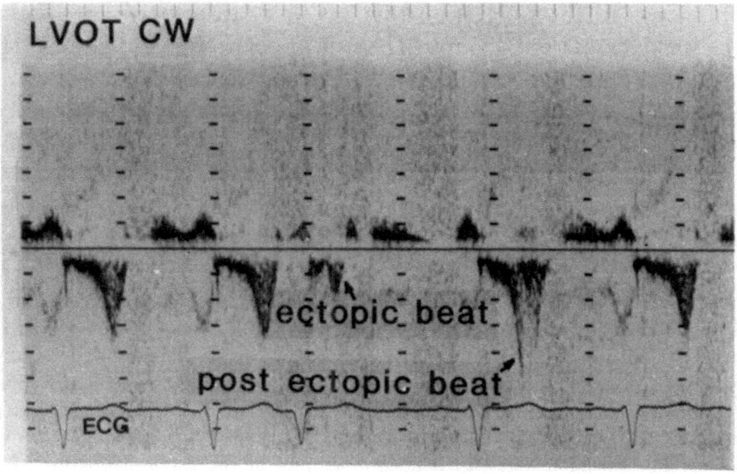

Figure 7. Maximal blood flow velocities in the left ventricular outflow tract (LVOT) are recorded with continuous wave Doppler in a patient with hypertrophic obstructive cardiomyopathy and premature ectopic beats. The velocity is 3.2 m/s representing a calculated pressure difference across the left ventricular outflow tract of 40 mmHg. With the premature ectopic beat a lower velocity is recorded and in the following beat the velocity is increased to approximately 5 m/s, yielding a pressure difference in the LVOT of 100 mmHg.

time, and an increased atrial systolic velocity and flow. This pattern, however, is highly variable since its results by a complex interplay of factors which affect relaxation and stiffness. Mitral regurgitation had confounding effects as well as age and heart rate. When the disease progresses, a restrictive filling pattern may become apparent (see Doppler assessment of restrictive cardiomyopathy).

4. Clinical implications and problems

Echocardiography and Doppler studies are invaluable in the detection and management of patients with hypertropohic cardiomyopathy, since virtually all aspects of the disorder can be evaluated. All patients should undergo complete M-mode, cross-sectional, standard Doppler and colour Doppler flow imaging studies to define the extent of hypertrophy, the hemodynamic subgroup, quantitation of left ventricular outflow obstruction, mitral regurgitation and the assessment of diastolic function. The pathophysiologic abnormalities caused by left ventricular hypertrophy and, in particular, to the diastolic dysfunction, have indicated the wide heterogenecity within a given clinical setting although abnormal left ventricular relaxation prevails in most patients. Hypertrophic cardiomyopathy has been reported with increasing frequency in the elderly and presents with a much broader spectrum of septal morphologic abnormalities and a greater symmetrical LV hypertrophy resulting in a large variability of LV shape [26, 27]. Nair et al. demonstrated that mitral annulus calcification increases with age, is independent of coronary artery disease and is more often accompanied by cardiac conduction disturbances [28]. This leads to the suggestion that HCM of the elderly is different from HCM in younger patient groups. Thus, it appears that the clinical spectrum of HCM grows more and more diverse, including heterogenicity of age, natural history, mitral valve structure, type of LV hypertrophy, electrophysiology abnormalities, and progression of severity.

REFERENCES

1. Report of the World health Organisation WHO/ISFC (1980) Task force on the definition and classification of cardiomyopathies. *Br Heart J* 44:672–673
2. Roberts WC (1976) The structural basis of abnormal cardiac function: A look at coronary, hypertensive, valvular, idiopathic myocardial, and pericardial heart disease, pp. 1–56 in: HJ Levine (ed.) , *Clinical Cardiovascular Physiology*. Orlando, Fla.: Grune & Stratton
3. Waller BF (1988) Pathology of the cardiomyopathies. *J Am Soc Echo* 1:4–19
4. Ten Cate FJ, Roelandt J (1983) Echocardiography of the cardiomyopathies: Congestive, hypertrophic and restrictive types, pp. 157–172 in J. Roelandt (ed.), *The Practice of M-mode and Two-dimensional Echocardiography*. The Hague/Boston: Martinus Nijhoff Publishers (Kluwer Academic Publishers) (DICM 23)
5. Gardin JM, Serie LT, Alkayam U, et al. (1983) Evaluation of dilated cardiomyopathy by pulsed Doppler echocardiography. *Am Heart J* 10:1057–65
6. Frederick H, Nanda NN, Hsiung M, et al. (1987) Colour Doppler assessment of mitral regurgitation with orthogonal planes. *Circulation* 75:175–183
7. Hatle L, Angelsen B (1985) pp 170–174 in: *Doppler Ultrasound in Cardiology: Physical Principles and Clinical Applications*, 2nd ed. Philadelphia: Lea & Febiger
8. Curry PJ, Seward JB, Chan KL, et al. (1985) Continuous wave Doppler determination of right ventricular pressure: A simultaneous Doppler-catheterization study in 127 patients. *J Am Coll Cardiol* 6:750–6
9. Masuyana T. Kodoma K, Kitabatake A, et al. (1986) Continuous wave Doppler echocardiography detection of pulmonary regurgitation and its applications to non-invasive estimation of pulmonary artery pressure. *Circulation* 74:484–92
10. Smith TJ, Kyle RA, Lie JT (1984) Clinical significance of histo-pathologic pattern of cardiac amyloidosis. *Mayo Clin Proc* 59:547–55
11. Roberts WC, Waller BF (1983) Kijack amyloidosis causing kijack dysfunction: Analysis of 54 necropsy patients. *Am J Cardiol* 52:137–46
12. Sequieira-Fiho AG, Cunha LP, Tajik AJ, et al. (1981) M-mode and two-dimensional echocardiographic features in cardiac amyloidosis. *Circulation* 63:188–96
13. Cueto-Garcia L, Reeder GS, Kyle RA, et al. (1985) Echocardiographic findings in systemic amyloidosis: Spectrum of cardiac involvement and relation to survival. *J Am Coll Cardiol* 6:737–43
14. Appleton CP, Hatle LK, Popp RL (1988) Demonstration of restrictive ventricular physiology by Doppler echocardiography. *J Am Coll Cardiol* 11:757–68
15. Appleton CP, Hatle LK, Popp RL (1988) Cardiac tamponade and pericardial effusion: Respiratory variation in transvalcular flow velocities studied by Doppler echocardiography. *J Am Coll Cardiol* 11:1020–30
16. Seward JB (1988) Restrictive cardiomyopathy: The assessment of definitions and diagnosis. *Cur Op Cardiol* 3:391–5
17. Marron BJ, Sato BN, Roberts WC, et al. (1979)Quantitative analysis of cardiac muscle cell disorganisation in the ventricular septum: Comparison of fetusses and infants with and without congenital heart disease and patients with hypertrophic cardiomyopathy. *Circulation* 60:685–96

18. Marron BJ, Wolfson JK, Ebstein ES, et al. (1986) Intramural ('small vessel') coronary artery disease in hypertrophic cardiomyopathy. *J Am Coll Cardiol* 8:545–57
19. Ten Cate FJ, Hugenholtz PG, van Dorp WG, et al. (1979) Prevalence of diagnostic abnormalities in patients with genetically transmitted asymmetric septal hypertrophy. *Am J Cardiol* 43:731
20. Maron BJ, Gottdiener JS, Epstein S (1982) Patterns and significance of distribution of left ventricular hypertrophy in assessment of cardiomyopathy. *Am J Cardiol* 48:418
21. DeMaria AN, Bommer W, Lee J, et al. (1980) Value and limitations of two-dimensional echocardiography in assessment of cardiomyopathy. *Am J Cardiol* 46:1224
22. Wigle ED, Sasson Z, Henderson MA, et al. (1985) Hypertrophic cardiomyopathy: The importance of the site and teh extent of hypertrophy. A review. *Prog Cardiovasc Dis* 28:1–83
23. Wigle ED (1987) Hypertrophic cardiomyopathy: A 1987 viewpoint. *Circulation* 75:311–22
24. Stewart WJ, Schiavone WA, Salcedo EE, et al. (1987) Intraoperative Doppler echocardiography in hypertrophic cardiomyopathy: Correlations with the obstructive gradient. *J Am Coll Cardiol* 10:327–35
25. Grimer PF, Mayewski RJ, Mushkin AI, et al. (1981) Selection and interpretation of diagnostic tests and procedures. *Ann Int Med* 94 (suppl):581
26. Whiting RB, Powell WJ, Dinsmore RE, Saunders CA (1971) Idiopathic hypertrophic subaortic stenosis in the lederly. *N Engl J Med* 285:196–200
27. Cooper MM, Mclntosh CL, Tucker ER, Clark RE (1987) Operation for hypertrophic subaortic stenosis in the aged. *Ann Thorac Surg* 44:370–78
28. Nair CK, Kudesia V. Hansen D, Thomson W, Pagano T, Ryschon K, Sketch MH (1987) Echocardiographic and electrocardiographic characteristics of patients with hypertrophic cardiomyopathy with and without mitral annular calcium. *Am J Cardiol* 59:1428–30

13. Can ultrasound reliably predict acute rejection in heart transplant recipients?

H. F. J. MANNAERTS,* J. R. T. C. ROELANDT,
G. R. SUTHERLAND, A. H. M. M. BALK & J. H. SMYLLIE

INTRODUCTION

We will review the echo-Doppler techniques and methods used for diagnosing acute rejection in heart transplant recipients. These methods range from the demonstration of functional changes by (Doppler) echocardiography during a rejection episode, to the determination of rejection related changes in LV mass and the visualization of rejection-related structural changes in the myocardium. The advantages and disadvantages of the currently used techniques will be discussed, as well as the clinical prospects based on our experience and on recently published studies.

PRESENT PRACTICE OF REJECTION DIAGNOSIS

At present the diagnosis of acute rejection and decisions on the intensification of immunosuppressive therapy in heart transplant recipients, are based on histological examination of endomyocardial biopsies[1,2]. Such biopsies can be graded according to a histological classification proposed by Billingham[3]. This classification is used in our hospital. It is our practice to treat acute rejection only when in addition to mononuclear infiltration myocytolysis is demonstrated (Billingham class 2 and 3).

There are a number of inherent disadvantages of the use of the endomyocardial biopsy technique for diagnosing and monitoring of allograft rejection. Its main disadvantage is the invasive nature of the procedure which leads to patient discomfort. Moreover, there is a small complication rate (less than 1%), which includes cardiac tamponade, air embolism, arrhythmias, cervical plexus lesions and pneumothorax. The number of biopsy procedures is limited because they are time consuming and require facilities in the catheterization laboratory as well as in the pathology department. In addition

* Supported by grant nr. 88.110 of the Dutch Heart Foundation.

E. Andries & R. Stroobandt (eds.), Hemodynamics in Daily Practice, 185–209.

Table 1. Classification of biopsies proposed by M. Billingham, Stanford University [3].

Class 0	*No rejection* Normal myocardium.
Class 1	*Mild acute rejection* Interstitial edema, and perivascular or sparse interstitial infiltration with round mononuclear cells.
Class 2	*Moderate acute rejection* Besides perivascular, predominantly interstitial infiltration of pyroninophilic lymphocytes. Focal myocytolysis.
Class 3	*Severe acute rejection* Markedly increased and mixed interstitial infiltrate. Usually vasculitis and interstitial hemorrhages. Usually more widespread myocytolysis.
Class 4	*Resolving phase* Active fibrosis. Some small non-pyroninophilic lymphocytes, plasma cells and hemosiderin. Abnormalities due to ischaemia or infiltration due to cyclosporin are also categorized within this class.

there is always the potential of sampling error [4]. This means that an estimated 2% to 5% of all biopsies may show normal findings during an acute rejection episode. This results from patchy distribution of inflammatory cell infiltration and myocytolysis. As a consequence the development of a noninvasive method for diagnosing the grades of acute rejection, which need specific anti-rejection treatment, and for monitoring after treatment, has a high priority. Early detection is very important because the outcome of the acute rejection process after treatment is presumed to be better in the early stage. It is in this stage that clinical symptoms of acute rejection are often lacking or are aspecific (a slight fatigue or subfebrile body temperature). The acute rejection process in later stages might, even with appropriate therapy, be irreversible and will then lead rapidly to death.

A number of recently published ultrasound studies have suggested that echo-Doppler techniques may allow the diagnosis of acute rejection in an early stage [5–11]. However, data are confusing and there is no agreement on which is the optimal ultrasound method to be used. There are also considerable differences in reported sensitivities and specificities, even if identical methods and parameters are used.

A significant reduction in summated R wave voltage on a standard 12 lead ECG used to be a useful criterion for the diagnosis of acute rejection in azathioprine treated heart transplant recipients. However, these ECG changes are not sensitive enough for predicting episodes of acute rejection in patients maintained on cyclosporine immunosuppressive therapy [8].

Other non-invase diagnostic modalities, like Nuclear Magnetic Resonance Imaging, Cine CT, or nuclear labeling techniques (e.g. antimyosin antibodies) which also might have the potential for diagnosing acute rejection, will not be discussed here because of practical limitations: they are not yet widely available and moreover, for several reasons, they cannot be repeated unlimitedly.

Radionuclide angiography, although it cannot be repeated unlimitedly, is widely available and therefore has been discussed in some detail. Controversy exists in literature whether measurement of LV function by this technique can be valuable to predict acute rejection [12–14]. One study (by means of serial evaluation) reported a significant decrease in LV ejection fraction only in case of severe rejection (Billingham class 3) [14]. Diastolic function deterioration in case of acute rejection (Billingham class 2) assessed by radionuclide angiography is reported by another study [12].

ALTERATIONS IN LV SYSTOLIC AND DIASTOLIC FUNCTION IN ACUTE REJECTION

General aspects of pathophysiology

Rejection diagnosis (e.g., by ultrasound) could be made from pathophysiological changes in either *systolic or diastolic LV function*. Impairment of systolic ventricular performance occurs, if at all, in a relatively late stage during the process of acute rejection. Diastolic function indices become abnormal at an earlier stage, and have been shown to be more sensitive for the early diagnosis of acute rejection.

Systolic LV function in cardiac transplant recipients both at rest and during exercise has been found to be within normal limits in the absence of acute rejection. Even increased myocardial contractility can be found in the early postoperative period [15–20].

During acute rejection, in cyclosporine treated heart transplant recipients, a marked decrease in global systolic function (by using various techniques) has been reported by some [11, 14], whereas others could not find a significant change in systolic function [9, 13, 19]. During acute rejection an altered sequence in contraction and relaxation events is reported whereby the peak rates of contraction and relaxation, both determined from two-dimensional echo short axis area change, are reached in a later stage within the cardiac cycle [11]. As far as the contraction phase is concerned, this may reflect loss of myocardial tissue due to myocytolysis and an impairment in excitation-contraction coupling during acute rejection.

The *diastolic LV function* is a complex interrelation of factors mainly determined by ventricular relaxation and ventricular compliance.

Ventricular relaxation is an active, energy requiring process, and predominantly influences the last part of left ventricular ejection, isovolumic relaxation and the rapid filling phase [21]. Ventricular compliance is the inverse of stiffness and mainly affects the slow filling period (also called diastasis) and atrial contraction[21].

Ventricular relaxation abnormalities are non-specific. They occur in all types of myocardial disease, and they reflect impairment in the uptake of intracellular calcium (from the myofilaments to the sarcoplasmatic reticulum) [22]. During acute rejection, ventricular relaxation deterioration will be accompanied by ventricular compliance deterioration. The latter is presumed to be caused by a stiffening of both ventricles, due to a combination of edema, cellular infiltration and myocytolysis. In our opinion edema and the amount of infiltration are the major determinants of the diastolic dysfunction, especially in the late post-transplantation period when edema due to ischemia has disappeared. This is important, since the decision to treat with additional immunosuppressive drugs in most centers is based on the finding of infiltration plus myocytolysis. The extent of myocytolysis is unknown, and can range from a few cells only, to a considerable amount leading to concomitant systolic dysfunction. It would seem reasonable to assume that the presence of only a few necrotic myocytes with only slight cellular infiltration and edema cannot be detected reliably by any currently available ultrasound technique.

It might be possible that a considerable amount of infiltration and edema precedes the onset of myocytolysis and is already decreasing when myocytolysis is present. This would fit in with our preliminary findings that there might be a significant decrease in isovolumic relaxation period (IVR, defined by the time-interval between aortic valve closure and mitral valve opening, in our opinion the best index to assess diastolic function with Doppler) one or two weeks before myocytolysis is found in the biopsy specimen. At the time of demonstration of myocytolysis changes in IVR are much less, while after treating the acute rejection, a considerable improvement in IVR values was found. Deterioration of diastolic function might not always be accompanied or followed by myocytolysis. This has important implications for giving anti-rejection treatment, if this is to be based on deterioration of diastolic function assessed by ultrasound. Overtreatment with immunosuppressive drugs is potentially harmful to the patient, because of a high risk of inducing infections and malignancies.

In the following section the available echo-Doppler techniques for determination of both systolic and diastolic LV function will be discussed.

Alterations of *systolic LV function* for the diagnosis of acute rejection determined by echo-Doppler (Table 2)

In heart transplant recipients two different echocardiographic methods which provide quantitative data on LV systolic function have been evaluated: digitized M-mode echocardiography and two-dimensional echocardiography.

Table 2. Summary of the systolic and diastolic function indices, used for the echo-Doppler diagnosis of acute rejection.

Methods used	Systolic function	Diastolic function
Digitized M-mode of the LV short axis	- Peak reate of thickening of LVPW - Peak rate of shortening of LVID	- peak rate of thinning of LVPW - Peak rate of lengthening of LVID - t max dD/dt - RT - MDMVO - ACP - RFP - SFP
Mitral M-mode		- IVR by dual M-mode or M-mode/phono
2D-echocardio-graphy	- Area change of LV short axis cross section (global LV function)	- Area change of LV short axis cross section (global LV function)
Doppler echo-cardiography		- PW Doppler of mitral of tricuspid inflow

A. *Digitized M-mode echocardiography of left ventricular systolic function using the left ventricular parasternal axis (at the level of the mitral chordae)* [9, 19, 23]

1. Peak rate of thickening of the left ventricular posterior wall (LVPW), normalized for instantaneous LVPW thickness (1/sec).
2. Peak rate of shortening of left ventricular internal dimension (LVID), normalized for instantaneous LVID (pSR, 1/sec). (Synonymous with peak velocity of circumferential fiber shortening (peak Vcf max).
3. Fractional shortening (FS). LV end diastolic internal diameter minus LV end systolic internal diameter, divided by LV end diastolic internal diameter (%).

The principal parameters obtained from digitized M-mode echocardiography are diagrammatically presented in Figure 1. The major disadvantage of this technique is that it is a one-dimensional technique which does not necessarily reflect the global behaviour of the LV. However, it remains a useful echo technique for determination of contraction and relaxation events in the cardiac cycle, because it adequately reflects posterior wall dynamics which has been shown to be sensitive for assessment of both systolic and diastolic function.

Two studies in heart transplant recipients however, using the above mentioned indices, could not demonstrate a significant decrease in systolic function during biopsy proven rejection episodes [9, 19].

B. *Two-dimensional (2D) echocardiography*

Global LV function [11]. This method is based upon computerized evaluation of the endocardial border in two-dimensional echocardiographic parasternal short axis views (by means of frame to frame analysis), with quantitations

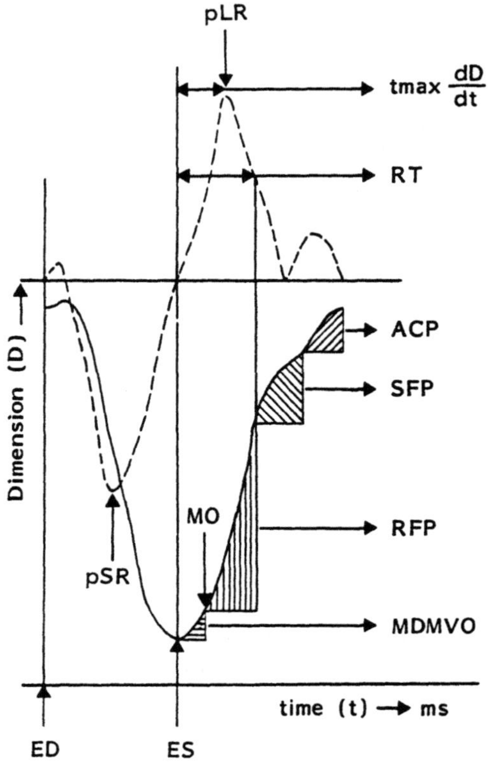

Figure 1. Diagrammatic representation of digitized M-mode echocardiogram of the LV. Instantaneous LV dimension (D) in mm plotted versus time (t) in ms (solid line) and its first derivative normalized for instantaneous dimension (broken line), are shown by digitized M-mode analysis. Timing of end systole (ES), end diastole (ED) and mitral valve opening (MO) are indicated. See text for further abbreviations and explanation.

of the extent and velocity of area change throughout the cardiac cycle. The principle is presented diagrammatically in Figure 2. This method is an approximation of global LV function since absolute end systolic and end diastolic volumes and ejection fraction are not determined. However, since this is a two-dimensional technique, it provides a better reflection of global LV function in comparison with digitized M-mode. Moreover, a decrease in LV diastolic area might be indicative of myocardial edema during acute rejection (in case of unchanged loading conditions). The technique provides a continuous plot of contraction and relaxation throughout the cardiac cycle. A disadvantage, compared to digitized M-mode echocardiography, is that the intra- and interobserver variability of an area measurement is larger and time resolution

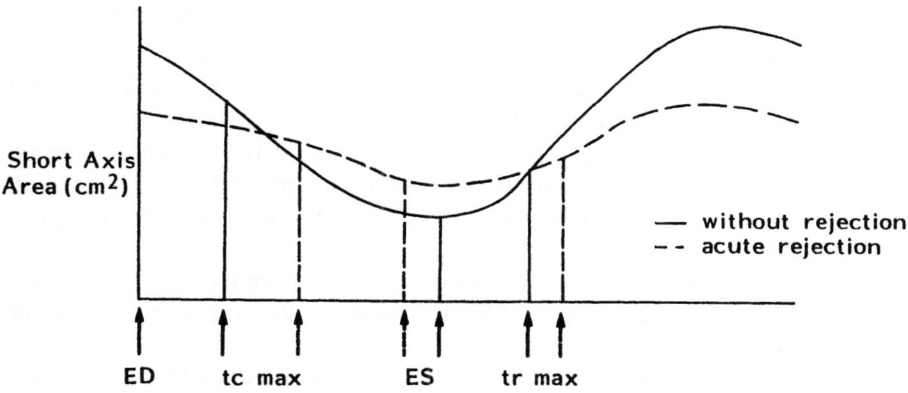

Figure 2. Two-dimensional echocardiogram. Short axis area change in time by frame to frame analysis. The solid line represents the normal short axis area change. The broken line represents the short axis area change in case of acute rejection.
Tc max is defined as the peak rate of area change during systole. Tr max is defined as the peak rate of area change during diastole. Note that both tc max and tr max occur in a later stage of the cardiac cycle in case of acute rejection.

is less than that of linear dimension measurement, requiring a more pronounced change to reach significance.

Angermann reported the following results of global LV systolic function assessment from two-dimensional echocardiography [11]: The percentage of systolic area change yielded a sensitivity of 61% and a negative predictive value of 36%. The systolic rate of area change yielded a sensitivity of 45% and a negative predictive value of 38%. These results are not good enough to reliably diagnose acute rejection in clinical practice.

Alterations of *diastolic LV function* for the diagnosis of acute rejection determined by echo-Doppler (Table 2)

A. *Mitral valve M-mode indices for the measurement of isovolumic relaxation time (IVR)* [8–11]

1a. IVR can be derived from the *mitral M-mode* echocardiogram when recorded in combination with a phonocardiogram. IVR is the time-interval between aortic valve closure on phono and the opening point (D point) on the mitral valve M-mode. However, the D point is sometimes difficult to discern, indicating the limitation of this method.

1b. IVR can also be measured using *simultaneous dual M-mode* registrations. IVR is the time-interval between the closure line of the aortic M-mode and the opening point of the mitral M-mode. This method is cumbersome and outdated with the use of Doppler.

B. *Digitized M-mode echocardiopgraphy of left ventricular diastolic function using the parasternal axis (at the level of the mistral chordae)* [19, 28, 30–32]
These measurements (except the first one) are presented in *Figure 1.*

1. Peak rate of thinning of left ventricular posterior wall (LVPW), normalized for instantaneous thickness of LVPW (1/sec).
2. Peak rate of lengthening (dimension increase) of left ventricular internal dimension (LVID), normalized for instantaneous LVID (pLR, 1/sec). Synonymous with peak velocity of circumferential fiber lengthening (peak Vcf min).
3. t max dD/dt (ms). This is the time-interval from endsystole to maximal rate of dimension increase of LVID. Synonym: Relaxation time to peak rate of dimension increase.
4. Relaxation time (RT, ms). (Not to be confused with IVR.) This is the time-interval from endsystole to 50% decrease in rate of dimension increase (50% dD/dt) of LVID (ms).
5. Interval from minimum cavity dimension to mitral valve opening (MDMVO, ms) (and relative dimension increase during this period as a percentage of the total dimension change during the cardiac cycle (DCMVO, %)) [28].
6. Duration of, and dimension increase during the rapid filling period (RFP, ms and mm).
7. Duration of, and dimension increase during the slow filling period (SFP, ms and mm). Synonym: Diastasis.
8. Duration of, and dimension increase during atrial contraction period (ACP, ms and mm).

In patients treated with maintenance immunosuppressive therapy consisting of prednisone and azathioprine, Paulsen [19] reported diastolic function abnormalities during moderate or severe acute rejection. A significant prolongation of the rapid filling period and decreased normalized peak rates of LV lengthening and posterior wall thinning were found.

Also other investigators [33–35] have reported diastolic dysfunction by means of several techniques in similarly treated heart transplant recipients during acute rejection.

No reports have yet appeared about the value of this technique in cyclosporine treated patients, in whom diastolic dysfunction during an acute rejection might be more difficult to detect. This is due to the more insiduous course of acute rejection in patients treated with cyclosporine.

Since volume (and dimension) derived indices provide a better characterization of relaxation than pressure- and interval-derived ones [22], digitized M-mode might be an additional technique for diastolic function assessment to transmitral Doppler or mitral M-mode echocardiography.

C. *Pulsed wave (PW) Doppler characteristics of transmitral flow*
Measurement of diastolic LV function measured by Doppler is based upon (patho)physiological concepts of mitral flow. The transmitral Doppler characteristics reflect the driving force (pressure) across the mitral valve. Diastolic

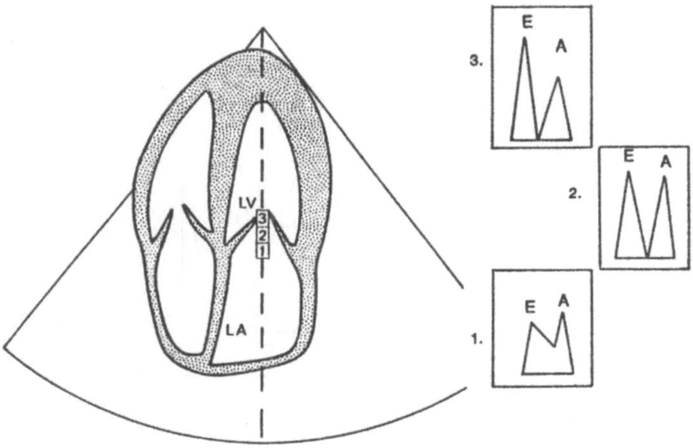

Figure 3. The PW transmitral waveforms obtained from an apical four chamber view. Sample volumes at level 1 (mitral annulus), at level 2 (halfway between levels 1 and 3), and at level 3 (tips of mitral leaflets) show an increase in flow velocities of both the E and A waves, as well as an increase in E/A ratioes.

filling of the heart is a complex sequence of interrelated events. These include: relaxation, passive stiffness and viscoelastic properties, coronary filling, ventricular interaction (Bernheim effect), atrial contraction, and pericardial constraints. Loading conditions (pre- and afterload), contractility, electrical (in)activation sequence and the nonuniformity of these conditions in the ventricles are other determinants [22]. Moreover, these interrelationships are influenced by heart rate.

The method of measurement of Doppler velocity indices of mitral inflow sampled within the apical four chamber view is illustrated in Figure 3.

The transmitral diastolic flow velocity waveforms can be measured at different levels within the mitral valve apparatus by changing the position of the PW Doppler sample volume. The velocity waveforms are dependent on the sample volume position. As the mitral valve is funnel-shaped, the velocities increase progressively across the mitral valve apparatus towards the outlet of the mitral funnel. The ratio of the (early) rapid filling (E) to late atrial (A) filling also progressively increases when the sample volume is positioned closer to the outlet of the mitral funnel [25].

For reasons of reproducibility, all PW Doppler measurements of the transmitral flow should always be made with the same sample volume in the same position in a given patient, preferably at the tips of the mitral leaflets, either from an apical long axis or four chamber view. In the majority of orthotopic heart transplant recipients, the position at the tips of the mitral leaflets is halfway the transducer and the back of the left atrium in the four chamber

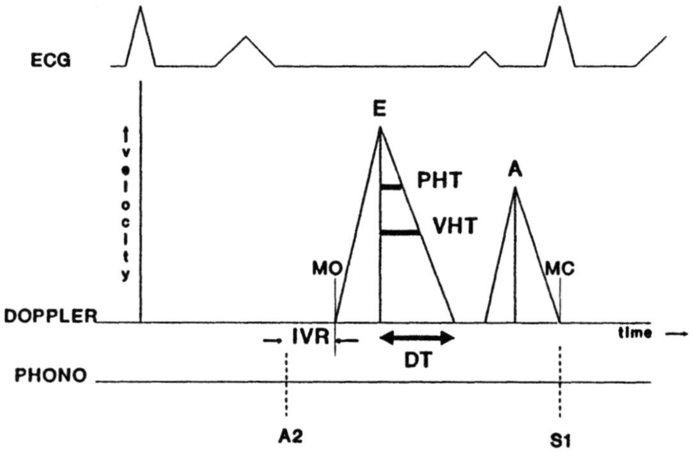

Figure 4. PW transmitral Doppler recordings at the tips of the mitral leaflets from an apical four chamber view with simultaneous phono and ECG recordings.
Indices of diastolic function are indicated. These are PHT (pressure half time), VHT (velocity half time), DT (deceleration time), IVR (isovolumic relaxation time). A2 is the aortic closure component of the second heart sound, S1 is the representation of the first heart sound on the phonocardiogram.

view (due to longitudinally enlarged atria). With high pulse repetition frequency transmitral Doppler interrogation, velocities in the posterior area of the left atrium which result from pulmonary venous inflow, are picked up simultaneously, and may give rise to 'baseline noise'.

Figure 4 diagrammatically illustrates the transmitral Doppler flow parameters which can be measured. The normal reference values [26, 27, 28] in normal healthy subjects (± 1 SD) are indicated in Table 3. However, it must be stressed that individual changes in diastolic function parameters are more important than absolute values when patients are monitored to detect acute rejection.

Table 3. Normal values (± 1 SD) – for normal healthy subjects – are indicated for PW transmitral Doppler/phonocardiographic indices of diastolic function.

E	(early rapid filling)	0.69 (0.12) m/s
A	(late artrial filling)	0.27 (0.07) m/s
IVR	(isovolumic relaxation time)	72 (12) ms
VHT	(velocity half time)	62 (14) ms
PHT	(pressure half time)	53 (8) ms

For abbreviations and their explanation see text and Figure 4. Although normal values for PHT are indicated, this parameter is theoretically only applicable in case of a stenotic atrioventricular valve.

The PW Doppler measurement of mitral inflow reflecting the *initial part of LV relaxation*, is determined by IVR

1. *Isovolumic relaxation time* (IVR, ms). This is a measurement defined by the time-interval between aortic valve closure (A2) on the phonocardiogram and the onset of the mitral inflow on the PW Doppler curve (extrapolated to the baseline). IVR reflects the speed of the initial part of LV relaxation, which is an active energy requiring process. However, it is also influenced by the endsystolic aortic pressure and by the left atrial pressure at the time of mitral valve opening. In the setting of cardiac transplant patients IVR can be regarded as the most important index of LV relaxation.

   Another way of measuring IVR is by positioning the sample volume of the PW Doppler halfway between the anterior mitral leaflet and the left ventricular outflow tract (LVOT). The time-interval between the end of the left ventricular outflow velocity waveform and the onset of the mitral inflow velocity waveform represents IVR[6]. When compared to PW Doppler used in combination with the phonocardiogram, this last way of measuring IVR seems to be inaccurate in our experience.

PW Doppler measurements of mitral inflow reflecting *the second part of LV relaxation* (i.e., the rapid filling phase) are described by numbers 2 to 6.

2. *Height of the E peak* (cm/s). The E peak ensues from the rapid filling phase. In this part of the cardiac cycle LV relaxation is still occurring causing a progressive drop in LV pressure. There will be a pressure crossover between left atrial and left ventricular pressure, which causes the mitral valve to open and rapid filling to occur.

   Usually the peak of rapid filling is represented by a single E velocity peak. In cardiac transplant patients however, often bifid E waves can be discerned. This may be due to the superimposed effects of acceptor atrial contraction and relaxation, to be discussed later. The area under the E wave is the time velocity integral (TVI, cm) of the E wave, and reflects the contribution of the rapid filling phase in the LV diastolic filling.

The following indices of PW transmitral Doppler are based on measurements of time-intervals, derived from the descending slope of the transmitral E wave. A common disadvantage of these indices in transplant patients is that the descending slope of the transmitral E wave often is only partially visible, or not at all. This is due to a marked sinus tachycardia, usual in denervated hearts, which causes a shift of E and A waves into each other, thereby obscuring the descending slope of the E wave. Another problem is created by acceptor atrial contraction, the effects of which may be superimposed on the E wave, thereby distorting its shape and making measurement of the descending E wave slope impossible.

Therefore, in cardiac transplant patients only beats where acceptor atrial contraction occurs in either late diastole or early systole can be used for measurement of velocity half time. Moreover, only in these cases, measurement of IVR, E wave and its descending slope will be less affected by the effects of acceptor atrial contraction, or not at all.

Of the following indices velocity half time, if measurable, will be the best reproducible and theoretically justifiable index.

3. *Pressure half time* (PHT, ms). This is defined to be the time-interval between the E peak and a point on 71% of the descending limb of the E peak, as calculated by the modified Bernouilli equation, which relates velocity to a calculated pressure gradient across the valve. Theoretically the PHT-measurement can only be applied in mitral valve stenosis, since the modified Bernouilli equation requires kinetic energy loss which does not occur in a normal mitral valve without hardly any pressure gradient.
4. *Velocity half time* (VHT, ms). This is the time-interval between the E peak and a point on 50% of the descending limb of the E peak envelope (when the velocity has decayed to half its maximal value). Since the modified Bernouilli equation is not involved in this measurement, this measurement can be applied to the normal atrioventricular valve without theoretical restraints.
5. *Deceleration rate* (DR, cm/s^2). This is defined as the tangent of the slope of the descending limb of the E peak. This is not a time-interval. Since deceleration is non-linear in a normal mitral valve, the DR is calculated by the best linear fit of the descending E wave slope. This may be an explanation of its larger variability as compared to VHT.
6. *Deceleration time* (DT, ms). This is a measure of how rapidly early diastolic filling stops. It is represented by the time-interval between the E peak and a point on the baseline where the descending limb crosses the baseline. This measurement requires extrapolation of the transmitral E wave slope with the same restraints as already discussed.

PW Doppler measurements of mitral inflow reflecting *LV compliance* are described by 7 and 8.

7. *Diastasis* (ms). This is defined as the interval between the E and A waves. It is only present in slower heart rates and therefore it usually is not measured. It represents the slow filling period, in which probably passive filling occurs. Alternatively this interval might be a reflection of flow within the left atrium itself, due to pulmonary venous drainage, picked up by high Pulsed Repetition Frequency (high PRF) Doppler when the sample volume is positioned at the level of the tips of the mitral leaflets in the apical four chamber view.
8. *Height of atrial contraction* (A peak, cm/s). This is an important index of diastolic function. In cardiac transplant patients there will be two atrial contractions, one of the donor atrium and one of the acceptor atrial remnant. The two atrial rhythms are completely dissociated, so their mechanical events (contraction as well as relaxation) are independent from each other.

This causes an important measurement variability of all diastolic function indices mentioned. The onset of the donor A wave occurs about 60 ms after the onset of the donor P wave. This allows identification of the donor A wave, in case of a double A wave. The area under the donor A wave is the time velocity integral (TVI, cm) of the A wave, and reflects the atrial contribution to LV diastolic filling.

The most practical and reproducible indices of LV diastolic function are IVR, the E and A wave velocities and their time velocity integrals. The measurements related to the descending E wave slope in transplant patients will for several reasons only be reproducible, when acceptor atrial contraction occurs in either late diastole or early systole.

D. *Pulsed Wave (PW) Doppler indices of the tricuspid inflow*
Virtually the same indices as recorded from the mitral inflow can be measured for transtricuspid diastolic flow (except for IVR since the exact determination of the closure of the pulmonic valve (P2) on the phonocardiogram is in practice not possible). In the setting of cardiac transplant patients this method has been used for the diagnosis of acute rejection [29].

In serial measurements a significant variability in the maximal E wave velocities and pressure half time of tricuspid PW doppler (from the apical four chamber view) in patients with and without mild acute rejection (Billingham class 1) was found. Results were not significantly different during mild acute rejection episodes. So this technique is not useful in monitoring the individual patient for acute rejection.

THE RELATION BETWEEN ACUTE REJECTION, TRANSMITRAL DOPPLER CHARACTERISTICS AND HEMODYNAMICS

Acute rejection causes stiffening of both ventricles. This is due to cellular infiltration, edema and myocytolysis and will directly result in a decrease of left as well as right ventricular relaxation and compliance [36]

Rejection induced changes in the PW Doppler curve of the mitral inflow might include a decrease in the isovolumic relaxation period, pressure half time and velocity half time, with an increase in E/A ratio, compared to a non-rejection episode when measured in the same patient. The PW Doppler waveform in case of acute rejection is illustrated in Figure 5.

The pattern shown in Figure 5 reflects restrictive diastolic filling hemodynamics, which has also been described as pattern 2 in Figure 6.

A hypothesis put forward by Appleton about the *sequence of appearance of different transmitral Doppler waveforms* is presented in Figure 6 [36]. Each of these waveforms is related to a certain severity of diastolic dysfunction. *A normal PW Doppler waveform* (in the center of the figure) reflects the situation without any relaxation abnormality and with normal hemodynamics. *Pattern*

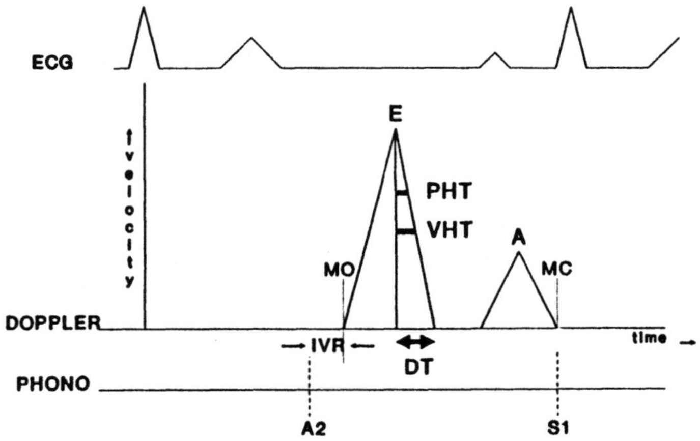

Figure 5. PW transmitral Doppler at the tips of the mitral leaflets from an apical four chamber view with simultaneous ECG and phono recordings.
Diastolic function indices as explained in Figure 4. Acute rejection causes a shortening of PHT, VHT, IVR and DT. The E wave velocity has increased, as compared to normal, resulting in a taller E wave. The A wave shows the opposite effect.

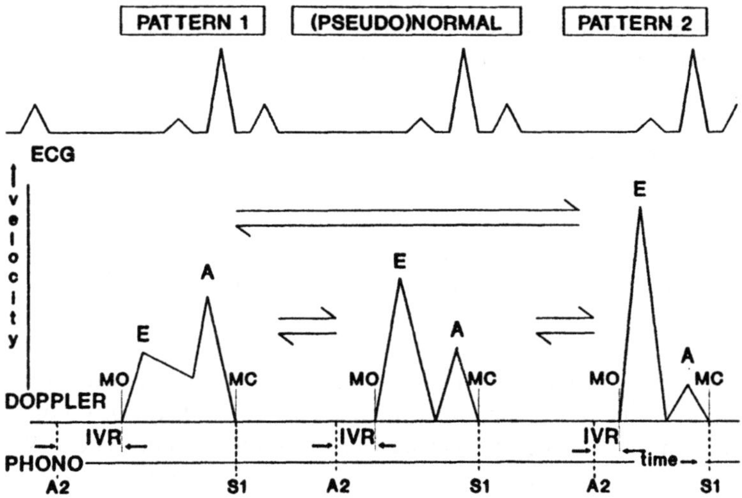

Figure 6. Transmitral Doppler – Sequential diastolic abnormalities. The sequential abnormalities in diastolic function of the PW transmitral Doppler at the mitral leaflet level of the apical four chamber view. With deterioration of diastolic function, the presumed sequence of patterns can be described as follows: The normal pattern (in the middle of the figure) changes in pattern 1 (left), followed by a pseudonormalized pattern (in the centre) with virtually the same waveforms as in the normal pattern, and eventually by pattern 2 (right). Abbreviations as in the previous figures.

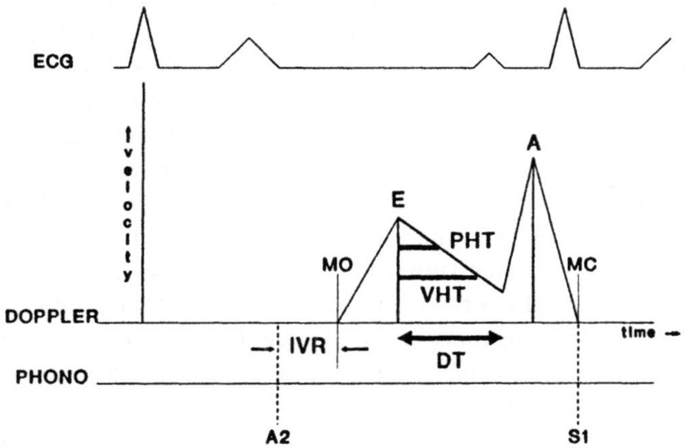

Figure 7. PW transmitral Doppler at the level of the tips of the mitral leaflets from an apical four chamber view. Early diastolic dysfunction is presumed to manifest itself by a relaxation abnormality, called pattern 1. Abbreviations as in previous figures. A prolongation of PHT, VHT, DT and IVR is found. Simultaneously there is a diminuition of the E wave and an increase of the A wave, reflecting a compensatory increase in the atrial contribution in diastolic filling of the left ventricle.

1 is a reflection of a mild relaxation abnormality with a normal or only slightly increased mean pulmonary capillary wedge pressure and LV diastolic pressure, and a slightly prolonged Tau (i.e., a hemodynamic relaxation constant). A decrease in the E peak and an increase in the A peak are indicative of this pattern, the latter being a reflection of compensatory increase in atrial contribution to diastolic filling. This is also shown in Figure 7. *A pseudo-normalized pattern* occurs if there is a further determination of LV relaxation with a beginning LV compliance abnormality. The Doppler waveform is a duplicate of a normal waveform, but left ventricular and left atrial filling pressures will be much higher. Thus, a marked relaxation and beginning compliance abnormality could be masked by a normal PW Doppler curve of mitral inflow. *Pattern 2* is the ultimate result of a sequence of increasing diastolic abnormalities and is presumed to be present in case of a moderate or severe acute rejection. There is a definite LV relaxation and compliance abnormality if this pattern is present. High pulmonary capillary wedge pressures and LV diastolic pressures can be measured together with a marked prolongation of time constant (Tau) and an increase in -dP/dt (i.e., a less steep descending limb of the LV pressure tracing). The low A peak has been explained as a result of atrial dysfunction due to a longstanding elevated atrial pressure.

FACTORS MODIFYING DIASTOLIC FUNCTION INDICES

Diastolic transmitral inflow velocities result from complex interaction of load, (in)activation sequence and non-uniform distribution of load and (in)activation sequence in space and time [22]. In the setting of orthotopic heart transplant recipients there are a lot of modifying factors, beside acute rejection, which may influence the diastolic function indices. These are systemic hypertension [37], pulmonary hypertension [38], changes in preload (diuretics, nitroglycerin) [39], mitral regurgitation [40], ischemia (early postoperatively or later on as a manifestation of progressive coronary artery disease) [37], heart rate[41], pericardial effusion which induces respiratory variability [42, 43], interstitial fibrosis (occuring in a later stage) [44] and a phenomenon unique to these patients: recipient atrial contraction in late systole [45]. Complete left bundle branch block is also presumed to influence LV relaxation, because of the alteration in electrical and mechanical activation and inactivation sequences [22]. The modifying factors are illustrated in Table 4.

The recipient atria are electrically and mechanically dissociated from the donor atria. Recipient atrial contraction in late systole just prior to the normal timed mitral valve opening causes an increase in left atrial pressure, resulting in an earlier opening of the mitral valve. This is reflected by a shortening of IVR. The opening of the mitral valve occurs at a moment when LV pressure is still relatively high, but is declining rapidly. This causes an increase in the E peak velocity. Also a shortening of VHT and PHT will occur.

These changes are observed only with recipient atrial contraction in late systole. In early systole recipient atrial contraction is associated with a longer pressure half time and a lower E peak velocity, isovolumic relaxation time is reported to be unchanged. Recipient atrial contraction in early diastole

Table 4. The effects of modifying factors on diastolic function indices in post transplant patients. The direction of changes is indicated with ↑ for increase, ↓ for decrease, – for no change.

	IVR	VHT
Heart rate ↑	↓	↓
Age ↑	↑	↑
RR + afterload ↑	↑	↑
LV hypertrophy ↑	↑	↑
Mitral regurgitation ↑ (moderate to severe)	↓	↓–
Preload ↑	↓	↓
Acceptor atrial contraction in late systole	↓	↓
Ischemia ↑	↑–↓	↑–↓
Pulmonary hypertension ↑	↑	?
Pericardial effusion ↑ (inspiratory beats)	↑	↑
Interstitial fibrosis ↑	↓	↓

IVR = isovolumic relaxation time; VHT = velocity half time.

resulted in a lower A wave than in systole, whereas simultaneous contraction of recipient and donor atria in late diastole resulted in an increase in the A wave [42]. Recipient atrial P waves on the ECG, as recorded simultaneously with the echo (Doppler) tracings, are in our experience only clearly discernable in a minority of transplant patients, especially in the late postoperative period (even if there are prominent donor atrial P waves). However, in those cases, the Doppler transmitral waveforms may strongly suggest the presence of recipient atrial contraction. Since the second half of the left ventricular ejection, together with the isovolumic and rapid filling periods are known to be load dependent, recipient atrial contraction in these parts of the cardiac cycle could be of major influence on left and right ventricular relaxation [12]. Therefore the isovolumic relaxation period, and E peak transmitral velocity with its velocity half time and pressure half times will be influenced by recipient atrial contraction occuring in these parts of the cardiac cycle. So changes in these indices might be more a reflection of the increase in atrial pressures rather than of a change in intrinsic myocardial relaxation. Theoretically the latter would be best represented by beats where recipient atrial contraction occurs in late diastole or early systole (in the early ejection phase).

Because of the many modifying factors, changes in diastolic function indices of PW Doppler mitral inflow (as compared to the previous measurements in the same patient) are not specific for acute rejection. The continuous interplay among these factors could obscure the effects of an episode of moderate acute rejection especially when those factors work in the opposite direction, preventing the establishment of a full blown restrictive filling pattern. It is thus conceivable that a rejection episode is missed on PW Doppler because a 'normal' pattern is found, which is in fact a 'pseudonormalized' pattern. Likewise a pattern 1 could be indicative of acute rejection, because modifying factors prevented it to become a pattern 2.

Even though Appletons hypothesis of the four patterns of PW mitral inflow is tempting and corroborated by hemodynamic measurements, it does not entirely exclude the possibility that IVR (early diastole), VHT and E peak (mid diastole) and A peak (late diastole) could vary independently from eachother, since they occur in different parts of diastole, and especially IVR is known to be very preload dependent [22]. It may be possible that there is no continuum in the transmitral Doppler patterns in contrast to what has been described by Appleton. A marked increase in E/A ratio has only been observed if left ventricular end-diastolic pressure (LVEDP) exceeded 17 to 20 mmHg in volume load dogs, whereas in normal to moderate elevated LV diastolic pressures E/A ratio was unchanged [28]. It may be conceivable that such a threshold in LVEDP exists in case of moderate acute rejection in orthotopic heart transplant recipients. Only if acute rejection is hemodynamically severe enough, and hence preload and LVEDP are high enough, the increased E/A ratio characteristic of restrictive filling would appear.

THE RESULTS OF RECENT REPORTED STUDIES OF DIASTOLIC LV FUNCTION IN RELATION TO ACUTE REJECTION

Major studies concerning this matter have been performed by Dawkins [8–9] and Valantine [7] from Stanford, USA; Desruennes [63] from Paris, France; Angermann [11] and Spes [29] from Munich, FRG; and Forster [5, 10] Thoraxcenter Rotterdam, The Netherlands. All six studies were designed to be prospective. The number of orthotopic heart transplant recipients in each study ranged from 20–55. Mean age: 37 (12–60). Gender: 19–41 men, 3–14 women. The commencement of follow-up after orthotopic heart transplantation ranged from 2 days to 2 months (even up to 65 months: Angermann[11], with a follow-up period after transplantation of 16 weeks to 19 months. Table 5 shows the methods which have been used. In each study the diagnostic criteria of the diastolic function indices, as compared to the biopsy results, were set at those levels which yielded the highest specificity and sensitivity. The results for IVR, PHT and E vs. endomyocardial biopsy are shown in Table 6, except for 2 studies in which no significant differences were observed between the presence and absence of moderate acute rejection. Acute rejection is defined as Billingham class 2.

Forster, Desruennes and Valantine excluded all beats influenced by acceptor atrial contraction in late systole from analysis. A paperspeed of 100 mm/sec was used except in the study of Desruennes, who used a paperspeed of 50 mm/sec. All studies, except the second study of Forster with CW Doppler, are based on longitudinal follow-up of diastolic function indices in individual

Table 5. Summary of the methods used in the 7 major studies. Indicated are respectively the author, the parameter(s) used for LV diastolic function determination with the corresponding technique, the number of consecutive beats analysed, and the diagnostic criteria for moderate acute rejection.

Author	Parameter	Technique	Beats	Diagnostic criteria
Angermann[11]	IVR	Dual M-mode	3	⩾10% reduction
Dawkins[8]	IVR	MV M-mode/phono	3	⩾23% reduction
Desruennes[6]	IVR	MV PW Doppler	10	⩾20% reduction
	PHT	MV PW Doppler	10	⩾20% reduction
Forster[5]	IVR	MV M-mode/phono and dual M-mode	10	⩾23% reduction
Forster[10]	VHT	MV CW Doppler	10	None*
Spes[29]	PHT	PW Doppler	?	None*
Valantine[7]	IVR	MW CW Dop./phono	10	⩾15 ms reduction
	PHT	MV CW Dop./phono	10	⩾12 ms reduction
	E	MV CW Dop./phono	10	⩾.33 ms increase

* Results were found not to be significant. MV = mitral valve.

Table 6. Review of results of studies relating IVR and PHT to biopsy results of acute rejection.

Author	Index	n	Sensitivity (%)	Specificity (%)	Predictive value	
					+ (%)	− (%)
Angermann[11]	IVR	15	77	-	-	-
Dawkins[8]	IVR	20	87	90	77	94
Desruennes[6]	IVR	55	60	87	79	72
	PHT		88	87	85	90
Forster[5]	IVR	26	56	79	21	95
Valantine[7]	IVR	22	88	68	58	92
	PHT		88	68	58	92
	E		71	71	55	83

patients (individual trend detection). These indices were independently compared to histological biopsy results. It should be noted that different techniques as well as different diagnostic criteria, were used for the echo-Doppler diagnosis of acute rejection. The number of patients and the number of analysed beats, was small (especially when considering the great beat-to-beat variability that exists, even when beats with acceptor atrial contraction in late systole are eliminated). When interpreting the results, this has to be taken into account. With respect to IVR, the methods of Dawkins and Forster can be compared, with respect to the CW Doppler method Valantine and Forster can be compared. In our opinion CW Doppler should not be used to measure diastolic function indices because it not only measures transmitral flow velocities, but in certain cases also intraventricular flow signals. An example of the latter is 'isovolumic relaxation flow' which can potentially be confused with the onset of the E peak of transmitral flow [46]. Beside this, longer deceleration times are measured in comparison with the PW Doppler transmitral flow [36]. PW Doppler for measurement of IVR, by positioning the sample volume halfway the mitral inflow and LV outflow tract, has in our experience proven to yield different results as compared to its measurement at the level of the mitral leaflets and thus IVR measured in combination with phono. Also IVR determined by mitral M-mode/phono is different in the same patient at the same occasion, as compared to the Doppler/phono method (the former is almost invariably shorter than the latter), indicating that these methods cannot be interchanged. IVR determined by mitral M-mode/phono is also different depending whether the long parasternal or short parasternal axis is used. The studies of Spes [29] and Desruennes [6] can be compared with respect to PHT. Differences in immunosuppresive therapy among different cardiac transplantation centres may provide an additional explanation for the discrepancies in results with regard to the diagnosis of moderate acute rejection in the 7 above mentioned studies. Although in all patients cyclosporine A in combination with prednisone was used as maintenance immunosuppressive therapy, in some centres patients received additional azathioprine (triple therapy). Moreover the maintenance dose of prednisone differs from centre to centre, as is the case for the indication of anti-rejection treatment (sometimes the prednisone dose is already increased if there is only mild acute rejection). It would seem reasonable to assume that if moderate acute rejection occurs in non-infiltrated myocardium, in spite of 'high dose' maintenance immunosuppression the corresponding ultrasonic changes will be more pronounced, than if they occur in myocardium which is already chronically infiltrated with lymphocytes. The latter is more likely if a 'low dose' immunosuppressive regimen is used.

Measurement variability of PW Doppler of mitral inflow in non-transplant cardiac patients proves to be sufficiently low to allow good reproducibility, except for E/A ratio, which showed a random variation coefficient of 22%, whereas for IVR this was 11% [47]. With CW Doppler Valantine found similar results for IVR, PHT, and E wave of about 10% in orthotopic heart transplant patients. The A wave had a variation coefficient of up to 23% [7]. The 95% confidence limits for random variation ranged for IVR from 9.4% [11] to 23% [47]. This means that only changes greater than these values can be detected if they are measured by the same observer.

From an epidemiological point of view the best strategy for the non-invasive diagnosis of moderate or severe acute rejection (Billingham class 2–3) by means of echo-Doppler will be to try to *exclude* acute rejection. Because there is a low pretest likelihood of finding a biopsy-specimen positive for acute rejection (in our hospital about 13% a year), there is even with the best diagnostic test with a sensitivity and specificity of both 90% (Dawkins, Desruennes) a post-test likelihood of only about 50% of detection of acute rejection (theorem of Bayes). However, to *exclude* acute rejection, the *same test will result in a calculated negative predictive value of about 99%* in our patient population. This means that in only 1% of all cases acute rejection will be missed on the basis of little or no varying diastolic function indices, and that acute rejection can then be excluded with a certainty of 99%.

CHANGES IN LV MASS IN RELATION TO THE DIAGNOSIS ACUTE REJECTION

Significant increase in wall thickness (of the interventricular septum and the LV posterior wall) and of LV mass was found in azathioprine-treated heart transplant recipients at times of acute rejection [19, 48]. However, with the introduction of cyclosporine as maintenance immunosuppressive treatment, the determination of LV mass and wall thickness has become much less valid [9]. This might be explained by the fact that under cyclosporine therapy the course of acute rejection is more insiduous with less striking edema. As a single sign, either total wall thickness or the determination of LV mass, has been reported by several authors to be too insensitive and nonspecific for the diagnosis of acute rejection [9, 49].

Ciliberto et al.[49] recently presented a 'multiparametric' evaluation of serial changes in myocardial structure and function in heart transplant recipients in order to differentiate between rejection and non-rejection episodes.

Using M-mode and two-dimensional echocardiography, changes in RV and LV diameters, interventricular septum plus posterior wall thickness, LV mass and LV ejection fraction were measured quantitatively. Deterioration of RV wall motion, increase in pericardial effusion and increased echogenicity were measured qualitatively (with all inherent limitations for the reproducibility of these measurements). All of these parameters were considered to be criteria for possible rejection. If at least one of these criteria was present sensitivity was 94%, if at least 2 criteria were present it dropped to 83% with a rise in specificity to 100%. None of the single criteria was sensitive enough to be of clinical value for the diagnosis of moderate acute rejection. The sensitivity of increases in total wall thickness (of $\geqslant$ 4 mm.) was only 61%, its specificity only 55%. This study only allows differentiation to some extent between no rejection (Billingham class 0) and rejection (Billingham class 1 and 2). Even with this 'multiparametric approach' this study cannot differentiate mild (class 1) from moderate (class 2) acute rejection in the individual patient.

Since in our experience a class 1 biopsy specimen is commonly found in heart transplant recipients and in most clinics specific anti-rejection treatment is only given to patients with a class 2 or 3 biopsy specimen, the results of this study will be of limited value.

TISSUE CHARACTERIZATION FOR THE DETECTION OF MYOCARDIAL CHANGES DURING ACUTE REJECTION

To differentiate moderate acute rejection episodes which need treatment from non-rejection episodes it is theoretically possible to look for changes in myocardial tissue morphology by means of tissue characterization. The rationale for ultrasound tissue characterization is that ultrasound energy interacts differently with normal and abnormal myocardium and that sufficient information may be available in the ultrasound signal returning from the myocardium to identify specific underlying abnormalities.

One approach is *amplitude analysis* [50,51]. Its validity has been tested in studies aiming at differentiating ischemic from non-ischemic regions in the heart and to detect fibrosis or scar formation after myocardial infarction.

With spectral and amplitude analysis the acoustic property of chief interest has been integrated backscatter. In broad terms this is the measurement of the amount of reflected ultrasound energy from a given volume of tissue. The echo-intensity is expressed in decibels or displayed as different gray scale levels and can be color encoded. Another acoustic property is attenuation (signal loss as sound passes through tissue).

Increased backscatter results from fibrotic and scarred tissue (when there will also be increased attenuation), and from myocardial edema or ischemia (in the latter decreased attenuation). However, integrated backscatter is influenced by the aperture and the focusing properties of the transducer and ultrasonic attenuation of the chest wall. Other factors which influence the results, are transducer frequency, cyclic variation within the cardiac cycle (increased backscatter due to wall thinning in diastole, which requires ECG gating techniques) and variation in the imaging characteristics as a function of the position of the region of interest within the sector field of view. This means that variation both in the depth and lateral resolution of the region of interest may result in backscatter results, which do not reflect the structural abnormalities of the underlying tissue. Recently two precordial studies have appeared in literature using different aspects of ultrasonic backscatter analysis for the diagnosis of moderate acute rejection. Increases in myocardial echo amplitude were used in one study [52], whereas the other study assessed moderate acute rejection by the demonstration of reduced cyclic variation in integrated backscatter [53]. Sensitivities of 90% and 86%, and specificities of 85% and 70% respectively were reported in these studies. The use of transoesophageal echocardiography may even improve these results, because of its higher signal to noise ratio and decreased attenuation, as a result of the proximity of the heart. In addition higher frequencies can be used, which provide better acoustic properties for backscatter analysis.

CONCLUSIONS AND RECOMMENDATIONS FOR THE ECHO-DOPPLER DIAGNOSIS OF ACUTE REJECTION

The aim is reduction of the number of biopsies by exclusion of acute rejection. Most profit is to be gained from individual trend detection of diastolic function indices, instead of using absolute values. In case of acute rejection diastolic function has been shown to deteriorate in an earlier stage compared to systolic function. Since decisions on the treatment of acute rejection are made on the finding of a Billingham class 2 or 3 biopsy specimen, the greatest challenge in the echo-Doppler diagnosis of acute rejection lies in its ability to differentiate these histological classes from class 1 biopsy results.

The seven hitherto published major studies concerning changes in diastolic function are to a large extent controversial in methods, diagnostic criteria and results. Diastolic function indices are not specific for acute rejection, because of the continuous interplay of many modifying factors in the post transplantation period. Different immunosuppressive treatment regimes among cardiac transplantation centres may provide another possible explanation for the controversy in the results of the 7 major studies with regard to diastolic function assessment by ultrasound. The presence and severity of modyfying factors might also differ among centres, providing a third explanation.

PW Doppler of mitral inflow has the advantage of assessing global LV function, whereas digitised M-mode or the two-dimensional area method essentially provide an assessment of regional function of the basal portion of the left ventricle. However a problem could arise in the interpretation of PW Doppler patterns, which might be due to the concomitant action of modyfying factors. Since peak posterior wall thinning rate (by digitised left ventricular M-mode) provides an assessment of intrinsic myocardial function it might be a complementary technique to PW transmitral Doppler in these cases.

If the ECG of the recording demonstrates clearly the recipient atrial P-waves, the beats in which recipient atrial contraction occurs in late diastole or early systole will better reflect the 'true' intrinsic myocardial relaxation without superimposed effects of the recipient atrial contraction or relaxation. Because of the considerable beat to beat variability in PW transmitral Doppler, enough (e.g. 20) consecutive beats, both in in- and expiration, should be analysed to average out the effects of acceptor atrial contraction and respiration.

A combination of several appropriate echo-Doppler cardiographic measurements of diastolic and systolic function, together with measurements of wall thickness, may prove to be more sensitive and specific, than the determination of diastolic or systolic function. In our opinion the present role for ultrasound is to serve as an adjunct in the diagnosis of moderate acute rejection. It may be useful to set the timing of biopsies, and in some centres with good results even to reduce the number of biopsies. However yet to much controversy exists in literature, and in general results are not good enough, to use it as a substitute for endomyocardial biopsy. Tissue characterization has already shown promising results for the noninvasive diagnosis of moderate acute rejection, and may well be the preferred technique in the near future.

REFERENCES

1. Caves PK, Stinson EB, Graham AF, et al. (1973) Percutaneous transvenous endomyocardial biopsy. *JAMA* 225:288–91
2. Mason JW (1978) Techniques for right and left endomyocardial biopsy. *Am J Cardiol* 41:887–92
3. Billingham ME (1988) Cardiac Surgery: State of the Art Reviews; 2:641–646 (editors- RW Emery, MR Pritzker)
4. Spiegelhalter DJ, et al. (1983) An analysis of repeated biopsies following cardiac transplantation. *Statistics in Medicine* 2:33–40
5. Forster T, et al. (1988) Can we assess the changes of ventricular filling resulting from acute allograft rejection with Doppler echocardiography? *J Heart Transplant* 7:430–4
6. Desruennes M, et al. (1988) Doppler echocardiography for the diagnosis of acute cardiac allograft rejection. *JACC* 12:63–70
7. Valantine HA, et al. (1987) Changes in Doppler echocardiographic indexes of left ventricular function as potential markers of acute cardiac rejection. *Circulation* 76:V:86–92
8. Dawkins KD, et al. (1984) Changes in diastolic function as a noninvasive marker of cardiac allograft rejection. *Heart Transplantation* 3:286–294
9. Dawkins KD, et al. (1985) Noninvasive assessment of cardiac allograft rejection. *Transplantation Proceedings* 17:215–217
10. Forster T, et al. (1988) Does the measurement of left ventricular isovolumic relaxation time allow early prediction of cardiac allograft rejection? *In press.*

11. Angermann CE, et al. (1989) Echokardiographische Diagnose akuter Abstossungsreaktionen bei herztransplantierten Patienten unter Cyclosporintherapie. *Kardiologie* 78:243–252.11
12. Thompson JA, et al. (1986) Radionuclide diastolic dysfunction: parameter of human cardiac rejection. *Circulation* 74 (suppl II):160 (abstract)
13. McGiffin DC, et al. (1984) Results of radionuclide assessment of cardiac function following transplantation of the heart. *The Annals of Thoracic Surgery* 37:382–386
14. Follansbee, et al. (1986) Acute rejection in the cardiac allograft is associated with measurable decreases in left ventricular ejection fraction. *Circulation* 74 (Suppl II):160 (abstract)
15. Borow KM, et al. (1985) Left ventricular contractility and contractile reserve in humans after cardiac transplantation. *Circulation* 71:866–872
16. Corcos T, et al. (1988) Early and late hemodynamic evaluation after cardiac transplantation: A study of 28 cases. *JACC* 11:264–269
17. Kemkes BM, et al. (1987) First pass radionuclide scintigraphy for long-term follow-up after heart and heart-lung transplantation. *Transplant Proc.* 19:2543–2545
18. Reid CJ, Yacoub MH (1988) Determinants of left ventricular function one year after cardiac transplantation. *Br Heart J* 59:397–402
19. Paulsen A, et al. (1985) Left ventricular function of heart allograft during acute rejection: an echocardiographic assessment. *J Heart Transplant* 4:525–529
20. Hastillo A, et al. (1983) Long-term prospective evaluation of cardiac allograft function utilizing exercise. *Circulation* 68(suppl III):183
21. Brutsaert DL, et al. (1984) Triple control of relaxation: Implications in cardiac disease. *Circulation* 69:190–196
22. Danford DA, et al. (1986) Doppler echocardiographic approaches to ventricular diastolic function. *Echocardiography* 3:33–40
23. Bahler RC, et al. (1983) The relation of heart rate and shortening fraction to echocardiographic indexes of left ventricular relaxation in normal subjects. *JACC* 2:926–933
24. Lewis JF, et al. (1984) Pulsed Doppler echocardiographic determination of stroke volume and cardiac output: Clinical validation of two new methods using the apical window. *Circulation* 70:425–431
25. Pearson AC, et al. (1988) Effect of sample volume location on pulsed Doppler-echocardiographic evaluation of left ventricular filling. *Am J Card Imaging* 2:40–46
26. Hatle L, et al. (1979) Noninvasive assessment of atrioventricular pressure half-time by Doppler ultrasound. *Circulation* 60:1096–1104
27. Spirito P, et al. (1988) Influence of aging on Doppler echocardiographic indices of left ventricular diastolic function. *Br Heart J* 59:672–679
28. Myreng Y, et al. (1990) Left ventricular filling at elevated diastolic pressures: Relationship between transmitral Doppler from velocities and atrial contribution. *Am Heart J* 119:620–626
29. Spes CH, et al. (1989) Serial Doppler echocardiography is not useful for diagnosis of mild cardiac allograft rejection. Abstract, *International Journal of Cardiac Imaging* 4:52
30. Ten Cate EJ, et al. (1983) Effects of short-term administration of verapamil on left ventricular relaxation and filling dynamics measured by a combined hemodynamic-ultrasonic technique in patients with hypertrophic cardiomyopathy. *Circulation* 68:1274–79
31. Spirito P, et al. (1986) Noninvasive assessment of left ventricular diastolic function: Comparative analysis of pulsed Doppler ultrasound and digitized M-mode echocardiography. *Am J Cardol* 58:837–843
32. Hanrath P. (1979) Abnormal left ventricular relaxation and diastolic filling patterns in left-sided heart disease, pp. 137–145 in: *Echocardiology*, ed. by Charles T. Lancee
33. Schroeder JS, et al. (1969) Acute rejection following cardiac transplantation: Phonocardiographic and ultrasound observations. *Circulation* 40:155–164
34. Leachman RD, et al. (1971) Serial hemodynamic study of the transplanted heart and correlation with clinical rejection. *J Thorac Cardiovasc Surg* 61:561–569
35. Griepp RB, et al. (1971) Acute rejection of the allografted human heart. *Ann Thorac Surg* 12:113–126

36. Appleton CP, et al. (1988) Relation of transmitral flow velocity patterns to left ventricular diastolic function: New insights from a combined hemodynamic and Doppler echocardiographic study. *JACC* 12:426–440
37. Lewis BS, et al. (1980) Isovolumic relaxation period in man. *Am Heart J* 100:140–499
38. Louie EK, et al. (1986) Doppler echocardiographic assessment of impaired left ventricular filling in patients with right ventricular pressure overload due to primary pulmonary hypertension. *JACC* (1986) 8:1298–1306
39. Choong CY, et al. (1987) Preload dependence of Doppler-derived indexes of left ventricular diastolic function in humans. *JACC* 10:800–808
40. Stevenson LW, et al. (1987) Mitral regurgitation after cardiac transplantation. *Am J Cardiol* 60:119–122
41. Lavine SJ, et al. (1988) Effect of heart rate alterations produced by atrial pacing on the pattern of diastolic filling in normal subjects. *Am J of Cardiol* 62:1098–1102
42. Appleton CP, et al. (1988) Cardiac tamponade and pericardial effusion: Respiratory variation in transvalvular flow velocities studies by Doppler echocardiography. *JACC* 11:1020–1030
43 Vandenberg BF, et al. (1988) Clinical significance of pericardial effusion after heart transplantation. *J Heart Transplant* 7:128–134
44. Appleton CP, et al. (1988) Demonstration of restrictive ventricular physiology by Doppler echocardiography. *JACC* 11:757–768
45. Valantine HA, et al. (1987) Influence of recipient atrial contraction on left ventricular filling dynamics of the transplanted heart assessed by Doppler echocardiography. *Am J Cardiol* 59:1159–1163
46. Sasson Z, et al. (1987) Intraventricular flow during isovolumic relaxation: description and characterization by Doppler echocardiography. *JACC* 10:539–546
47. Myreng Y, Ihlen H (1988) Reproducibility of transmitral flow velocity parameters measured by pulsed Doppler echocardiography. *J Cardiovasc Ultrasonography* 7:257–261
48. Sagar KB, et al. (1981) Left ventricular mass by M-mode echocardiography in cardiac transplant patients with acute rejection. *Circulation* 64 (Suppl II):216–220
49. Ciliberto GR, et al. (1981) Echocardiographic assessment of cardiac allograft rejection. *Eur Heart J* 10:400–408
50. Miller JG, et al. (1985) Ultrasonic Characterization of Myocardium. *Progress in Cardiovascular Diseases* 28:85–110
51. Skorton DJ (1989) Ultrasound tissue characterization: Can the state of the myocardium be assessed directly yet noninvasively? *JACC* 13:92–94
52. Lythall D, et al. (1989) Quantitative analysis of myocardial echo amplitude – a useful marker of cardiac rejection. *Circulation* 80 (suppl II):677 (abstract)
53. Masuyama T, et al. (1990) Serial measurement of integrated ultrasonic backscatter in human cardiac allografts for the recognition of acute rejection. *Circulation* 81:829–839.

14. Cardiac transplantation

F. WELLENS

INTRODUCTION

In the last ten years cardiac transplantation has progressed to a routine procedure for a subgroup of patients with end stage cardiac disease. In 1988 nearly 2000 heart transplants were registered at the Registry of the International Society for Heart Transplantation. The number of centers performing heart transplantation increased from 10 in 1979 to 173 in 1988. The 30 day mortality was 9%. The increasing number of transplant centers and potential recipients introduced quickly the problem of adequate donor resources. One of the most important developments in cardiac and other intrathoracic transplantation will be the extension and optimalisation of the scarce resource of donor organs. During the last six years nearly three hundred hearttransplants have been performed in Belgium (population, 10,000,000) in five transplant centers. The overall results were comparable to the results of the International Registry.

1. SELECTION OF TRANSPLANT CANDIDATES

Due to the accumulated experience, criteria (see Table 1) have become less restrictive, mainly for age and diabetic patients. In general we have to deal with patients with end stage disease without any outlook for improvement with classical medical or surgical means. Estimated life expectancy is around 6 to 12 months. The most frequent diagnosis is ischaemic heart disease in our country, followed by idiopathic dilated cardiomyopathy. A few patients suffer from valvular or congenital heart disease.

Every potential recipient is admitted at the cardiac surgery department during one week for complete evaluation (Table 2). If there are no contraindications, the patient is accepted as a potential candidate on the listing of Eurotransplant, an international organization to optimize organ distribution.

Hemodynamic measurements are very often the decision making factors in the evaluation of a potential transplant candidate. Transplantation of a

E. Andries & R. Stroobandt (eds.), Hemodynamics in Daily Practice, 211–224.

Table 1. Primary criteria for recipient selection.

Criteria

1. New York Heart Association Class III-IV: estimated life expectancy of 6 - 12 months.
2. Maximum age: 60 to 65 years.
3. Normal or reversible hepatic and renal function.
4. Acceptable medical compliance.
5. Emotional and familial stability.

Contraindications

1. Pulmonary hypertension $\geqslant$ 6 U. Wood (*or* TPG > 15 mmHg) without response to O_2 or vasodilator therapy.
2. Active infection.
3. Systemic disease (except for insulinodependent diabetes).
4. Disabling chronic obstructive lung disease.
5. Extreme obesity.
6. Recent pulmonary embolism.
7. Alcohol- or drugabuse.
8. Significant peripheral or cerebrovascular disease.

Table 2. Pretransplant screening tests.

A. - Complete bloodanalysis: bloodgroup, RBC, WBC, reticulocytes, coagulationtest, Coombs, cold agglutinines, immunoelectrophoresis.
- HLA: A, B, C and DR; anti HLA antibodies.
- Glucose + profile, ureum, creatinine, electrolytes.
- Liver function tests.
- Viral serology: EBV, CMV, Herpes, Varicella, Toxoplasmosis, Legionella, HIV, Hepatitis.

B. Check-up: (1) ophtalmology, (2) dentistry, (3) nose, ear, throuth, (4) urology - gynaecology, and (5) urinanalysis.

C. (1) Chest X-ray, (2) X-ray abdomen, and (3) Echo: *liver*, *galbladder*, *kidneys*, *pancreas*, *spleen*, and *abdominal aorta*.

D. (1) ECG, (2) Echocardiogram, (3) MUGA-scan, (4) Left and right heart catheterization + coronary angiography, and (5) Manipulation of pulmonary pressure (with vasodilator therapy and inotropes).

E. Pulmonary function test, perfusion ventilation lungscan.

patient with high pulmonary vascular resistance will very often lead to acute right heart failure of the non-adapted donorheart. Standard criteria for very precise and comparable measurements between transplant centers are not yet well established.

In our center pulmonary vascular resistance (PVR) and transpulmonary gradient (TGP) are measured in baseline conditions and expressed as:

$$\text{PVR} = \frac{\text{Mean pulmonary artery pressure} - \text{Wedge pressure}}{\text{Cardiac output}} \quad \text{in Wood units}$$

$$\text{TPG} = \text{Mean pulmonary artery pressure} - \text{Wedge pressure} \qquad \text{in mmHg}$$

In case of normal PVR and/or TPG no further measurements are performed. In case of borderline or high PVR, manipulation with drugs is undertaken in order to examine the reversibility of PVR. Cardiac output and/or vascular resistance are corrected by means of Dobutamine, Amrinone, Nitroprusside or calciuminhibitors. With borderline results, a trial with IV prostaglandines can even be undertaken as a screening test for its possible peroperative use. Patients with borderline results (PVR ± 6 - 8 U.Wood or TPG 15 - 18) can be accepted with some higher operative and early postoperative risk. In addition there remains an incremental risk of premature death in this high risk group.

2. SELECTION OF DONORS

With the increasing success of organ transplantation, restricted donor availability has become the main problem over the recent years. Potential donors have to be optimally treated in order to maximize donor sources (Table 3). Education of medical and paramedical personnel in all hospitals dealing with brain death patients is therefore a must. Better organ preservation to extend donor ischemia is another issue for research in the near future.

Recently, donor criteria have become much more liberal and older age, previous hypotension or thoracic trauma are no longer contraindications anymore. Actually local donor retrival accounts for 40% of our donor resources. Long distance procurement (40% outside the country) has become routine and needs perfect organization. In order to reduce donor ischemic time, one

Table 3. Criteria for donor selection.

Criteria

1. Brain stem death.
2. Age: 10 to 55 years: coronary angiography/when possible in patients (female ⩾ 50 years; male ⩾ 45 years).
3. Stable haemodynamics (restricted use of Dopamine ⩽ 10 Gamma/kg/min).
4. Absence of major cardiovascular disease.
5. Absence of important infectious disease.
6. Absence of systemic disease.

Screeningtests

1. Complete blood control:
   - Creatinine, ureum, glucose.
   - Bloodgroup.
   - Hepatitis, CMV, HIV, Toxoplasmosis, EBV, Herpes, Varicella, Legionella.
2. Chest X-ray.
3. ECG.
4. Cardiac echo.

After procurement

1. Lymphocyte crossmatch.
2. HLA.

needs to have easy access to fast ground transport, helicopter and/or aeroplane and is organized by the transplant coordinator. A safe ischemic time up to 4 hours is generally accepted. For practical reasons only ABO compatibility will be taken in account in the choice between donor and recipient. Prospective HLA matching is actually not yet possible for organizational reasons.

3. OPERATION AND POSTOPERATIVE TREATMENT

Orthotopic hearttransplantation is now considered as a routine cardiac procedure and is performed by the staffmember on call. The Lower-Shumway technique is used with double septal connection (Figures 1–4).

1. *Cardiopulmonary bypass* is initiated as in routine cardiac surgery except for the posterior placement of the venous cannulae. The recipient heart is removed by transsection of the right atrium at the level of the atrio-ventricular groove up to the coronary sinus on one hand and to the aorta on the other hand. The aorta and pulmonary artery are transsected just above their valvular level. The roof of the left atrium is incised and the left atrium is divided at the level of the atrioventricular groove. Finally the interatrial septum is transsected and the heart removed. At this stage the posterior part of the right atrium with its caval junctions and the recipient's sinus node remain in place together with the interatrial septum and the posterior aspect of the left atrium containing the orifices of the four pulmonary veins (Figure 1).

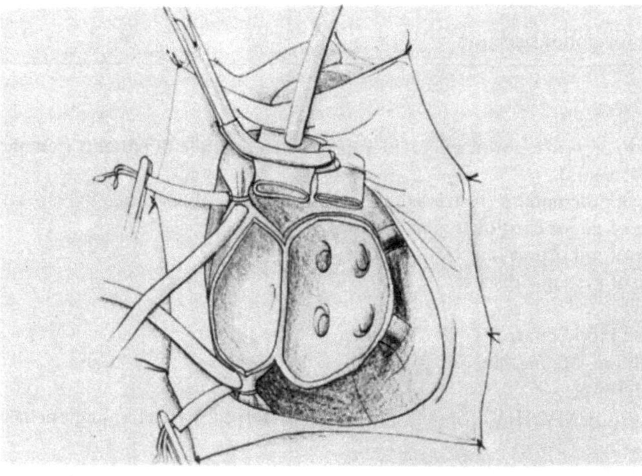

Figure 1. Anatomical situation after recipient's cardiectomy. Transsection of ascending aorta (with aortic cannula and crossclamp) and Pulmonary artery. Posterior aspect of right atrium (with cannula in superior and inferior vena cava), interatrial septum and left atrium with orifice of the four pulmonary veins.

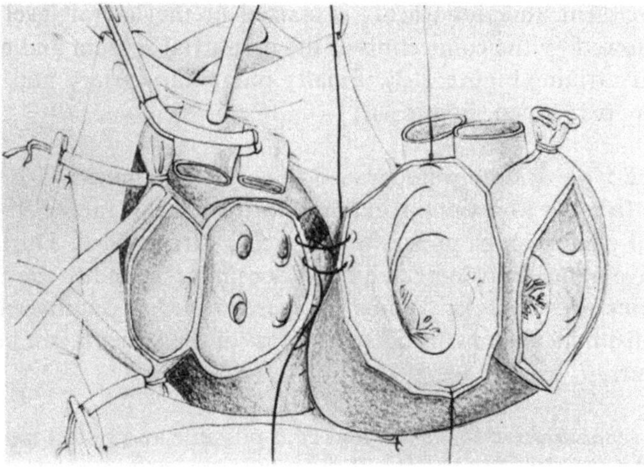

Figure 2. First phase in orthotopic heart transplantation: Posterior view of the donor heart with wide open left and right atrium. Anastomosis between donor and recipient's left atrium is started at the lateral site.

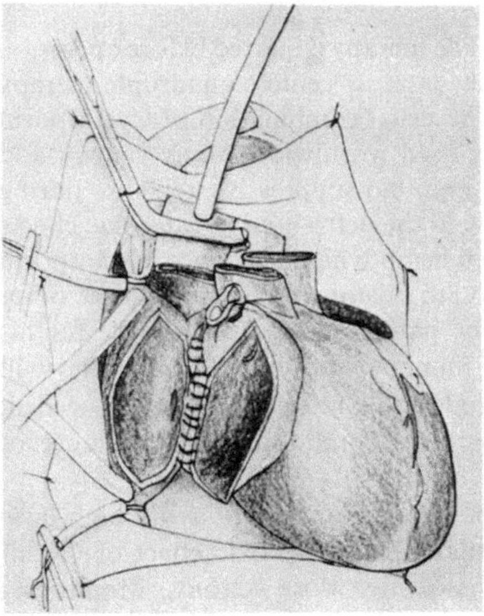

Figure 3. Second phase: Anastomosis of the interatrial septum and right atrium.

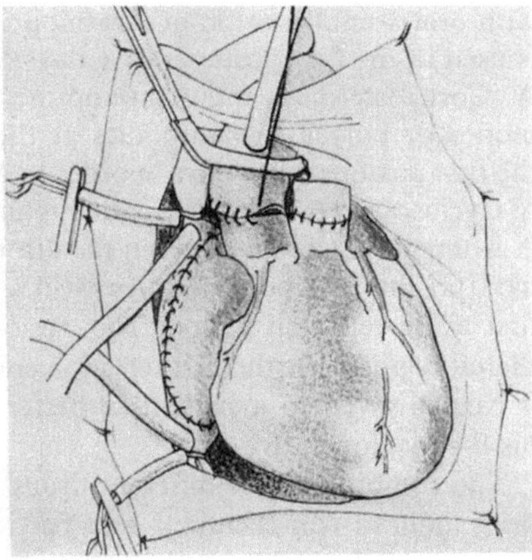

Figure 4. Third phase: Anastomosis of aorta and pulmonary artery between donor and recipient and completion of the orthotopic heart transplantation.

The donorheart is prepared at the level of both atria (Figure 2). Connection between recipient and donorheart is started at the lateral level of the left atrium, followed by the connection of the interatrial septum and anastomosis of the right atrium (Figure 2–3). Finally pulmonary artery and aortic anastomoses are performed (Figure 4).

2. *At the end of the operation* moderate doses of Dobutamine and/or Dopamine are started. In order to maintain an adequate donorheart rate (± 95–100 beats/min.), atrial pacing or Isoprenaline (Isuprel®) can be used. During the first postoperative hours the denervated heart does not respond to the Starlinglaw, and maintains a fixed stroke volume. Increase in cardiac output will be mainly dependant from increased chronotropy. Most of the patients can be extubated after 24 hours.

3. *Cardiac rehabilitation* starts as quickly as possible and a stationary bicycling program is begun after 8 to 10 days. Besides the immunosuppressive medication, a local oral antiseptic and a prophylactic agent for stress and gastritis are administered. Most of the patients will have some fluid restriction and daily use of diuretics (Lasix®) is routine. Due to the immunosuppressive therapy (Cyclosporin and Corticosteroids) many patients develop quickly arterial hypertension. Administration of drugs as diuretics, calciuminhibitors and Minoxidil is therefore very common in transplant patients even on a chronic basis.

4. *Immunosuppressive therapy* (Table 4). The therapy is started before operation with oral administration of Azathioprine. In most centers quadruple therapy is used in the first postoperative days. The usual combination of Cyclosporin A, Corticosteroids, and Azathioprine is used worldwide. Many centers add mono- or polyclonal antibodies at the immuno-suppressive regimen during the first postoperative days in order to avoid the nefro- and hepatotoxic effects of Cyclosporin A in patients with impaired hemodynamic balance. Cyclosporin A is therefore started between the 4th to 8th postoperative day. On the other hand in the first postoperative weeks the patient is most vulnerable for his first acute rejection period. The use of mono- or polyclonal antibodies will therefore postpone the first rejection episode and if rejection therapy is needed, it can be given to a patient in better general condition and at distance of his first postoperative days.

The combination of different drugs has the advantage to avoid high dose drug induced complications and particularly the nefrotoxic effect of Cyclosporin and the wellknown complications of high dose steroids. Monitoring of Cyclosporin levels, renal function, white blood cell counts remain imperative throughout the follow-up period, as well as concentration of OKT3, T3-cells and OKT3 antibodies during their administration. Cyclosporin levels have to be closely monitored in case of combination with other drugs, which will in- or decrease the Cyclosporin bloodconcentration. Ketoconazole, macrolides,

Table 4. Immunosuppressive therapy.

Preoperative: Azathioprine 2 mg/kg.
Peroperative: 500 mg Methylprednisolone IV at the end of extracorporeal circulation.
Postoperative:

a) OKT3: 5 to 10 ml IV/day during 15 days.
   First dose 4 – 6 hours postoperatively when stable haemodynamics.
   2 × / week: OKT3 serum concentration, T3 cells concentration, OKT3 antibodies.
b) Azathioprine
   Day 0 – Day 14: 2 mg/kg/day (adapt to WBC count).
   As off Day 15: 1 à 1.5 mg/kg/day.
c) Prednisolone
   Day 0: 3 × 125 mg IV.
   Day 1 – Day 14: 0.5 mg/kg/day.
   Day 15 – Day 30: 0.5 mg/kg/day to 0.15 mg/kg/day.
d) Cyclosporine
   Day 5/7 : 5 mg/kg/day (adapt to serumthrough levels).

barbiturates and Rifampicine are the most common drugs used in a cardiac transplant service with an interaction on the Cyclosporin blood concentration. Tables 5 and 6 indicate respectively the drugs which have a proven and potential interaction with the Cyclosporin level. With the drugs actually used, acute rejection is monitored via endomycardial biopsies performed via the right internal jugular vein with a specially designed cardiac bioptome.

Table 5. Cyclosporin (Sandimmun®): Substantiated drug interactions.

Drugs increasing the concentration of Cs	Drugs reducing the concentration of Cs	Drugs causing additive nephrotoxicity	Miscellaneous (described effect)
Calcium channel antagonists (incl. diltiazem, nicardipine, verapamil)	Barbiturates & derivatives (incl. phenytoin and phenobarbitone)	Aminoglycosides (incl. gentamycin and tobramycin)	Nifedipine (gingival hyperplasia)
Corticosteroids (incl. prednisolone and methylprednisolone)	Carbamezepine Metamizole	Amphotericin B Melphalan	
Doxycycline	Nafcillin	Trimethoprim (incl. co-trimoxazole)	
Ketoconazole	Rifampicin		
Macrolide antibiotics (incl. erythromycin and josamycin)	Sulphadimidine with trimethoprim (IV)		
Oral contraceptives/ Androgenic steroids (incl. danazol, levonorgestrel, northisterone)			

Source: I. Cockburn and P. Krupp – Drug Monitoring Center, Sandoz Ltd (1988).

Table 6. Cyclosporin (Sandimmun®): Suspected drug interactions.

Drugs increasing the concentration of Cs	Drugs reducing the concentration of Cs	Drugs causing additive nephrotoxicity	Miscellaneous (described effect)
Alcohol (heavy intake)	Anticonvulsants, others (incl. mesuximide, primidone)	Acyclovir (incl. ganciclovir)	1,25 Dihydroxy-vitamin D3 (immunomodulation)
Acetazolamide			
Coumarine anticoagulants (incl. dicoumarin, warfarin)	Metoprolol	Adriamycin	
Dioctyl sodium sulfosuccinate	Omeprazole	Captopril	Atracuronium (potentiation of neuromuscular blocking)
H2–antagonists (incl. cimetidine and ranitidine)	Somatostatin analogues	Cephalosporins (incl. ceftazidine and latamoxef)	
Imipenem/cilastatin	Sulfinpyrazone	Digoxin	Chlorpropamide/Disulfiram/metronidazole (antabuse-effect)
Itraconazole		Disopyramide	
Metoclopramide		Furosemide	
Norfloxacin		Metolazone	Etoposide (immunomodulation)
Pentazocine		NSAID's (incl. diclofenac and indomethacin)	Lovastatin (myopathy)
Pristinamycin			Hizoribine (immunomodulation)
Tanoxifen			Verapamil (immunomodulation)
Ticarcillin			

Source: I. Cockburn and P. Krupp – Drug Monitoring, Sandoz Ltd (1988).

Histologic classification of the myocardial biopsies, originally described by Billingham and coworkers from Stanford, will define the strategy of rejection treatment. At this moment only histology of the cardiac biopsy is the golden standard for the diagnosis of rejection. Clinical signs, E.C.G., echo-Doppler or immunologic monitoring are inconsistent and therapeutic strategy is difficult without histologic diagnosis. Biopsies are taken weekly for 4 weeks. The rhythm of biopsies is high up to three months postoperatively, when the thread for acute rejection is high and also in a doubtful situation or during a period of rejection therapy. In case of acute rejection, general accepted antirejection protocols are followed as described in Table 7. However, in a desperate situation with intreatable acute rejection and haemodynamic impairment, acute retransplantation is the only alternative. Early mortality is high (40 à 50%) in this subgroup of critical ill patients.

Table 7. Cardiac rejection: Treatment.

1. *Prednisolone* Pulse therapy
   Day 1 - 2 - 3: 1 g IV
   Day 4 - 7: 0.5 mg/kg/day orally
   Day 8 - 14: 0.4 mg/kg/day orally
   Day 15 - 21: 0.3 mg/kg/day orally
   As off day 22: 0.3 → 0.15 mg/kg/day

If unsuccesful, then:

2. OKT3
   Day 1 - 15: 5 to 10 ml/IV/day

If unsuccesful, then:

3. a) Antithymocyteglobulins (via central venous catheter)
   Day 1 - 14: 3 mg/kg
   + 250 mg Prednisolone IV before first injection.

   or

   b) Antilymphocyteglobulins
   Day 1 - 14: 1 ampulla /10 kg body weight
   + 250 mg Prednisolone IV before first injection.

4. RESULTS

The introduction of Cyclosporin in 1981 opened a new era in hearttransplantation and induced an exponential increase in the number of hearttransplants. Increased experience and refinements in immunosuppressive therapy account for the excellent results in cardiac transplantation with a one year survival of approximately 80% and a five year survival of 65% to 70% worldwide. The highest mortality is still within the first three months after the operation, mainly due to acute rejection and infection. Mortality is low between one up to five years after transplantation. Afterwards the thread of progressive diffuse coronary atherosclerosis appears and becomes the main cause of late death in a transplant patient. The pathophysiological mechanism of this diffuse atherosclerosis is probably multifactorial, but it could reflect the evolution of a longstanding chronic rejection process. Recently, cytomegalovirus infection has been suspected to play a role in this accelerated coronary artery disease process.

Infection remains the other main cause of death in transplant patient even with the evolution in the immunosuppressive regimen to a low dose triple therapy. Every patient remains prone to either sort of infection throughout his life and careful infection monitoring is imperative. Opportunistic infections account for a great number of severe and lethal infections in this patients. Most frequent opportunistic infections are herpes, CMV, Ebstein-Bar virus, Legionella, Nocardia, Toxoplasma, Pneumocystis and Fungi. The incidence of lymphoma's is somewhat higher than in a general population and is probably due to immunosuppressive therapy which includes polyclonal or monoclonal antibodies for a long period of time. In general, transplant patients return to a very acceptable and near-normal life style. Besides the standard chronic immunosuppressive therapy, many patients will need a treatment for arterial hypertension. Those patients are submitted to a combined treatment of diuretics, Calcium antagonists or α_1-blockers as prazorine (Minipress®) or Minoxidil. Some centers add an antiplatelet drug to the daily treatment and a cholesterol lowering diet to prevent early and agressive coronary atherosclerosis.

5. CARDIAC REHABILITATION

The ultimate goal of heart transplantation remains the restoration of a near-normal activity level with the opportunity for social, recreational and professional reintegration for the majority of the transplanted patients. Early postoperative rehabilitation is mostly spectacular in the majority of this very sick patient group. Rehabilitation starts already in the intensive care unit after extubation of the patient with passive mobilization of the extremities (antiembolic effect). After 2 to 3 days orthostatic stress is added 2 to 3 times a day when the patient is allowed to leave his bed. After the transfer to the cardiac surgical unit, the rehabilitation program is continued, adapted to the degree of preoperative disability. Normally the patient will have assisted stand and ambulation activities in his room for the following 2 or 3 days, combined with the initial passive mobilization. After approximately 8 days the program resembles close to the usual cardiac surgical rehabilitation program.

Training with the bicycle ergometer is started and resistance and duration is progressively increased. The patient is allowed to have in hall walking activities at ± 10 days after his operation.

The patients will leave the hospital already after ± 3 weeks with an outpatient cardiac rehabilitation program which is adapted to their predischarge bicycle ergometer testing results. For the majority of transplant patients, the program will be very similar to this of the standard cardiac surgical patient. The home program contains bicycle ergometer exercice with monitoring of heart rate and blood pressure. Later on increase of arm ergometer training is also allowed and even encouraged. Very quickly the patient will start unmonitored sessions to increase exercice activity and compliance. Young patients will quickly restart recreational and sports activities. During the outpatient clinic controls, regular bicycle ergometer tests are performed by the transplant rehabilitation team in order to adapt the exercice program when needed.

6. PHYSIOLOGY OF THE TRANSPLANTED HEART
CLINICAL IMPLICATIONS OF THE DENERVATED HEART

Due to the surgical technique of orthotopic heart transplantation, cardiac innervation of the donor heart is completely absent. Extensive longterm clinical and histological studies could never demonstrate any sign of cardiac reinnervation up to 14 years post-transplant. Most of the patients have an excellent functional result after their transplantation, indicating that even in the denervated state, the donor allograft has sufficient adaptive mechanism to support a near-normal circulation. Borrow and his coworkers demonstrated also that the chronically denervated transplanted non-rejecting left ventricle had normal contractile characteristics and reserve. Most of the patients will have normal to near-normal hemodynamics but the response to exercise (Table 8) and also to cardioactive drugs (Table 9) will be totally different due to the absence of autonomic cardiac innervation.

Table 8. Clinical findings related to the denervated heart.

	Resting conditions	Exercise
Symptoms:	NO CARDIAC PAIN	
Heart rate	High normal and loss of nocturnal decline	Slow in- and decrease
Bloodpressure	– High normal/elevated – Loss of nocturnal decline	Slow in- and decrease
ECG	– P-wave: donor + recipient – Sinus rate: high normal – Normal AV-conduction	Slow in- and decrease
Cardiac output	Normal to low normal	Normal exercise factor

Table 9. Response to cardioactive drugs of the denervated heart.

Drug	Sinus rate	AV-conduction	BP	CO
Digoxin				
Acute	–	–	–	–
Chronic	–	↓	–	↑ ?
Atropine	–	–	–	–
Norepinephrine	↑↑	↑	↑	↑
Isoproterenol	↑↑	↑	↓	↑
Propranolol	↓	↓	– or ↓	↓↓

Cardiac function is normally regulated by both neural and humoral factors. Afferent fibers from the baroreceptors in the carotid sinuses and in the aortic arch and direct central nervous stimulation will stimulate the cardioregulatory center. From this center direct vagus efferent fibers go mainly to the sinoatrial node and will decrease heart rate and conduction. On the other hand sympathetic efferent fibers will stimulate betareceptors at both atrial and ventricular sites with consequent increase in heart rate and contractility. The second, but slower regulating pathway is sympathetic stimulation of the suprarenal medulla with consequent release of catecholamines in the circulation and β-receptor stimulation. The totally denervated heart will lose its first regulatory pathway with absence of direct neural vagal and/or sympathetic stimulation.

Blood pressure is thus primarily maintained by the preserved control of peripheral vascular resistance by means of the arterial baroreceptors. The clinical impact of this phenomenon must be taken in account by every physician dealing with transplant patients, as it influences clinical and electrocardiographic findings, response to exercise and to vasoactive drugs.

Cardiac transplant patients exert no cardiac pain. In the setting of progressive coronary atherosclerosis and myocardial ischemia, no warning symptoms will reveal a possible myocardial infarction and sudden death is not uncommon as the first clinical sign of an underlying myocardial ischemic process. Noninvasive tests and routine coronary angiography during the annual complete check-up are the only means to detect and/or to predict possible ischemic complications. In resting conditions heart rate is in the high normal range due to the lack of physiologic vagal inhibition. This is reflected on the electrocardiogram in rest where a normal high sinusrate is noticed. The AV-conduction is normal and two P-waves both from donor and recipient heart can be identified. The recipient P-wave is still submitted to the normal cardiovascular autonomic function and its rate will differ completely from the donor sinus rate in rest and in exercise. Immediately after the operation ECG signs of right ventricular strain and right bundle branch block are very common findings. Blood pressure is also higher probably due to a combination of increased peripheral vascular tone and water and salt retention and the pharmacological effects of Cyclosporin A. The effect of Cyclosporin is probably due to a combination of its direct action on the peripheral vessels and to its effect on kidney function.

In a prospective study Reeves and coworkers [5] demonstrated also the loss of normal nocturnal decline in blood pressure and heart rate in heart transplant patients and is probably also related to the definitive loss of autonomic function of the transplanted allograft. The hemodynamic respons to exercice differs also in transplant patients due to the lack of immediate response of the autonomic nervous system on the sinus node and on the myocardial β-receptors. The initial response to exercise is only mediated via the increased venous return and subsequent preload augmentation with increased muscular activity. Subsequent increase in cardiac output is finally mediated by humoral stimulation with increase of circulating catecholamines which will increase heart rate and myocardial contractility. This explains clearly why heart transplant patients present a slow increase in heart rate and blood pressure followed by a more graduate decrease, as would be expected by the direct effect of the circulating catecholamines and the absence of a fast autonomic nervous feedback mechanism. However, peripheral circulatory reflexes remain intact as demonstrated by the normal increase in heart rate and blood pressure during exercise. Before starting vigourous exercise 'a warming up' period is therefore advisable to transplant patients with heavy professional or recreational activities. Another consequence of the denervated status of the transplanted heart is the different response of a number of drugs (Table 9). All specialities dealing with cardiac transplant patients and mainly cardiology and anesthesiology have to apply to this pharmacological principles.

CONCLUSION

Orthotopic heart transplantation is now an accepted therapeutic modality for end-stage heart disease. Clinical results have been encouraging over the last years. In order to keep heart transplantation as a successful treatment, we have to solve many problems for which close collaboration between all transplant centers is mandatory. (1) Increase of the number and optimal use of donor organs is one of the most urgent problems in view of the increasing recipient's demand. Prolonged donor heart preservation is another unresolved issue which could optimize the actual donor sources. (2) Besides the problem of donor scarcity, the second greatest problem to resolve is the continuous thread of progressive coronary atherosclerosis of the transplanted heart with the ultimate loss of graft function. This is another unexplored field and research is hardly needed to improve the longterm outcome of hearttransplant patients. (3) Enormous progress, however, has been made over the last nine years and this procedure has offered to many patients an excellent rehabilitation, which has led to a renewed interest in their lives. These results should provide inspiration, ideas and courage to those involved in the difficult issue of a cardiac transplant program.

REFERENCES

1. Myerwitz PD (1987) *Heart Transplantation.* Mount Kisco, New York: Futura Publishing Company Inc.
2. Heck CF, Shumway SJ, Kaye MP (1989) The registry of the International Society for Heart Transplantation: Sixth Official Report. *J Heart Transplant* 8(4):271–280
3. Greenberg ML, Uretsky BF, Sudhakar Reddy P, Bernstein RL, Griffith BP, Hardesty RI, Thompson ME, Bahnson HT (1985) Long-term hemodynamic follow-up of cardiac transplant patients treated with Cyclosporine and Prednisone. *Circulation* 71(3):487–494
4. Borow KM, Neumann A, Arensman FW, Yacoub MY (1985) Left ventricular contractility and contractile reserve in humans after cardiac transplantation. *Circulation* 71(5):866–872

5. Reeves RA, Shapiro AP, Thompson ME, Johnsen AM (1986) Loss of nocturnal decline in blood pressure after cardiac transplantation. *Circulation* 73(3):401–408
6. Billingham ME (1981) Diagnosis of cardiac rejection by endomyocardial biopsy. *J Heart Transplant* 1(1):25–30
7. Frist WH, Stinson EB, Oyer PhE, Baldwin JC, Shumway NE (1987) Long-term hemodynamic results after cardiac transplantation. *J Thoracic Cardiovasc Surgery* 94:685–693
8. Gay WA, O'Connell JG, Burton NA. Karwande SV. Renlund DG, Bristow MR (1988) OKT3 monoclonal antibody in cardiac transplantation: Experience with 102 patients. *Ann Surgery* 1988:287–290
9. Kirklin JK, Naftel DC, Kirklin JW, Blackstone EH, White-Williams C, Bourge RC (1988) Pulmonary vascular resistance and the risk of heart transplantation. *J Heart Transplant* 7(5):331–336

Subject index

MIX
Papier aus verantwortungsvollen Quellen
Paper from responsible sources
FSC® C105338

If you have any concerns about our products,
you can contact us on
ProductSafety@springernature.com

In case Publisher is established outside the EU,
the EU authorized representative is:
Springer Nature Customer Service Center GmbH
Europaplatz 3, 69115 Heidelberg, Germany

Printed by Libri Plureos GmbH
in Hamburg, Germany